Jewish refugees and the British nursing profession

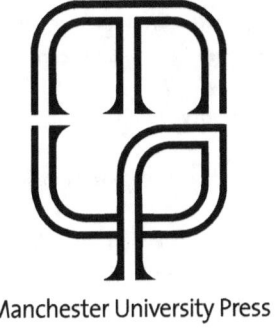

Manchester University Press

NURSING HISTORY AND HUMANITIES

Series editors: Christine E. Hallett and Jane E. Schultz

This series provides an outlet for the publication of rigorous academic texts in the two closely related disciplines of Nursing History and Nursing Humanities, drawing upon both the intellectual rigour of the humanities and the practice-based, real-world emphasis of clinical and professional nursing.

At the intersection of Medical History, Women's History and Social History, Nursing History remains a thriving and dynamic area of study with its own claims to disciplinary distinction. The broader discipline of Medical Humanities is of rapidly growing significance within academia globally, and this series aims to encourage strong scholarship in the burgeoning area of Nursing Humanities more generally.

Such developments are timely, as the nursing profession expands and generates a stronger disciplinary axis. The MUP Nursing History and Humanities series provides a forum within which practitioners and humanists may offer new findings and insights. The international scope of the series is broad, embracing all historical periods and including both detailed empirical studies and wider perspectives on the cultures of nursing.

Previous titles in this series:

Mental health nursing: The working lives of paid carers in the nineteenth and twentieth centuries   Edited by Anne Borsay and Pamela Dale

Negotiating nursing: British Army sisters and soldiers in the Second World War   Jane Brooks

One hundred years of wartime nursing practices, 1854–1953   Edited by Jane Brooks and Christine E. Hallett

'Curing queers': Mental nurses and their patients, 1935–74   Tommy Dickinson

Histories of nursing practice   Edited by Gerard M. Fealy, Christine E. Hallett and Susanne Malchau Dietz

Nurse writers of the Great War   Christine Hallett

Beyond Nightingale: Nursing on the Crimean War battlefields   Carol Helmstadter

African nurses and everyday work in twentieth-century Zimbabwe   Clement Masakure

Who cared for the carers? A history of the occupational health of nurses, 1880–1948   Debbie Palmer

Colonial caring: A history of colonial and post-colonial nursing   Edited by Helen Sweet and Sue Hawkins

Ellen N. La Motte: Nurse, writer, activist   Lea M. Williams

Jewish refugees and the British nursing profession: A gendered opportunity   Jane Brooks

Jewish refugees and the British nursing profession

A gendered opportunity

Jane Brooks

MANCHESTER UNIVERSITY PRESS

Copyright © Jane Brooks 2024

The right of Jane Brooks to be identified as the author of this work has been asserted in accordance with the Copyright, Designs and Patents Act 1988.

Published by Manchester University Press
Oxford Road, Manchester, M13 9PL

www.manchesteruniversitypress.co.uk

British Library Cataloguing-in-Publication Data
A catalogue record for this book is available from the British Library

ISBN 978 1 5261 6742 2 hardback
ISBN 978 1 5261 9490 9 paperback

First published 2024
Paperback published 2026

The publisher has no responsibility for the persistence or accuracy of URLs for any external or third-party internet websites referred to in this book, and does not guarantee that any content on such websites is, or will remain, accurate or appropriate.

EU authorised representative for GPSR:
Easy Access System Europe – Mustamäe tee 50,
10621 Tallinn, Estonia
gpsr.requests@easproject.com

Typeset
by Cheshire Typesetting Ltd, Cuddington, Cheshire

Contents

List of figures	vi
Preface	vii
Acknowledgements	ix
Abbreviations	xiii
Introduction: Nursing: gender, migration and opportunity	1
1 Escape	39
2 The nursing world	85
3 War nurse	127
4 From the post-war world to a nursing legacy	171
Conclusion	218
Bibliography	231
Index	258

Figures

0.1 Susan Charles's (Ingelore Czarlinksi's) identity document for young person admitted under the Inter-Aid Committee for Children. 12
0.2 Hortense Gordon (*right*) and her younger sister, Beate, with the family dog, c. late 1920s? 23
1.1 Ruth Rawraway with a cradle of babies, probably during her employment at the Berlin B'nai Brith mother and baby home, c.1930–34. 40
1.2 Maria Fuchs's (Mia Ross's) passport. 54
2.1 Aviva Gold in her Princess Margaret Rose Hospital uniform. 93
2.2 Cartoon showing the push and pull between Communist Russia and Nazi Germany, *Nursing Times*, Christmas edition, 1935. 99
3.1 Lisbeth Hockey in her London Hospital uniform, c.1938–39. 131
4.1 Annie Altschul with her Fellow of the Royal College of Nursing (FRCN) medal, 1978. 198

Preface

In February 2022, I was privileged to attend a masterclass with the eminent Holocaust historian, Professor Marion Kaplan. In the introduction to this fascinating workshop, she asked all the participants about their research interests. I informed her that I was writing a book about female Jewish refugees who fled Nazi Europe and entered the nursing profession in Britain. She admitted that whilst she knew about domestic service as a means of escape and employment, she did not know about nursing. I hope that I did not bore her and the other participants when I briefly outlined the story. The profession of nursing provided a critical opportunity for escape, valued work and financial independence for this group of women. The offer of nursing as employment was also opportunistic on the part of the Government and the profession's elite. As the war approached, Britain's hospitals were in the grip of severe nursing shortages. The refugees could help alleviate that crisis.

As I spoke, the critical rationale for the research I was undertaking became clearer. In the middle years of the twentieth century the nursing profession and its members were beset by multiple challenges. These included difficulties in recruitment and even worse problems with retention, alongside criticisms of petty discipline, poor pay and harsh working conditions, all of which will be examined throughout this text. Yet, despite this, nursing was a useful vehicle for this cohort of women refugees to regain some self-respect, self-worth and independence. The personal testimonies of the refugees whose stories comprise this book tell of the camaraderie of the Nurses' Home, the joy of working with patients and the wide variety of opportunities the profession offered once qualified.

They also identify antisemitic and anti-German sentiments and at critical moments a complete lack of sympathy to their plight. Nevertheless, working as a nurse gave the women the chance to recoup a sense of social justice after the persecution of their co-religionists in Germany, Austria and Czechoslovakia. It was also a highly gendered opportunity. For those who had been doctors or medical students prior to their escape it also offered the chance to retain an interest in healthcare. Nursing may not have had the status of medicine, but at least women refugees were given the chance of escape and a future supporting the health of the community. Male refugee doctors were offered no such option. I hope I can do justice to their stories.

Acknowledgements

I should like to thank the Eleanor Crowder Bjoring Center for Historical Nursing Inquiry at the University of Virginia, USA for supporting this project through its Barbara Brodie Fellowship which I was awarded for 2019–20. My sincere thanks also to the American Association for the History of Nursing (AAHN) for honouring me with the H15 research grant in 2020 which also supported this project. These grants were invaluable in my ability to access relevant archives and libraries and to attend the Florence Nightingale Bicentenary International Conference in Italy in 2020. It was just after this conference that the world went into lockdown for two years as the COVID-19 pandemic reeled through the globe. Both the Eleanor Crowder Bjoring Center and the AAHN were generous enough to extend the timeline of my grants until the world returned to near-normal. I should also like to extend my thanks to the School of Health Sciences at the University of Manchester for awarding me pump-priming funding. This money enabled me to carry out all my oral history interviews and to attend archives in the UK.

I am grateful to the following archives, museums and libraries and their staff for preserving the oral histories and documents which have been so central to *Jewish Refugees and the British Nursing Profession: A Gendered Opportunity*. The British Library, the Friends Meeting House Library, the Imperial War Museum, the Jewish Museums in both Manchester and London, King's College London Archives, the London Metropolitan Archives, the People's History Museum, the Royal College of Nursing Archives, Tower Hamlets Local History Library and Archives and the Wiener

Library in the UK. My thanks also to the Barbara Bates Center for the Study of Nursing History, Philadelphia, the Leo Baeck Institute for their online oral history archive and Holocaust Memorial Museum, Washington, DC, in the USA. Much of the material used in this monograph comes from the archives in these institutions. I have reproduced extensive quotations from both their printed and oral sources, all of which have been vital to my research. I am most grateful to the Board of Jewish Deputies for permitting me to view their restricted access material at the LMA. These documents have been critical to my understanding of the work of the Jewish Refugee Committee.

My profound thanks to all those retired refugee nurses and their families who enabled me to conduct some of the most powerful and moving interviews of my academic life. To Heidi Cowen (pseudonym), Lee Fischer, Hortense Gordon, Cilly Haar, Susi Loeffler, Leonore Lowton (pseudonym), Kitty Schafer and Ruth Shire. My sincere thanks to all their family members who supported the interviews and the relationships that were built around them. I remain deeply grateful also to all those family members whose late mothers and aunts had been refugee nurses and who sent me details of their lives, documents about their nursing work and images related to them. To Susi Loeffler's nephew Cameron Woodrow and Aviva Gold's daughter, Dina, to the families of Susan Charles, Eva Flatow, Charlotte Hoxter, Ruth Rawraway and Mia Ross. Several of the images donated to me are reprinted in this book with their kind permission. The contributions of all those who spoke to me and sent me documents have played a crucial role in any success this book may find. Their generosity will support the legacy of the women about whom I have written. My thanks also to Dina and her husband for taking care of me in Washington and inviting me to the Jewish Film Festival as their guest – it was delightful.

I should like to thank several academic colleagues who have offered advice and archival material which have proved essential to the book. My thanks to Professor Paul Weindling at Oxford Brookes University for giving me complete access to his Biographical Database of European Medical Refugees in Great Britain, 1930s–1950s. Not only has this archive enabled me to engage with the biographical information related to a number

Acknowledgements

of refugee nurses, it also contains the memoirs of Trudie Moos, Marianne Parkes and Margaret Marflow. My sincere thanks to Professor Peter Nolan for taking time to talk to me about Annie Altschul. An especial thanks to Dr Jennifer Craig-Norton for all her unfailing support and for facilitating my access to oral histories and written testimonies from her own archive and those of the Parkes Institute at the University of Southampton. I am most grateful to Professor Eva-Marie Ulmer for her advice on the Jewish nurses from Frankfurt am Main. A huge thanks to my colleagues at the University of Manchester Centre for Jewish Studies, Professor Emeritus Philip Alexander and Professors Alex Samely and Daniel Langton, for their support and assistance with my studies and to Laura Mitchell, the previous Centre administrator. My gratitude to Professor Michael Berkowitz at University College London for his kindness and enthusiasm towards my project. Finally, my thanks to Martin Sugarman, the archivist for AJEX – the Association of Jewish Ex-Servicemen and Women, who helped me locate a number of narratives and documents in their archive.

This book would not have been possible without the support of Professors Christine Hallett and Jane Schultz, the editors for the Nursing History and Humanities series published by Manchester University Press. This is the third book of mine in the series. Their unfailing enthusiasm and dedication to promote the best of academic nursing history is essential to the discipline across the globe. My thanks also to Meredith Carroll, the commissioning editor at MUP, for her patience and excellent advice throughout the process. I am grateful to the whole production team for making this monograph possible.

I am indebted to the anonymous reviewers for the book. Their critical eye and constructive advice have been invaluable in helping me make the volume worthy of the memory of the refugee nurses. My thanks to Dr Helen Sweet for acting as my critical reader. I should also like to thank my dear friend Katherine Wackerbarth for proofreading the book for me. Her keen eye has saved me many long hours correcting bizarre syntax.

I should finally like to thank all my colleagues and friends in the Division of Nursing, Midwifery and Social Work for supporting my work in the history of nursing. To Professor Dawn Dowding, my manager and to Professor Hilary Mairs, the head of the division, both my good friends. My thanks to all my colleagues and friends who form the global community of historians of nursing. Thank you to my friends and family for your love and support. Finally, my most special thanks go to my husband James Campbell for his love, support and patience throughout the writing of this book.

Abbreviations

FRCN   Fellow of the Royal College of Nursing
NHS   National Health Service
QNI   Queen's Nursing Institute
RCN   Royal College of Nursing
SMA   Socialist Medical Association

Introduction:
Nursing: gender, migration and opportunity

Hortense Gordon fled Nazi Germany for England at the end of May 1939, just three months before the start of the Second World War. In her oral history Gordon recalled that she had suggested to her parents she emigrate to England on a domestic service visa: 'And to seek, or help, work on my parents and sister also coming out.'[1] She was never able to rescue her parents or younger sister, all of whom perished in the Holocaust. Gordon was fortunate to find work with a family, even though it was work for which she was totally unsuited.[2] Having been brought up in a household with servants, Gordon was now required to become one herself. On 3 June 1939, she took the train to Surrey to take up employment as the 'cook general ... And I stayed with the family until October 1941 when I was able to start training as a nurse.'[3]

Gordon's story is in many ways typical of Jewish and 'non-Aryan' refugees whose narratives comprise this book.[4] Most refugees had least one family member who was murdered in the Holocaust. Gordon came from a relatively affluent background and had ambitions to become a medical doctor. Other refugees had similar professional aspirations. Trudie Moos and Annaliese Pearl, like Gordon, had wanted to study medicine. Lisbeth Hockey and Josephine Bruegel were medical students when they were forced to escape. Annie Altschul was studying mathematics with a view to teaching. Eva Flatow wished to be a concert pianist. Margaret Marflow's interest was chemistry. Despite Charlotte Kratz's assertion that nursing was a 'non-job' in Germany, several of the refugees whose stories are told in this book either had ambitions to be nurses or were already nurses before they escaped.[5]

Cilly Haar and Kitty Schafer stated that nursing had long been their ambition. Ruth Rawraway, Elisabeth Katz and Margot Hodge were all nursing in Jewish hospitals in Germany before they fled. Erna Harding's parents had given her permission to train as a nurse during the First World War, although they had refused to allow her to work full-time on qualifying. In this her parents followed the accepted position of middle-class domesticity in which men went out into the public world of work and women's domain was firmly that of the home environment.

Jewish Refugees and the British Nursing Profession: A Gendered Opportunity explores the personal and professional lives of female Jewish refugees who chose nursing as their method of gaining independence and for some, escape. Having fled Nazi Europe for Britain, many young women refugees found themselves without family, friends or financial security. At the most fundamental level, nursing offered a pragmatic method of escape and independence. It provided accommodation, training and a ready-made family in the environment of the Nurses' Home. Even those refugees who had not considered nursing before arriving in Britain could see the opportunity it offered as the country faced the imminent threat of war. When conscription was extended to women in 1941, nursing also became one of a limited number of jobs that were accepted as war work.[6] As will be discussed in Chapter 2, nursing was seen as positive action in support of the Allied effort against Nazism.[7] It gave refugees the chance to help the sick and in need.[8] Gertrude Roberts's analysis of nursing's liberating purpose is clear: 'I was kind of making up for not nursing my parents; I was at last able to help someone.'[9]

The purpose of the book is to give a voice to women who supported our healthcare system during the war and gave service as nurses in the early years of the National Health Service (NHS). It bears witness to the gendered nature of 'refugeedom' and the determination of women refugees to forge successful careers into the latter half of the twentieth century. Finally, it foreshadows their legacies to the profession and the nation's health. The courting of refugees by the profession and encouragement by the British Government, was not, however, entirely altruistic.

From the reforms of the nineteenth century, nursing had been highlighted as work that could offer women geographical and social mobility, independence and a professional future. Anne Summers argues that by the 1850s, middle-class women's philanthropic zeal led them to value their place in the public arena, which had hitherto excluded them from agency. Middle-class and upper-class women started to care for the poor as lady visitors, members of religious sisterhoods and nurses.[10] Some 'lady nurses', anxious about the loss of social status which a salary would engender, continued to refuse remuneration for their 'work'.[11] The changing demographic of Britain led to a growing disparity in the number of women requiring a husband to support them and the number of men available. These changes meant that for many women seeking nursing work, a salary was a necessity.[12] As medical science and hospital expansions gathered apace in the latter years of the nineteenth century, more nurses were needed.[13]

The influx of thousands of young Voluntary Aid Detachment recruits (VADs) into nursing during the First World War might have heralded a golden age for the profession. But the end of the war also ended their interest in nursing work.[14] Only a few VADs decided to undertake formal training for the newly regulated profession.[15] Despite ongoing rhetoric by the nursing elite as to the profession's value, it never managed to recruit and retain sufficient women to staff the nation's hospitals. Reports conducted in the 1930s into the staffing crises that beset nursing highlighted multiple problems with the profession.[16] However, none were able to suggest strategies for improvement that were acceptable to government finances, the medical profession's desire for hegemony or the matrons' determination to maintain control of their nursing staff. Most of the Jewish refugees whose narratives comprise this book came from educated and cultured homes and were keen to forge professional careers for themselves. Once in Britain, their options were severely curtailed by limited finances, gender restrictions and their alien status.[17] The nation's need for nurses opened an occupational route that could lead to a professional future, or at least a useful training during hostilities. They would therefore comprise a small but significant pool of recruits from the late 1930s and throughout the war.

Of the 55,000 Jews who fled to Britain, 20,000 were women, the majority of whom entered domestic service.[18] As historian Jennifer

Craig-Norton argues, they comprised the 'largest single bloc of refugees' who were admitted to Britain.[19] The number of refugees who became nurses was never as large as those who worked in other people's homes. In 1940, the Home Office recorded that there were 941 nurses, probationer nurses and midwives working in hospitals across the country.[20] Nurse historian John Stewart argues, however, that even at this early juncture of the war there were probably more.[21] By the middle years of the war, nursing was advocated as a valuable destination for the most able women refugees. While male refugee doctors and dentists struggled to gain access to their respective professions, women doctors and medical students were encouraged to retrain as nurses and midwives.[22] The story of Jewish refugee women who became nurses in Britain thus informs the gendered space between the elite male refugee and the female servant. Nurses theoretically had a professional training. It was, however, one that was founded in a highly disciplined and harsh apprenticeship system, away from the exalted world of the university. Whilst all hospital nurses were notionally under the auspices of the matron, the medical staff and hospital committee held the ultimate authority. The expectation was that nurses would be obedient and subservient. The long-heralded vocational element meant that the profession was imbued with a religious dedication to service. As one British nurse who trained at St Thomas's Hospital in London maintained, 'students in 1938 were told to "polish their brasses to the glory of God"'.[23] These attributes perpetuated the ambivalent nature of the professional status of nursing and made it unpopular with British women.

By the 1930s the crisis in nurse recruitment and retention was at a critical point. The 'courting' of female refugees by the profession and the Government was an undeniable case of opportunism. The nation needed nurses. Neither the country, nor the Committee of the Central Office for Refugees – the organisation established to support Jewish refugees – could afford to finance all those fleeing Nazi Europe. Nursing was essential work for a nation facing war and female refugees were ideally placed to care for the sick and needy of Britain. What could not be predicted in the 1930s was that despite the relatively low numbers of refugees who became nurses, they would contribute significantly to nursing practice, education and research. The book therefore reflects on the contribution of female Jewish refugees to nursing in a century of conflict and considerable scientific and professional change.

Migration past and present

As I began writing this book in 2020, the world was facing refugee crises on multiple fronts. Five years earlier, in 2015, it was estimated that there were 65 million refugees across the globe, a figure that approximates to one in every 113 people world-wide.[24] Across the African continent people fled hostile regimes and famine. Europe and its many constituent nations faced a refugee crisis, by which it meant 'a crisis for European states, rather than a crisis for refugees'.[25] As historian of Jewish refugees Tony Kushner argues in the Preface to *Journeys from the Abyss*, 'Isolationism and the attack of the "enemy within" and the "enemy without" in the form of the illegal/criminal "alien"' were critical features in the successful 'Brexit' campaign in the UK.[26]

The nursing profession itself has not been immune from such divisive tropes. Both the *Nursing Times* and *Nursing Standard* published reports revealing the nascent racism in the nursing profession and the nation's cared-for population.[27] Significantly for the purposes of *Jewish Refugees and the British Nursing Profession*, the profession needs to understand the impact of an anti-migrant narrative that fails to acknowledge the multiplicity of diasporic identities, especially if we are charged with caring for, and with those who might discriminate against migrant nurses.

In 2015, the British Conservative Government introduced the Immigration Health Surcharge to all migrant workers from outside Europe for their access to the National Health Service (NHS). The surcharge was instituted as part of the 'Hostile Environment' legislation, enacted to discourage illegal immigration, but which in a number of cases also adversely affected those whose immigration was legal.[28] Calls to waive the fee – originally set at £200 and increased to £400 in 2018 – for healthcare workers were refused.[29] The disproportionate number of COVID-19 deaths among healthcare workers from black and minority ethnic backgrounds, including those who were recent migrants, increased the calls for the surcharge to be waived. On 22 May 2020, the Government finally agreed to scrap the fee for all health and social care staff. Dame Donna Kinnair – then General Secretary of the Royal College of Nursing – welcomed the volte-face, but commented, 'it is a shame it took this pandemic for the Government to see sense'.[30] The ambivalence of the Government to those who come to Britain to work in the NHS and social care sector, bound as it is in a trope of both recruitment and repudiation, is not new.

Pertii Ahonen, a historian of modern Europe, argues that there are significant problems with taking a diachronic approach to understanding the current refugee crises through the lens of the Holocaust.[31] However, we can use the past to signal ways in which the present can be understood. There are perennial problems facing refugees. First, as a body of people, refugees face the risks of being 'denied sanctuary and continuing uncertainty'.[32] Second, the necessity to escape and the influx of refugees into countries of refuge are often met with a simultaneous hardening of immigration regulations.[33] Third, and importantly for this book, refugees face ongoing difficulties in gaining access to paid employment, specifically professional employment, because of language, culture and reciprocity of registration.[34] Qualified migrant nurses frequently end up in 'direct care-worker jobs' that are not commensurate with their qualifications and experience.[35] In fleeing conflict and disaster, refugees may suffer the loss of documents that can prove professional qualifications.[36] However, as the eminent human geographer Linda McDowell argues, once they are able to re-access professional nursing, the female migrant considers that she has re-established herself in her middle-class family origins.[37]

Current immigrants to the UK are not all victims of forced migration and it is acknowledged that there are fundamental differences in the experiences of migrants and refugees.[38] Nevertheless, whether economic migrants or refugees, the situation for those not living in their country of origin was, and remains, perilous. Finally, the gendered aspect of refugee crises resonates across time. There are currently 232 million women living outside the country of their birth.[39] Women are more likely to have suffered interpersonal violence and precarious living conditions and work choices.[40]

The situation for those female Jewish refugees who escaped to Britain in the 1930s was also precarious. As I explore in Chapter 1, most were young women on their own, and most had left family and friends behind and were aware of the sort of regime under which they were living. Whilst some were cared for in their new homes, many faced exploitation at best and at worst, abuse. The opportunity to enter the nursing profession in Britain meant that refugees moved into the Nurses' Home – a place of relative safety, despite the suspicion and unkindness sometimes experienced. In her exposition of refugees who escaped on domestic service visas, Craig-Norton describes the movement from houses where the women were treated badly, to homes where they were treated as members of the family, as being 'pulled from the margins and into the centre of family life'.[41] Those who left domestic service for nursing often saw the change in the same positive terms. Edith Menkes Wolloch maintained that the sisters in the hospital:

> Were marvellous because they were understanding. I was so exhausted one day, I came off duty, I had my own room. I shared a bathroom with a group of girls, of probationary nurses. I fell asleep in the bathtub and it overran and the sister just helped me mop up the bathroom, but I never heard anything, she was really so nice.[42]

Migrant nurses, refugee voices

Not all hospitals and their staff were sympathetic to the refugees' plight.[43] Admissions from refugees about the harshness of nurse training tended to be sanguinary, acknowledging that nursing was hard for all. As Lee Fischer recalled in her oral history, 'We were all nurses. We were all young. You know, most of us started at age 18 or 19, and the war was on.'[44] Despite Fischer's assertion that they were 'all nurses', personal narratives do identify antisemitic, anti-refugee and anti-German prejudices directed at the refugees by hospital authorities and fellow nurses. Although it is difficult to decipher the specific cause of the discrimination in each case, the refugees' 'otherness' marked them.[45] The image of nurses as single, white women pervaded and still pervades the profession. As Julia Hallam argues, 'as long as nursing is presented as white, middle-class and feminine those who do not fit this ideal, even if they are 25 per cent of the nursing workforce, are marginalised as outsiders, unlegitimised [sic] and lacking in status.'[46]

The nursing profession had courted immigrant nurses since before the Second World War. Whilst most of the sources discuss the use of Irish nurses to bolster the newly established NHS from 1948, Britain did employ Irish nurses during the conflict.[47] The struggle to recruit British women into nursing and the limited opportunities for women in Ireland rendered nurse training in Britain a valuable opportunity, if not an entirely attractive option.[48] In her oral history, Annie Altschul, who fled to Britain from Austria in 1938, identified the numerous Irish women at her nurse training school.[49]

As a cohort, Jewish refugees were significantly different to other migrant nursing recruits and therefore require a new and detailed analysis. First, the Jews who fled Nazi Europe were refugees and not economic migrants. Second, many had no family to turn to once in Britain, having left loved ones in Nazi Europe – the majority of whom then perished in the Holocaust. Third, whereas Irish and Caribbean recruits came specifically to nurse and saw nursing as social mobility, the youthful ambitions of female Jewish refugees were more wide-ranging.[50] Even some of those who specifically chose nursing as their route to escape had originally aspired towards university subjects or the arts. Fourth, the refugees came from markedly more cultured, educated and middle-class homes than many of their British colleagues, attributes that were appreciated by only a few hospital matrons at the time. Finally, whether from secular or religious households several of the refugees whose narratives comprise this book identify with a strong sense of social justice.[51] Although it is important not to overstate the case, this cultural tilt, according to Joachim Wieler, gave rise to a higher proportion of Jews than non-Jews entering the helping professions in pre-National Socialist Germany.[52] The inclination to help the less fortunate was transferred into the nursing profession in Britain by the refugees. Several of them came from families where the father or other family members were medical doctors and others from families that were acknowledged social democrats.[53] Lisbeth Hockey felt she was partly seen as an enemy of the State, not because of her Jewish ancestry, but because of her father's liberal political involvement.[54] In her oral history Lee Fischer maintained, 'my parents always told us to be helpful to others and share our life with other people, to be helpful'.[55] Trudie Moos admitted in her memoir that she understood she could be of 'service to my fellow human beings as a nurse'.[56]

An opportunity for female refugees

In 1938, the Government supported the creation of a Nursing and Midwifery Committee under the chairwomanship of Miss G. V. Hillyers, matron of St Thomas's Hospital. The remit of the Committee was to coordinate the recruitment of educated Jewish women into the nursing profession.[57] In a letter to the *Nursing Times*, Hillyers informed her fellow nurses that all candidates would initially be interviewed abroad and their personal and professional credentials reviewed. They would be required to complete a detailed questionnaire. Only the most suitable candidates would be brought to England to take up training places.[58] Given the nurse staffing crisis in Britain, this stringent process not only prevented escape for some women desperate to flee Nazi persecution, but also stymied the recruitment of adequate numbers of potential nurses for the nation's hospitals. Despite the coalition between the Government and the elite of the profession, not all hospitals were willing to take even these highly vetted refugees into their training schools. Not all nurses were keen to work alongside German and Austrian Jews. As I discuss in Chapter 3, following the invasion of France by Germany in the spring of 1940, fears of spies and fifth columnists led to all refugees being dismissed from their hospital appointments. As more British nurses volunteered for active service overseas, the nurse staffing crisis at home became increasingly critical. By early 1941, many of the restrictions placed on refugees had been lifted.[59] With the relaxation of regulations, hospitals could once again appoint refugees onto their nursing staffs.

In May 1941, E. N. Cooper, a Home Office official, wrote to the Central Office for Refugees recommending nursing as a professional choice for refugee women who had fled Nazi Europe.[60] Two months later in July, the Committee of the Central Office for Refugees reported on the vision of Florence Horsburgh, Parliamentary Secretary to the Ministry of Health. Horsburgh appealed for young women and girls in Britain to become nurses.[61] The Committee agreed that given the great need for nurses in a time of war, 'Nursing thus offers a special opportunity for following an urgent and present need at the same time of training for the future.'[62] Female Jewish refugees who had arrived in Britain on domestic service visas or who had fled via the Kindertransport and were now over 18 years old were encouraged to pursue nursing as a career. The Committee outlined for discussion the practicalities of entering a training school. Instructions were given to those who had trained previously as nurses 'abroad', who could take positions either as assistant nurses or retrain in a recognised training school. For those with no previous training there were directions on applying to training schools for a two-year course for 'Fever, Orthopaedic, mental or tuberculosis nurses or a three-year course for children's nursing'.[63] That is, those areas of nursing for which recruitment was the most challenging.

The government drive to recruit refugee women and girls into the nursing profession became more vigorous as the need for more nurses was fuelled by war. Those who had arrived on domestic service visas were encouraged to transfer to more useful war occupations. Nursing was just one of an increasing number of war-related jobs that female refugees could undertake alongside munitions factory work, the Land Army and joining the Auxiliary Training Service (ATS). Walter Laqueur argued that the widening of opportunities for women after 1941 'was a blessing', but only in so far as 'anything was better than returning to domestic service'.[64] However, the refugee narratives that comprise this study identified nursing as a genuine choice for war work. For some this was because they saw the alternatives as less attractive. Others felt they could contribute in a more meaningful way as nurses. For those who were already nurses in Germany and Austria, or who had always wanted to train as a nurse, the opportunity to do so in Britain was welcomed. There were others for whom it was likely that the vocational element of nursing added to its appeal, especially for those whose childhood ambitions had been medicine. What is apparent is that for specifically female refugees, nursing was understood to be a pragmatic choice of valuable war work and the chance to assimilate into their new country.

Refugee nurses, the Second World War and the Holocaust

Jewish Refugees and the British Nursing Profession is specifically about the contribution of female Jewish refugees to twentieth-century nursing and the impact that being a nurse had on them as individuals. As such it is not a book about the Holocaust, nor is it a book about the Second World War, but both are central to the ideas within it and the lives of the refugee nurses about whom it is written. The refugee nurses whose stories form the book only came to Britain because of the anti-Jewish programme of the Nazis. Their escapes discussed in Chapter 1 are understood through the lens of our modern understanding of the Holocaust and the murder of six million Jews. It is appreciated that they could not have known the full extent of the impending disaster for European Jewry. However, their families were sufficiently worried about the future to make the decision to send their daughters to safety.

Initially it had been thought that women and children would be spared the brutality of the Nazi regime. In most families, daughters were encouraged to stay to care for elderly relatives. Furthermore, it was not considered safe for girls and young women to travel alone, a belief that was brought into stark relief with the strip-searching of escaping female refugees.[65] Although only men and boys were arrested in the pogrom on 9 and 10 November 1938, known as *Kristallnacht*, it was clear to even the youngest of children that the event marked a dangerously violent shift in Germany.[66] From this point many of the refugees' testimonies described being told by their parents that they were being sent to Britain. Many also recalled hushed conversations between adult relatives about the dangers of Nazi Jewish policy.

Between the November pogrom and the outbreak of the Second World War, families clamoured to get their daughters out of Nazi-occupied territories. Many escaped only in the last months before hostilities began. Some, like Kitty Schafer, waited nearly a year for a visa. Schafer eventually escaped to England in June 1939. Lee Fischer and Susi Loeffler escaped on some of the last Kindertransport out of Germany and Czechoslovakia in July 1939. Susan Charles escaped and arrived in England on 5 July 1939, just two months before the declaration of war (see Figure 0.1).⁶⁷

The outbreak of the Second World War meant almost all escape routes were blocked. The testimonies are replete with stories of families and friends whose escape was planned for September 1939, but who were never able to leave and subsequently perished. Holocaust historian David Cesarani argues that the war was pivotal to the Holocaust and the murder of the Jews. First, he maintains, Hitler had long threatened to punish the Jews should Germany be plunged into a global conflict. When the United States entered the war in December 1941, the Jews became 'culprits who deserved sanguinary retribution'.⁶⁸ Second, as the progress of the war went against Hitler, removing far-flung spaces into which he could send the Jews, their fate was sealed. Hitler and his regime forced Jews from Germany and their occupied territories to render the

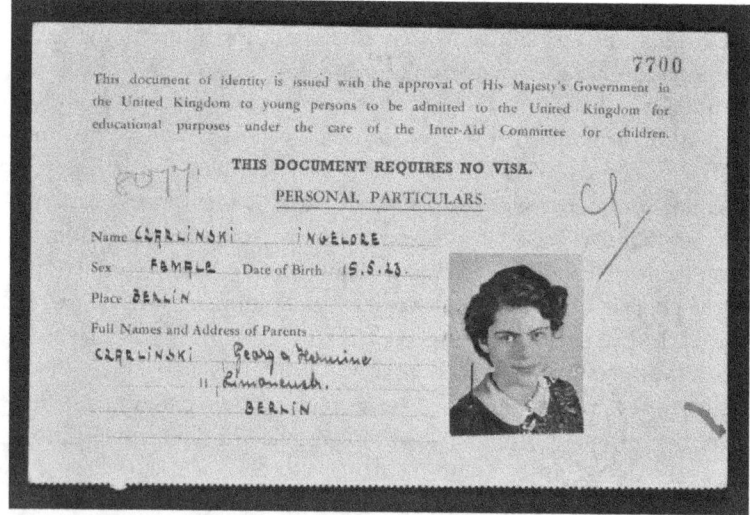

Figure 0.1 Susan Charles's (Ingelore Czarlinksi's) identity document for young person admitted under the Inter-Aid Committee for Children. Reproduced with kind permission of her family [fo. 13]

Greater Reich *Judenfrei*, or Jew-free. The failure to conquer Russia and North Africa meant there was now nowhere to send them; slave camps and ultimately death became the only destination.[69] Therefore, although the book is not about the war, the war was central to the fate of the Jews and is thus critical to the lives of the nurses and those they left behind. Furthermore, all the refugee nurses whose stories comprise this book worked during the war years, demonstrating their willingness to sacrifice themselves for their nation of refuge.

Secondary literature

This is the first book to consider the lives and work of female Jewish refugees who became nurses. It does so against a backdrop of the mid-twentieth-century nursing recruitment and retention crisis as the country faced imminent war. It is also the first book to consider the position of women refugees in a professional career. Given the presence of nurses in people's lives, their absence from the literature is peculiar. Nurses and midwives are there at birth and death. They are present when you visit your local medical centre and general practitioner. They are there at the bedside when you are ill in hospital. They have a presence in schools, older adult care facilities and in community health environments, yet they are often invisible, occupying a liminal space between the family carer and the physician. Their presence in the historiography is no less hidden. Historian of nursing Sioban Nelson argues: 'I, for one, like to remind colleagues that the history they are writing is in danger of gross distortion if the largest female professional group, the largest single workforce in some instances, is left completely out of the picture.'[70] The invisibility of nurses and nursing is made even more stark when those nurses are women of colour, especially migrants and refugees. Their liminality is as critical in the twenty-first century as it was in the mid-twentieth. It is hoped that *Jewish Refugees and the British Nursing Profession* can open the history of nursing to new audiences in Holocaust and refugee studies.

Although this is the first monograph to explore the lives of Jewish refugees who became nurses, there have been previous studies that have focused on this cohort of women. Paul Weindling's database of refugee nurses and doctors has enabled him to construct a broad history of the differing experiences for these two professional groups. His work also highlights the class and gender aspects of professional organisations' attitudes to the would-be recruits.[71] John Stewart's essay on refugee nurses has been a particularly important platform for the study.[72] His analysis of the responses of the General Nursing Council and individual hospitals brings into stark relief the motivations of those who would help refugees and those who would stymie attempts to support their recruitment. Whilst these studies have been critical to the development of my current research, their focus on the professional and organisational aspects has meant that the personal experiences have been less clearly delineated.

The interest in ordinary women's lives, especially those who lived in extraordinary times, has grown significantly since the last decades of the twentieth century. Penny Summerfield's *Reconstructing Women's Wartime Lives* marked an important shift in the historiography that focused on the personal experiences of women in war.[73] *Jewish Refugees and the British Nursing Profession* brings to the fore the individual perspectives of female Jewish refugees who supported the British nursing profession during the war and into the second half of the twentieth century. It therefore offers a subjective voice to the political and professional discussions of previous work.

Barbara Mortimer's anthology, *Sisters: Memories from the Courageous Nurses of World War Two*, provides some personal perspectives of Jewish refugee nurses.[74] This excellent text reproduces vignettes from oral histories of Second-World-War nurses that are held in the Oral History Collection of the Royal College of Nursing Archive in Edinburgh. Mortimer not only includes narratives from influential nurses such as Hockey and Altschul, but also from the less well-known, including Rosa Sacharin and Edith Bown. Although the book contains limited critical analysis, it has been invaluable as additional source material.

Many of the refugees who eventually became nurses arrived in Britain either on domestic service visas or the Kindertransport. Tony Kushner's and Jennifer Craig-Norton's analyses of the exploitative nature of domestic service as a means of escape are essential reading.⁷⁵ Given the number of women who arrived on domestic service visas, their work is critical to understanding the early months and years of young women refugees' lives in Britain. A minority of refugee servants, Kushner suggests, were treated with dignity; others with extreme callousness. The majority were treated with neutrality and a distinct lack of understanding, making the early months of their lives in Britain a misery.⁷⁶ These texts therefore provide a crucial precursor to the stories of those who later became nurses. *Jewish Refugees and the British Nursing Profession* takes the narratives of the refugees from the hidden world of those who work in other people's houses to professional service and valued war work. These personal testimonies identify a developing self-worth despite their being denigrated by domestic service employers.

Craig-Norton's work on female Jewish refugees who entered Britain on the Kindertransport provides another vital background to this study. In *The Kindertransport: Contesting Memory*, she offers a critical eye on the trope that Jewish refugees were often high achievers. Craig-Norton identifies the girls' option to train as a 'medical nurse', as opposed to a children's nurse, as the equivalent of refugee boys' opportunity to enter a profession, rather than a trade. Such ambitions were, she argues, frequently thwarted. Even when they were achieved, the Kinder faced difficulties from lack of money, demands they take menial work to pay for their board and lodging and poor treatment because employers were often suspicious of their foreign heritage.⁷⁷ As the book demonstrates, some used nursing as a method of escaping neglectful and unkind foster parents. Others discovered the possibility of entering nursing through caring foster parents, keen for them to settle into meaningful work. Significantly, *Jewish Refugees and the British Nursing Profession* builds upon Craig-Norton's assertion that nursing offered a genuine opportunity for clever refugee girls.

There is also a substantial body of literature that focuses on the experience of Jews as refugees across the globe, Bernard Wasserstein's *Britain and the Jews of Europe* being the seminal text from 1979. More recently, Frank Caestecker and Bob Moore's edited book *Refugees from Nazi Germany*, Louise London's *Whitehall and the Jews, 1933–1948* and Colin Holmes's *A Tolerant*

Country? critically consider global attitudes about Jewish refugees in the 1930s.[78] These texts have been invaluable to this book, providing context and background to the lives of refugees who left Nazi Europe for safer countries. However, whilst they offer some analysis of the experiences of women and to some extent children, they tend to take a male-centric approach, or one that treats refugee experiences as gender neutral. Given the gendered nature of 'refugeedom', this book that focuses specifically on women refugees contributes a critical voice to global refugee study.

According to historian Angela Davies, there is a growing appreciation by gender historians of the limitations of a male-centric focus.[79] Although, as Jillian Davidson maintains, there are several challenges in placing Jewish women's lives into Holocaust memory.[80] Women are, she argues, both visible – as the sacrificing mother taking her children to the gas chambers – and invisible – as the historiography focuses on the actions and rescues of great men. Women's invisibility is reproduced when their status as refugees is considered, both because of male-centric histories and because of the block domestic service visas under which most arrived. At the beginning of 1939, up to 400 visas for domestic service work were being given out each week.[81] The system, whilst enabling many to leave, engendered anonymity, which was then replicated as the women refugees entered the homes of the British middle class as a faceless mass of domestic servants. Nurses were less anonymous, existing as they did in the public eye, although the naming of all students 'Nurse' and the wearing of uniform for much of their time rendered them a homogenous group, rather than individuals.[82] *Jewish Refugees and the British Nursing Profession* offers a detailed and intimate focus on individual women refugees who came to Britain. It thus makes an important contribution to the literature by moving women out of the shadows and placing them centrally and visibly in the historical canon.

Most recent texts which explore the world of Jewish women focus on their lives in their country of origin, rather than in the countries of escape. In her essay, 'Jewish women in Nazi Germany before emigration', Marion Kaplan details the stark differences between the experiences of Jewish women and men living in Nazi Germany. Women were, she argues, much closer to the street and could better see the changes in society: 'Raised to be sensitive to interpersonal behaviour and social situations, women's social antennae were more finely tuned than those of their husbands. They registered the increasing hostility of their immediate surroundings.'[83] The prescience experienced by Jewish women, sadly, had little impact on their abilities to convince their husbands of the need to leave.

Esther Hertzog argues that in a crisis, the exclusions applied to women in politics and occupations are 'weakened', thus enabling them to take more direct action in a bid for survival.[84] Nevertheless, if gendered roles shifted from 1933 after many Jewish men lost their jobs, accepted patriarchy remained intact.[85] As heads of the households, many men ignored their wives' anxieties about the increasing dangers, and families remained in Germany.[86] Britain's acceptance of 20,000 women refugees as domestic servants may have enabled parents to eventually get their daughters to safety, but for those women who were left, many faced certain death. As Cesarani argues, women who were pregnant, who gave birth in the camps, women with infants and the elderly, 'stood no chance'.[87] *Jewish Refugees and the British Nursing Profession* offers a picture of Jewish women in which they succeed independently, rather than being embedded in a social system that failed to listen to their voices and placed them in danger of their lives. By focusing on the professional and personal lives of refugee women who entered the nursing profession, I place Jewish women survivors of the Holocaust as women with agency rather than victims of a murderous regime.

Personal testimony

This book uses a range of personal narratives, both oral and written, letters and articles from the nursing and medical press of the day and archival documents. The sources reveal a kaleidoscope of experiences that girls and young women, refugees, enemy aliens and nurses described. What is stark in much of the personal testimony that has been provided by survivors and refugees is that most had at least one parent who was murdered. Many lost both parents, as well as siblings and other family members. Using the personal testimony of Holocaust survivors enables them to bear witness to their lives and those who were murdered.[88] Jane Georges and Susan Benedict acknowledge the value of letters in this endeavour,[89] but this is also enabled through other forms of written narrative and oral history.[90] Probably the most famous of all written Holocaust testimonies is *The Diary of Anne Frank*, first published in 1952. The diary may only reflect one small space into which the Holocaust invaded, but it did at least humanise the suffering and horror.[91] Placed alongside the vast realms of testimony collected since the end of the Second World War, it adds to the essential witness-bearing of those who perished and those who survived. Jessica Wiederhorn argues that personal accounts of the Holocaust were created long before the end of the Second World War. The majority of diaries, letters and notes that were hidden have been lost. Some however, survived and these 'express a desperation to tell, to document, to bear witness, and to commemorate'.[92]

Written personal testimonies used in this book include the letters and diary of Edith Bown and several memoirs, some published and some created for the family audience. Like all personal testimony, these written accounts are deeply qualitative, reflecting the feelings, experiences and perceptions of the refugees as actors in their own stories. I acknowledge that there is a broad continuum on the theory of personal testimony. At one end is the belief that it should be given equal value to more objective forms of documentary evidence; at the other that its utility as source material should be rejected.[93] There is, however, a middle ground and it is this middle ground on which the testimony of this book rests. Whilst accepting that the experiences and feelings expressed may not reflect completely the objective reality, they are valued as the true experiences of the individual.

The letters and diary of Bown are particularly valuable as they begin before the war was declared and continue into the early war years when its outcome was not known. Framed within a memoir that was started in the 1990s, the document enables the reader to witness the shifts in Bown's life experiences and the manner in which she composed her world, as she 'tracks herself through time'.[94] Diaries are a valuable method for the non-elite young woman to explore the emotional experiences of her life.[95] They are also repository for feelings and experiences that are too traumatic to discuss in the open.⁹⁶ Michael Roper argues that narration can be a psychological process in which the author is able to make sense of their trauma and distress through words on the page.⁹⁷ Written testimony cannot be refuted, nor can it be challenged.⁹⁸ Bown's words thus rest on the page; they are highly personal thoughts and experiences which expose what was 'true' to her. Nevertheless, the employment of multiple sources of personal testimony and printed archival documents throughout this book support the validity of the claims made in such individual narratives.

The use of memoir is more complex, written, as it is, often many years after the event and with an audience in mind. Margaret Hodge, Edith Bown and Mia Ross all created memoirs specifically for their families, none of which have been published. Others, including Trudie Moos, Marianne Parkes, Cilly Haar and Margaret Marflow, published their memoirs. Rosa Sacharin summarised the reason for her memoir and in doing so highlights the challenges the reader faces when pursuing the veracity of its contents. Having admitted she was interested in history and particularly the history of the Jews, she stated that in her memoir that she attempted to piece together both 'what I have been told about events of the time' and also 'the events in my life – most of which are memories of personal experiences'.⁹⁹ This piecing together means that the narrative contain any number of inaccuracies, particularly as third-hand information is notoriously difficult to verify. However, this does not make her story necessarily any less valuable. Against the primacy of archival documents and perhaps even the oral history interview, memoirs have been called a 'debased currency', as their validity as a historical source is challenged.¹⁰⁰ Historian John Tosh goes further, arguing that memoirs are 'selective to the point of distortion', although he is reflecting on the use of memoir by politicians keen to justify their positions.¹⁰¹

Nevertheless, the limited number of written personal testimonies meant a pragmatic choice needed to be made. Memoir comprised the most created form of written personal testimony by refugee nurses. Furthermore, whilst I acknowledge all the possible criticisms of this literary form, the narratives in all the memoirs used for *Jewish Refugees and the British Nursing Profession* are remarkably similar. All the memoirs provide an image of life before National Socialism that was relatively safe and happy. They reflect on the growing persecution and then destruction of European jewry and the challenges all the women faced on their arrival in Britain. Their use therefore as a method of personal narrative has been essential to this book.

Oral history is able to tell the story in a way that written testimony cannot.[102] From the 1970s feminist oral historians have focused on the intersubjectivity of their work. Contemporary oral historians are concerned with both the power of truth when engaging with marginalised groups and working with the participant to interrogate their understanding of the past.[103] Penny Summerfield's analysis of 'composure' in the oral history interview is particularly salient. As Summerfield argues, in oral history, the participant not only composes their life story, but finds composure in its telling; they 'make sense of the subject matter they recall by interpreting it'.[104] Given the limited time allotted to an interview and the subsequently inevitable loss of the complexities of someone's life, the telling of one's life and the making sense of that life are all part of the narrative and its formulation.[105] Whilst oral historians acknowledge that narrators may make errors in their stories, such errors do not make the entire narrative aberrant.[106]

Minor factual errors are trivial compared to the value of the knowledge gained. When Ruth Shire, one of the participants for the study, was describing the employment of refugee nurses at the Staines Emergency Hospital during the war, she said that the matron, Miss Lang, took ten refugees.[107] Later, when Heidi Cowen, a friend and colleague since their nurse training days, joined the interview, she said that Lang employed thirty refugee nurses.[108] Clearly there is a considerable difference in the numbers remembered by two refugees who were in the same place at the same time. However, what is important here is not the precise number of refugee nurses employed, but that Lang was pleased to have a significant ratio of refugee nurses among their British counterparts. This is especially noteworthy given the government quota of refugees allowed in hospitals in the early years of the war.[109]

It is acknowledged that 'insider research', that is, when the researcher belongs to the same group as the participants, has its difficulties. As part of the group, it is easy to take the subjective view and lack criticality when analysing the data.[110] If the researcher is too close to the subject matter it is easy to forget to explore details, denying the reader the nuances of the story. Being an insider can, conversely, promote a sense of trust and collegiality between the interviewer and the participant, enabling the narrator to talk of things they may not tell someone outside the group. As I am a nurse, participants felt able to talk openly of their lives in nursing, the positive and the negative aspects, knowing that I would understand.[111] My insider status is not, of course, absolute. First, I do not speak German. However, all the interviews used for the project were in English and the participants' professional lives were in Anglophone countries. At least one stated that she refused to speak German. The decision to use English only is, arguably, a methodologically appropriate one for this book. Second, I am not Jewish, nor do I have any experience of genocide. Holocaust memories create additional difficulties for the oral history interview. Trauma, extreme sorrow, guilt at survival, the identity of the participant and the overlaying of eighty years of rescue narratives all impact the testimony. Within my multi-positionality, I hope that I was able to find a path in which I gained the trust of the women I interviewed and have made sense of their stories.

All the oral histories for the book were taken at least fifty years after the end of the Second World War and are therefore likely to be affected by inevitable compromises in human memory. I was able to interview eight surviving refugee nurses. Five of these women stayed in the UK; others emigrated, one to Canada, one to the United States and one to Australia. All of them were in their nineties except one. Most had previously talked about their escape and life in Britain, but none had specifically been asked about their professional nursing lives. I had also interviewed two refugees for a previous project in 2001. These two participants, Lisbeth Hockey and Annie Altschul, have a range of data related to their lives in the public domain as well. They were, respectively, the first director of nursing research and the first professor of mental health nursing in the UK. They both died early this century.

I was also fortunate to have been contacted by the relatives of deceased refugee nurses, who offered written testimonies which their mothers and aunts had created for them while still alive. Some family members simply had memories they wished to share and others had documents related to their relatives' escape, nursing lives and family stories. I am most grateful for the interest these families have taken in my research. Their insights into their relatives have been invaluable in building a picture of the refugee nurses' lives. Finally, there are several oral and written narratives in the public domain. All the narratives, oral and written, used for the book are deeply personal and constructed by individuals with a range of experiences both before and after fleeing Nazi Europe. Together they reveal a number of critical issues that I will go on to explore. Significantly, all the testimonies demonstrate a sense of fracture and loss. This sense of what was lost pervades the stories, from the loss of the security of a childhood home and the loss of education, to most profoundly the loss of friends and family members.

Remembering loss and trauma

Survival was a matter of luck.[112] But as well as luck, people survived because of their abilities.[113] This was undoubtedly true in the concentration and extermination camps. As Primo Levi argues, having a particular skill could engender certain privileges and thus more food: 'death by hunger, or by the diseases of hunger, was the prisoner's normal destiny. This could be avoided only with additional food, and to obtain it a large or a small privilege was necessary.'[114] The ability to escape from Nazi Europe would also involve certain attributes. Only about eleven per cent of Jews who were children when the war started survived.[115] As Craig-Norton argues, the children most likely to be saved via the Kindertransport were those who were the least Jewish-looking, with girls being more favoured than boys. Those with physical or mental defects were unlikely to be chosen.[116] Nevertheless, luck was also central to the moment of escape, with one family member's visa arriving on time and another's not.

Not all those refugee nurses whose personal narratives comprise this book were children when they escaped the Nazis, but most were either in their teens or very early twenties. Some, like Hortense Gordon and Edith Bown, escaped to Britain, but had siblings and cousins who were murdered.[117] Why Gordon should have been given the ability to live, whilst her younger sister perished with her parents, was sheer serendipity. Gordon held the memory of her sister's death until she died herself in 2019. One of her last requests was that she would like the photo of her with her sister to be preserved in the Holocaust galleries at the Imperial War Museum in London (see Figure 0.2). Judith Tydor Baumel argues that there were those who achieved physical survival but were left with permanent psychological trauma.[118] Whether Gordon's desire to preserve her sister's memory above all others was a product of trauma, extreme sorrow or an uninterrupted sense of loss is not known, but on meeting her there was no doubt that this loss left her with a permanent sense of rupture in her life.

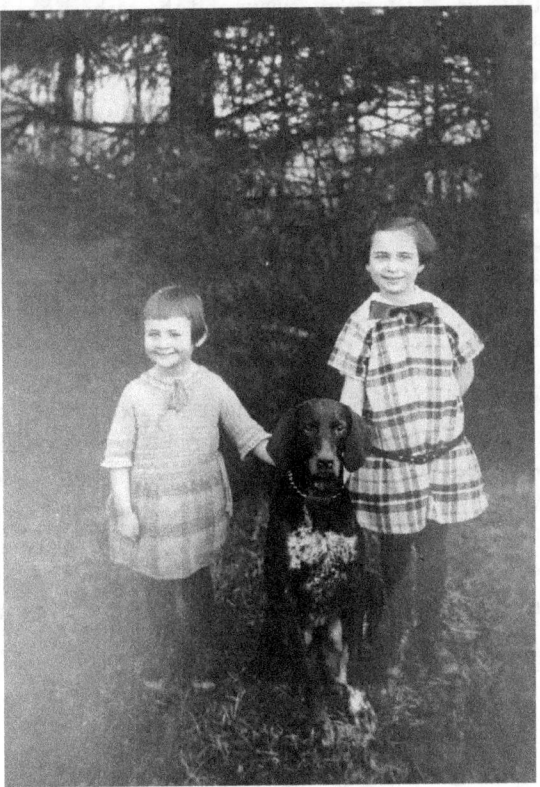

Figure 0.2 Hortense Gordon (*right*) and her younger sister, Beate, with the family dog, *c.* late 1920s? Reproduced with kind permission of her daughter, Yvonne Gordon [fo. 25]

In her essay 'Field notes on catastrophe: reflections on the September 11, 2001, Oral History Memory and Narrative Project', Mary Marshall Clark argues that the value of oral historians is partly in their ability to restore 'a sense of order in the telling of their [the participants'] life narrative'.[119] More than the myriad of professionals supporting victims, oral historians simply listened to the stories of trauma, loss and tragedy. Mahua Sarkar maintains that oral history narration brings meaning to the life of the participant.[120] However, whilst interviews can be cathartic, the 'relational dynamics already present … are compounded when trauma is involved'.[121] Lynn Abrams identifies the 'therapeutic' nature of the oral history interview and the cathartic construction of the self.[122] But we need to be mindful where we draw the line between research, catharsis and therapy.

In Deborah Dwork's monograph of Jewish children in Nazi-occupied territories, *Children with a Star*, one of her participants maintained that 'the past is always present'.[123] Traumatic memories can be triggered by seemingly insignificant events and moments. Cathy Caruth argues that these flashbacks can be themselves 'retraumatizing; if not life-threatening … and this would seem to explain the high suicide rate of survivors, for example, survivors of Vietnam or of concentration camps, who commit suicide only after they have found themselves completely in safety'.[124] The question of how safe survivors actually feel once they have found refuge is, of course, a moot point but something that I will consider later. Annie Altschul admitted to historian of mental nursing, Peter Nolan, 'sometimes when I am alone, I will turn round and I think I can see Hitler'.[125] In the absence of skilled psychologists, using such memories as a method of therapy can be harmful, and as a historian it is incumbent upon us to minimise that harm, not harness it for the narrative.[126]

Structure of the book

Jewish Refugees and the British Nursing Profession takes a broadly chronological structure. It follows the lives of the refugees from being young girls in Germany, Austria and Czechoslovakia prior to National Socialism and their escape to Britain and entrance into nursing. The book traces their experiences as nurses in the Second World War and the post-war world and finally explores their professional work and its legacy in the latter half of the twentieth century. Chapter 1 considers the ordinary and mainly happy lives of young Jewish girls and women in Germany, Austria and Czechoslovakia before the rise of Hitler. It considers their ambitions to be doctors, teachers and in some instances nurses. It follows the rise of Nazism, the increasingly draconian anti-Jewish laws and the arrests. The chapter considers the girls' move to Jewish schools and ghettos and finally the pogrom in November 1938, which raised the determination of parents to send their daughters to safety. The chapter then focuses on the methods of escape and the gendered nature of forced migration, especially for very young women and girls. The chapter reviews the experiences of those who travelled to Britain on nursing visas, some of whom were already certificated nurses in Germany, or were students of nursing, and others who chose nursing as a means of escape. It considers those young girls who were sent away on the Kindertransport, those who escaped on domestic service visas and those who were left behind. Within this exploration the chapter brings into stark relief the self-interest of the British Government in offering domestic service and nursing visas as escape routes. As Craig-Norton argues, 'British immigration policies were coldly pragmatic rather than humanitarian.'[127]

As the prospect of war increased, both the Government and nursing elite saw the potential of recruiting female refugees to staff the country's hospitals. Despite this opportunism and although nursing comprised hard work, long hours and harsh discipline, it was also understood to offer training, accommodation and a potential professional future, albeit not a well-paid one.

Chapter 2 explores 'The hospital world' and the refugees' place in it. The chapter begins with an analysis of the situation in British hospitals, the crisis in nurse recruitment and retention and comparisons with other professional groups, most especially physicians. The chapter considers the work of the Nursing and Midwifery Department located at Bloomsbury House and sets its recruitment drive for nurses alongside the medical profession's animosity towards potential Continental doctors. Finally, the chapter considers the responses of individual hospitals to Jewish refugee nurse recruits and the attempts of the refugees themselves to gain a place to train as a nurse.

Chapter 3 considers the refugees as 'War nurses'. It examines the role of refugee nurses as valuable and necessary war workers. However, this value was to be thwarted when, after the fall of France in spring 1940, refugee nurses were classed as 'enemy aliens' and dismissed from their hospital training programmes. As the Second World War progressed and more British nurses volunteered for active service overseas, the work of women not traditionally recruited into nursing became increasingly necessary and refugee nurses were invited back into the profession. As I argue, not all accepted this volte-face and some refused to return. Those who did became part of a system that accepted the help of married nurses, girl guides and male orderlies. The chapter then focuses on the experiences of refugees who were willing – either because they wanted to nurse, or because of the lack of alternatives – to return to hospital nursing. I consider the development of camaraderie and a new 'nurse' family in the face of wartime needs

Chapter 4, 'From the post-war world to a nursing legacy', turns to the latter half of the twentieth century. The refugees' dedication to nursing during the war meant that many were offered naturalisation in the very early years after the war. As the chapter demonstrates, many of the refugees accepted Britain as their home and were keen to become British citizens. The chapter examines the immediate post-war work of refugees. Some, like Alice Fink and Eva Minden, returned to Germany to support the relief of Bergen-Belsen before emigrating to the United States. Most stayed in Britain, keen to support the new NHS.

Four of British nursing's most influential nurses in the late twentieth century, Annie Altschul, Marion Ferguson, Lisbeth Hockey and Charlotte Kratz, were refugees. The chapter considers their professional and personal lives and discusses their lasting influence on the nursing profession. Not all refugee nurses had such illustrious careers. Nevertheless, several forged successful professional futures as nurse educators, public health nurses and one as an examiner for the General Nursing Council. Susan Charles was the nurse who assisted in the delivery of King Charles III.[128]

Like British women in the post-war milieu, many married and left the profession as hospitals reasserted regulations on 'living-in', which precluded the employment of married nurses.[129] Others were able to continue working as nurses, influencing their workplace in a number of small but significant ways. Cilly Haar and Hortense Gordon both returned to work when their children were young. Haar recalled that she could not remember any other married nurses working.

In the concluding chapter, the book's central thesis – that nursing offered a space in which female refugees could reassert themselves in the face of the horror of the Holocaust, is considered. It sets this analysis against a backdrop of crises in recruitment and retention and extensive criticism of the nursing profession both from within and without. The book also situates itself in the canon of refugee and migration studies, particularly of women migrants. As the first monograph to explore women refugees' experiences in a profession, it brings female migrants' stories out of the shadows and bears witness to their lives as they created a space for themselves in their new home. The book enables readers to view refugees not as victims or potential subversives, but women with agency.

Jewish Refugees and the British Nursing Profession acknowledges the gendered nature of nursing as opportunity. In this analysis, gender both constrained the refugees' opportunities for escape and work and was also the key. Nursing was poorly paid and maintained its corpus of students with petty discipline and harsh conditions, making it unpopular with British girls and young women. Nevertheless, it did provide training, a home and both social and geographic mobility on qualification. Furthermore, whereas male doctors and dentists struggled to find employment and therefore safe passage out of Nazi territories, female doctors and medical students were encouraged to escape through the nursing visa scheme. The book explores the value that these women offered the nursing profession at a time when most applicants were not from educated and cultured backgrounds. It reviews the notion, that for some, nursing was a redemptive pursuit, enabling the refugee women to care for humankind in a way that they could not care for their families who perished in the Holocaust. As I argue, these women understood the need to survive and chose nursing not only as a pragmatic method of escape and gaining independence, but also as an emerging profession with an increasing contribution to the health of the nation. In the final analysis, *Jewish Refugees and the British Nursing Profession* demonstrates the value that nursing, with all its challenges, offered these young women.

Notes

1 Hortense Gordon, oral history interview by Sharon Rapaport in London on 3 July 2004. Interview 65, Refugee Voices: Association of Jewish Refugees (AJR) Audio-Visual Testimony Archive, British Library, London.
2 Letter from H. Z. Oates at the Home Office, probably to the Chair of the Domestic Bureau. The issue of the suitability of refugees coming to Britain on domestic service visas was addressed: 'it must always be understood that the Bureau will recruit and place in domestic service only refugees who are suitable for such employment and likely to remain in it'. ACC/2793/04/05/01, London Metropolitan Archives (LMA) (original underlining). Although Gordon came over via private introduction, many refugees who came on domestic service visas continued to be wholly unsuitable. Many came from the professional and servant-employing echelons of German society, rather than the domestic servant strata. For further discussion on the suitability of refugees for domestic service, see for example, Jennifer Craig-Norton, 'Refugees at the margins: Jewish domestics in Britain 1938–1945', *Shofar: An Interdisciplinary Journal of Jewish Studies* 37, 3 (2019): 295–330.
3 Gordon, oral history interview, 2004.
4 The term non-Aryan refers to persons who were either only part-Jewish or came from families who had previously converted to Christianity. However, under Nuremberg Laws they were all marked as carrying Jewish blood and therefore enemies of the State. For the purposes of the book, therefore, I shall refer to all the refugees as Jews. This will include, for the sake of brevity, those who were non-Aryan and whose Jewish identity only became a matter of any importance after 1933.
5 Charlotte Kratz, oral history interview at her home in Eastbourne on 16 September 1988. Interview T37, Oral History Collection, Royal College of Nursing (RCN), Edinburgh.

6 Penny Summerfield, *Reconstructing Women's Wartime Lives: Discourse and Subjectivity in Oral Histories of the Second World War* (Manchester: Manchester University Press, 1998), 70.
7 Just an alien nurse, 'Alien nurse wishes to serve', *Nursing Mirror and Midwives Journal* (29 June 1940): 317.
8 Shmuly Yanklowitz, *The Soul of Jewish Social Justice* (Jerusalem: Urim Publications, 2014).
9 Gertrude Roberts, oral history interview by Alan Dein on 23 January 1982. Audio 184, Oral History Collection, Jewish Museum, London.
10 Anne Summers, *Female Lives, Moral States: Women, Religion and Public Life in Britain, 1800–1930* (Newbury: Threshold Press, 2000), 21.
11 Robert Dingwall, Anne Marie Rafferty and Charles Webster, *An Introduction to the Social History of Nursing* (London: Routledge, 1988), 40.
12 Sue Hawkins, *Nursing and Women's Labour in the Nineteenth Century: The Quest for Independence* (London: Routledge, 2010), 28.
13 Anne Marie Rafferty, *The Politics of Nursing Knowledge* (London: Routledge, 1996), 24.
14 Christine E. Hallett, *Veiled Warriors: Allied Nurses of the First World War* (Oxford: Oxford University Press, 2014), 255.
15 Nursing became a regulated and registrable profession in 1919 with the Nurses Registration Acts. Susan McGann, Anne Crowther and Rona Dougall, *A History of the Royal College of Nursing, 1916–90: A Voice for Nurses* (Manchester: Manchester University Press, 2009), 31.
16 Specifically, the Lancet Commission (1932) and the Athlone Report (1937). The state of British nursing in the 1930s and 1940s is discussed in full in Chapter 2 of this book.
17 Jennifer Craig-Norton, *The Kindertransport: Contesting Memory* (Bloomington: Indiana University Press, 2019), 190.
18 Tony Kushner, *The Holocaust and the Liberal Imagination: A Social and Cultural History* (Oxford: Blackwell, 1994), 81.
19 Craig-Norton, 'Refugees at the margins'.
20 Nursing and Midwifery Department, Central Office for Refugees, 'Brief survey of situation regarding nurse refugees' (29 August 1940), 2. Aliens Department – Home Office HO 213/521, National Archives, Kew, London.
21 John Stewart, 'Angels or aliens? Refugee nurses in Britain 1938–1942', *Medical History* 47 (2003): 157.
22 Central Council for Jewish Refugees, 'Report for 1939', 14, Central Council for Refugees. ACC/2793/S/A/84, LMA.

23 Anonymous military nurse, 'Frontline Females', BBC Radio 4 (11 April 1998), H9872/2, Sound Archive, British Library, London. This two-part radio programme, introduced by Claire Rayner, involved a number of Second-World-War nurses. It is not possible to identify individual women in the broadcast. For a full list of participants, see the Bibliography. 'Brasses' refer to the brassware in the wards that the probationer (student) nurses were required to clean.
24 Loredana Radu, 'More or less Europe? The European leaders' discourses on the refugees crisis', *Romanian Journal of Communication and Public Relations* 18, 2 (2016): 22.
25 Peter Gatrell, 'The question of refugees: Past and present', *Origins: Current Events in Historical Perspective* 10, 7 (2017) https://origins.osu.edu/article/question-refugees-past-and-present?language_content_entity=en [accessed 20 September 2023].
26 Tony Kushner, *Journeys from the Abyss: The Holocaust and Forced Migration from the1880s to the Present* (Liverpool: Liverpool University Press, 2017), ix.
27 Royal College of Nursing, 'London nurses experience the most racism', *Nursing Standard* 33, 8 (2018): 6; Steve Ford, 'Exclusive: High level of racial discrimination faced by nurses revealed', *Nursing Times* (2 October 2019). www.nursingtimes.net/news/workforce/exclusive-high-level-of-racial-discrimination-faced-by-nurses-revealed-02–10–2019/ [accessed January 2020].
28 Amelia Gentleman, 'Calls grow to scrap NHS surcharge for migrant health workers', *Guardian* (3 May 2020). https://www.theguardian.com/society/2020/may/03/calls-grow-scrap-nhs-surcharge-migrant-healthcare-workers-coronavirus [accessed 20 May 2020].
29 Gemma Mitchell, 'Minister rejects plea to waive NHS fee for overseas nurses', *Nursing Times* (14 November 2018). https://www.nursingtimes.net/news/policies-and-guidance/minister-rejects-plea-to-waive-nhs-fee-for-overseas-nurses-14–11–2018 [accessed 26 May 2020].
30 Mike Shallcross, 'Government u-turns on charging migrant healthcare workers to use the NHS', *Independent Nurse* (22 May 2020). www.independentnurse.co.uk/content/news/government-u-turns-on-charging-migrant-healthcare-workers-to-use-the-nhs [accessed 26 May 2020].
31 Pertti Ahonen, 'Europe and refugees: 1938 and 2015–16', *Patterns of Prejudice* 52, 2–3 (2018): 147.
32 Gatrell, 'The question of refugees'.
33 Jenny Phillimore and Lisa Goodson, 'Problem or opportunity? Asylum seekers, refugees, employment and social exclusion in deprived urban areas', *Urban Studies* 43, 10 (2006): 1715–36.

34 John Willott and Jacqueline Stevenson, 'Attitudes to employment of professionally qualified refugees in the United Kingdom', *International Migration* 51, 5 (2013): 120–32.

35 Robyn I. Stone, 'The migrant direct care workforce: An international perspective', *Generations: Journal of the American Society on Aging* 40, 1 (2016): 100.

36 Barbara Brush, 'Refuge and rescue: Jewish nurse refugees and the International Council of Nurses, 1947–1965', *Nursing History Review* 7 (1999): 113–25. Brush's analysis of the obsession of the International Council of Nurses with refugees' credentials and the organisation's failure to understand refugee nurses as part of 'forced migration' speaks directly to this current project.

37 Linda McDowell, 'Moving stories: Precarious work and multiple migrations', *Gender, Place and Culture: A Journal of Feminist Geography* 25, 4 (2018): 480.

38 Sofie Baarnhielm, Kees Laban, Meryam Schouler-Ocak, Cecile Rousseau and Laurence J. Kirmayer, 'Mental health for refugees, asylum seekers and displaced persons: A call for a humanitarian agenda', *Transcultural Psychiatry* 54, 5–6 (2017): 565–74; Ade Kearns, Elise Whitley, Matt Egan, Catherine Tabbner and Carol Tannahill, 'Healthy migrants in an unhealthy city? The effects of time on the health of migrants living in deprived areas of Glasgow', *International Migration and Integration* 18 (2017): 675–98; Kyriakos S. Markides and Sunshine Rote, 'The healthy immigrant effect and aging in the United States and other Western countries', *Gerontologist* 59, 2 (2018): 205–14.

39 McDowell, 'Moving stories'.

40 Dolores Vojvoda, Stevan M. Weine, Thomas McGlashan, Daniel F. Becker and Steven M. Southwick, 'Posttraumatic stress disorder symptoms in Bosnian refugees 3½ years after resettlement', *Journal of Rehabilitation Research and Development* 45, 3 (2008): 421–6; McDowell, 'Moving stories'.

41 Craig-Norton, 'Refugees at the margins', 318.

42 Edith Menkes Wolloch, oral history interview at her home on 21 March 2006. Interview 2297, AHC Oral History Archive, Leo Baeck Institute, Berlin and New York. https://digipres.cjh.org/delivery/DeliveryManagerServlet?dps_pid=IE2981299 [accessed 1 October 2023]. When Wolloch refers to 'sisters' these are the women who are in charge of wards, the senior nurses in a hospital. There is no religious affiliation.

43 Edith Bown recalled the hospital chaplains constantly trying to convert her. Edith Bown, oral history interview by Barbara Mortimer

in Maidstone on 24 May 2008. Interview T379, Oral History Collection, RCN, Edinburgh.
44 Lee Fischer (Liesl Einstein), oral history interview by Jane Brooks on 12 October 2017. Personal archive.
45 Rachel Pistol, '"Heavy is the responsibility for all the lives that might have been saved in the pre-war years": British perceptions of refugees, 1933–1940', *European Judaism* 40, 2 (2017): 41.
46 Julia Hallam, *Nursing the Image Media, Culture and Professional Identity* (London: Routledge, 2000), 118. Hallam highlights that in 1972 the *Nursing Times* published a paper that identified 25 per cent of the nursing workforce as being black. At this time there was no representation of black nurses in the media.
47 Henrietta Ewart, '"Coventry Irish": Community, class, culture and narrative in the formation of a migrant identity, 1940–1970', *Midland History* 36, 2 (2011): 225–44; Louise Ryan, 'Migrant women, social networks and motherhood: The experiences of Irish nurses in Britain', *Sociology* 41, 2 (2007): 295–312; Nicola Yeates, 'A dialogue with "global care chain" analysis: Nurse migration in the Irish context', *Feminist Review* 77 (2004): 79–95; Sean Glynn, 'Irish immigration to Britain, 1911–1951: Patterns and policy', *Irish Economic and Social History* (1981): 50–69. https://journals.sagepub.com/doi/10.1177/033248938100800104 [accessed 25 September 2023].
48 Ewart, '"Coventry Irish"', 230.
49 Annie Altschul, oral history interview by Jane Brooks at her home in Edinburgh on 7 August 2001. Personal archive.
50 For detail on the work and migration of Caribbean women as nurses, see for example, Karen Flynn, 'Proletarianization, professionalization and Caribbean immigrant nurses', *Canadian Woman Studies* 18, 1 (1998): 57–60; Karen Flynn, *Moving Beyond Borders: A History of Black Canadian and Caribbean Women in the Diaspora* (Toronto: University of Toronto Press, 2011); M. Shkimba and Karen Flynn, '"In England we did nursing": Caribbean and British nurses in Great Britain and Canada, 1950–70', in Barbara Mortimer and Susan McGann (eds), *New Directions in Nursing History: International Perspectives* (London: Routledge, 2004).
51 Rabbi Sidney Schwartz, *Judaism and Justice: The Jewish Passion to Repair the World* (Woodstock: Jewish Lights Publishing, 2006), xix; Peter Pulzer, 'Jews and nation-building in Germany 1815–1918', *Baeck Institute Year Book* 41, 1 (1996): 214.
52 Joachim Wieler, 'Destination social work: Émigrés in a women's profession', in Sibylle Quack (ed.), *Between Sorrow and Strength: Women*

Refugees of the Nazi Period (Cambridge: Cambridge University Press, 1995), 267.
53 For example, Dr Maximilian Liebstein, Josephine Bruegel's father, was a country doctor. He died in 1929.
54 Lisbeth Hockey, oral history interview by Helen Sweet at her home in Edinburgh on 13 August 1996. Interview T221, Oral History Collection, RCN, Edinburgh.
55 Fischer, oral history interview.
56 Gertrud (Trudie) Moos, 'I Remember: My Life Story' (printed 1995), 42. A biographical database of European Medical Refugees in Great Britain, 1930s–1950s, Oxford Brookes University, Oxford.
57 Stewart, 'Angels or aliens?',155.
58 G. V. Hillyers, 'Refugee nurses', *Nursing Times* (10 December 1938): 1310.
59 Walter Laqueur, *Generation Exodus: The Fate of Young Jewish Refugees from Nazi Germany* (London: I. B. Tauris, 2004).
60 E. N. Cooper to R. Clare Martin Esq., Central Office for Refugees, 'Dear Clare Martin' (23 May 1941) Report on the work of the Aliens War Service Department: Volume I: 1939–1944. HO 213/2093/3, National Archives.
61 Central Office for Refugees, 'Circular No. 100. B: Nursing and Medical Auxiliaries: Hospital Nursing' (6 June 1941). HO 213/523, National Archives.
62 Central Office for Refugees, 'Circular No. 100. B: Nursing and Medical Auxiliaries'.
63 Central Office for Refugees, 'Circular No. 100. B: Nursing and Medical Auxiliaries'.
64 Laqueur, *Generation Exodus*, 202.
65 Sibylle Quack, 'Introduction', in Sibylle Quack (ed.), *Between Sorrow and Strength: Women Refugees of the Nazi Period* (Cambridge: Cambridge University Press, 1995).
66 Marion Berghahn, *Continental Britons: German-Jewish Refugees from Nazi Germany* (Oxford: Berg, 1988), 73. For the purposes of this book I shall refer to the night of 9 November 1938 as the November pogrom, not as Kristallnacht. Current research considers the term to be wholly inadequate and apologist for the Nazi crime. The Holocaust Memorial Museum, Washington, DC states on its website: 'The Nazis came to call the event Kristallnacht ("Crystal Night," or "The Night of Broken Glass"), referring to the thousands of shattered windows that littered the streets afterwards, but the euphemism does not convey the full brutality of the event.'

www.ushmm.org/collections/bibliography/kristallnacht [accessed 10 August 2022].

67 Marion Charles, 'From Nazi Germany to Clarence House', *Association of Jewish Refugees Magazine* (date unknown): 4.

68 David Cesarani, *Final Solution: The Fate of the Jews, 1933–1949* (London: Pan Macmillan, Kindle edition, 2016), 31.

69 Cesarani, *Final Solution*, 393.

70 Sioban Nelson, 'The fork in the road: Nursing history versus the history of nursing', *Nursing History Review* 10 (2002): 185.

71 Paul Weindling, 'Medical refugees and the modernisation of British medicine, 1930–1960', *Social History of Medicine* 22, 3 (2009): 489–511.

72 Stewart, 'Angels or aliens?'

73 Summerfield, *Reconstructing Women's Wartime Lives*.

74 Barbara Mortimer, *Sisters: Extraordinary True-Life Stories from Nurses in World War Two* (London: Hutchinson, 2012).

75 Craig-Norton, 'Refugees at the margins'; Jennifer Craig-Norton, 'Servitude, displacement and trauma: Jewish refugee domestics in Britain, 1938–45', in Paula A. Michaels and Christina Twomey (eds) *Gender and Trauma since 1900* (London: Bloomsbury, 2021); Tony Kushner, 'Asylum or servitude? Refugee domestics in Britain, 1933–1945', *Bulletin of the Society for the Study of Labour History* 53, 3 (1988): 19–27; Kushner, *Holocaust in the Liberal Imagination*, 90–115.

76 Kushner, 'Asylum or servitude?; Kushner, *Holocaust in the Liberal Imagination*, 90–115.

77 Craig-Norton, *Kindertransport*, 205.

78 Frank Caestecker and Bob Moore (eds), *Refugees from Nazi Europe and the Liberal European States* (New York: Berghahn Books, 2010); Louise London, *Whitehall and the Jews, 1933–1948: British Immigration Policy, Jewish Refugees and the Holocaust* (Cambridge: Cambridge University Press, 2000); Colin Holmes, *A Tolerant Country?: Immigrants, Refugees and Minorities in Britain* (London: Faber & Faber, 1991).

79 Angela Davies, '"Belonging and unbelonging": Jewish refugee and survivor women in 1950s Britain', *Women's History Review* 26, 1 (2016): 131. http://dx.doi.org/10.1080/09612025.2015.1123028 [accessed 25 September 2023].

80 Jillian Davidson, 'German-Jewish women in England', in Werner E. Mosse, Julius Carlebach, Gerhard Hirschfield, Aubrey Newman, Arnold Pauker and Peter Pulzer (eds), *Second Chance: Two Centuries*

Introduction 35

    of German-Speaking Jews in the United Kingdom (Tübingen: J. C. B. Mohr, 1991).
81 Tony Kushner, 'An alien occupation – Jewish refugees and domestic service in Britain, 1933–1948', in Mosse et al. (eds), *Second Chance*, 562.
82 In her war memoir Ann Radloff (Reeves) complains about being known simply as N. Reeves, or Nurse Reeves, and not by her own name: 'The gruelling process of depersonalisation began on arrival at our destination. The dragon who met us (sister) thrust a tray of labels disdainfully at my front and without looking at me ordered me to "take one – it will show you where you are to sleep". It was marked N. Reeves. Naively, for I didn't realise I now had no identity, I protested that my initial was A. "Stupid girl, don't you know that N stands for Nurse?"' Ann Radloff, 'Going to Gooseberry Beach: Travels and adventures of a nursing Sister', 1, Private Papers: Documents 147, Imperial War Museum, London.
83 Marion Kaplan, 'Jewish women in Nazi Germany before emigration', in Sibylle Quack (ed.), *Between Sorrow and Strength: Women Refugees of the Nazi Period* (Cambridge: Cambridge University Press, 1995).
84 Esther Hertzog, 'Introduction: Studying the Holocaust as a feminist', in Esther Hertzog (ed.), *Life, Death and Sacrifice: Women and Family in the Holocaust* (Jerusalem: Gefen Publishing House, 2008), 2–3.
85 Mitchell G. Ash, 'Women émigré psychologists and psychoanalysts in the United States', in Sibylle Quack (ed.), *Between Sorrow and Strength: Women Refugees of the Nazi Period* (Cambridge: Cambridge University Press, 1995).
86 Kaplan, 'Jewish women in Nazi Germany before emigration', 37.
87 Cesarani, *Final Solution*, 771.
88 Primo Levi maintained that the true witnesses are those who were murdered, who were sent to the gas chambers, those who cannot bear witness. The survivors, of which he was one until his suicide in 1987, can only tell part of the story, and that, over time, becomes distorted by what they do not want to remember and what they do. Primo Levi, *The Drowned and the Saved* (London: Abacus, 2013).
89 Jane Georges and Susan Benedict, 'Nursing gaze of the Eastern Front in World War II: A feminist narrative', *Advances in Nursing Science* 31, 2 (2008): 140.
90 Deborah Dwork, *Children with a Star: Jewish Youth in Nazi Europe* (New Haven, CT: Yale University Press, 1991), xxiv.
91 Kushner, *Holocaust and the Liberal Imagination*, 245.

92 Jessica Wiederhorn, 'Case study: "Above all, we need the witness": The oral history of Holocaust survivors', in Donald A. Ritchie (ed.), *The Oxford Handbook of Oral History* (Oxford: Oxford University Press, 2011), 244.
93 Barbara A. Pickering, 'Women's voices as evidence: Personal testimony is pro-choice films', *Argumentation and Advocacy: The Journal of the American Forensic Association* 40 (Summer 2003): 1–22.
94 Irina Paperno, 'What can be done with diaries', *Russian Review* 63, 4 (2004): 561–73, at 571.
95 Alison Twells, '"Went into raptures": Reading emotion in the ordinary wartime diary, 1941–1946', *Women's History Review* 25, 1 (2016): 143–60.
96 Agatha Schwartz and Tatjana Takševa, 'Between trauma and resilience: A transnational reading of women's life writing about wartime rape in Germany and Bosnia and Herzegovina', *Aspasia: The International Yearbook of Central, Eastern, and Southeastern European Women's and Gender History* 14 (2020): 124–43.
97 Michael Roper, 'Splitting in unsent letters: Writing as a social practice and a psychological activity', *Social History* 26, 3 (2001): 318–39.
98 Walter Ong, *Orality and Literacy: The Technologizing of the Word*. 30th Anniversary Edition with John Hartley (London: Routledge, 2002), 78.
99 Rosa M. Sacharin, *The Unwanted Jew: A Struggle for Acceptance* (Tullibody: Diadem Books, 2014), Preface.
100 Emily Jane Haire, 'A debased currency? Using memoir: Material in the study of Anglo-French Intelligence Liaison', *Intelligence and National Security* 29, 5 (2014): 758–77.
101 John Tosh, *The Pursuit of History* (London: Pearson Education, 2002), 61.
102 Mahua Sarkar, 'Between craft and method: Meaning and inter-subjectivity in oral history analysis', *Journal of Historical Sociology* 25, 4 (2012): 578.
103 Anna Sheftel and Stacey Zembrzycki, 'Who's afraid of oral history? Fifty years of debates and anxiety about ethics', *Oral History Review* 43, 2 (2016): 338–66.
104 Penny Summerfield, 'Culture and composure: Creating narratives of the gendered self in oral history interviews', *Cultural and Social History* 1 (2004): 67. For a detailed analysis of 'composure' in oral history, see also Summerfield, *Reconstructing Women's Wartime Lives*.
105 Lynn Abrams, 'Liberating the female self: Epiphanies, conflict and coherence in the life stories of post-war British women', *Social History*

39, 1 (2014): 20; Judith Tydor Baumel, '"You said the words you wanted me to hear but I heard the words you couldn't bring yourself to say": Women's first-person accounts of the Holocaust', *Oral History Review* 27, 1 (2000): 23.
106 Dominick LaCapra, *Writing History, Writing Trauma* (Baltimore, MD: Johns Hopkins University Press, 2001), 88–9.
107 Ruth Shire, oral history interview by Jane Brooks at her home in the West Midlands on 13 February 2018. Personal archive.
108 Heidi Cowen (pseudonym) and Ruth Shire, oral history interview by Jane Brooks at Shire's home in the West Midlands on 13 February 2018. Personal archive.
109 Anonymous, 'Aliens may nurse again', *Nursing Mirror and Midwives' Journal* (9 November 1940): 121.
110 Christina Chavez, 'Conceptualizing from the inside: Advantages, complications, and demands on insider positionality', *Qualitative Report*, 13, 3 (2008): 474–94.
111 The value of insider research has been discussed elsewhere in relation to oral history projects in the history of nursing. See for example, Tommy Dickinson, *Curing Queers: Mental Nurses and their Patients, 1935–74* (Manchester: Manchester University Press, 2015).
112 Dwork, *Children with a Star*, xxiii.
113 Donald Bloxham and Tony Kushner, *The Holocaust: Critical Historical Approaches* (Manchester: Manchester University Press, 2005), 18.
114 Levi, *Drowned and the Saved*, 37.
115 Dwork, *Children with a Star*, xxiii.
116 Craig-Norton, *Kindertransport*, 243.
117 Gordon, oral history interview 2004; Hortense Gordon, oral history interview by Jane Brooks at her home in London on 27 October 2017. Personal archive; Bown, oral history interview.
118 Judith Tydor Baumel, *Double Jeopardy: Gender and the Holocaust* (London: Vallentine Mitchell, 1998), 57.
119 Mary Marshall Clark, 'Case study: Field notes on catastrophe: Reflections on the September 11, 2001, oral history and memory narrative project', in Donald A. Ritchie (ed.), *The Oxford Handbook of Oral History* (Oxford: Oxford University Press, 2011), 263.
120 Sarkar, 'Between craft and method', 578.
121 Robert Reynolds, 'Trauma and the relational dynamics of life-history interviewing', *Australian Historical Studies* 43 (2012): 78–88.
122 Lynn Abrams, 'Liberating the female self', 15.
123 Dwork, *Children with a Star*, xli.

124 Cathy Caruth, *Unclaimed Experience: Trauma, Narrative, and History* (Baltimore, MD: Johns Hopkins University Press, 1996), 63.
125 Personal communication with Peter Nolan on 22 September 2022. Altschul examined Nolan's PhD thesis and they remained friends until she died, with Nolan visiting her regularly at her home in Edinburgh.
126 Sheftel and Zembrzycki. 'Who's afraid of oral history?', 354.
127 Craig-Norton, 'Refugees at the margins', 298.
128 Charles, 'From Nazi Germany to Clarence House', 4.
129 Jane Brooks, *Negotiating Nursing: British Army Sisters and Soldiers in the Second World War* (Manchester: Manchester University Press, 2018), 179–80, 183.

1

Escape

Ruth Rawraway was a 31-year-old trained children's nurse in charge of the children's ward at the Jewish Hospital in Berlin.[1] She was clearly a most competent nurse, having once saved the life of the premature baby born to the wife of one of her medical colleagues. In August 1939, she received a telephone call whilst on duty at the hospital warning her not to go home as the Gestapo were waiting for her. The doctor whose child she had saved, greatly appreciative of her life-saving skills, was able to get Rawraway on a plane out of the country. Fortunately, she had all her exit papers on her. She arrived in Britain and sought nursing work. According to her family, Rawraway was employed by St Thomas's Hospital as a nurse, though what sort of nurse is unclear.[2] There was no reciprocity of registration between German and British nurses. Those refugees with nursing qualifications were expected to undertake further training and examinations to enter the British General Nursing Council Register.[3] Nevertheless, a testimonial from Lola Hahn-Warburg on 26 January 1939 attested to Rawraway's talents:

> I'd like to confirm that sister Ruth Rawraway has looked after the children's department of the Jewish Hospital as a nursing officer totally on her own. I hence had the chance – since both children had been lying in the ward to see them during the work [sic]. She had a delightful way to get on with children, exceptionally organisational [sic] talent and some medical knowledge which is out of the usual way (ordinary).
>
> I am convinced that she would master the work as nurse wherever she would be – with full satisfaction.[4]

In some ways Rawraway's story is unusual amongst the nurses who narratives comprise this book. She was a qualified nursing sister in charge of a ward and older than most when she fled – she was already in her thirties (see Figure 1.1). The danger and fearful nature of her escape was, however, not unusual. Once safely in Britain, Rawraway remained in nursing until 1941, when she had a daughter and, like all nurses at that time, was required to leave the profession. In recognition of their wartime work, refugee nurses gained naturalisation early. Rawraway became a British

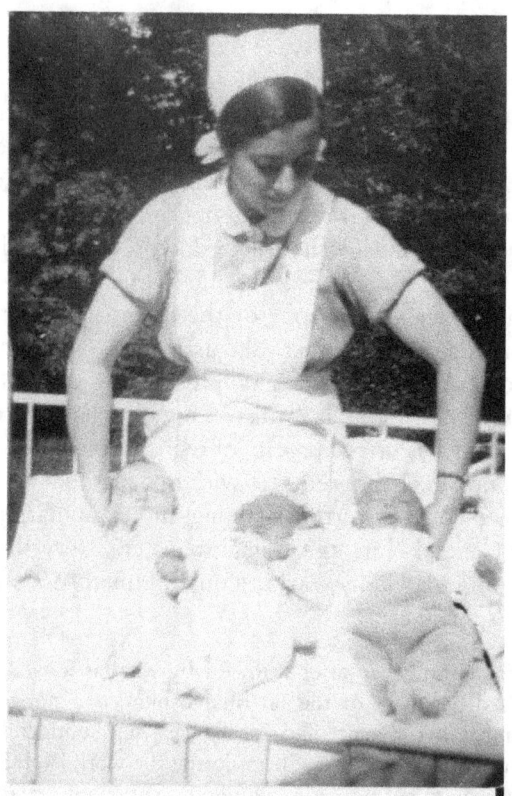

Figure 1.1 Ruth Rawraway with a cradle of babies, probably during her employment at the Berlin B'nai Brith mother and baby home, c.1930–34. Reproduced with kind permission of her daughter, Susan Zisman [fo. 46]

citizen on 14 June 1947, under her married name, Ruth Anneliese Simon.[5]

This chapter explores the experiences of Jewish refugee nurses, beginning with their lives in the period before National Socialism. It considers their family homes, schooling and ambitions, all of which were put into jeopardy when Hitler came to power in 1933. The focus then turns to the rise of National Socialism and the critical moment of the November pogrom. As I argue, the pogrom meant that Jews were finally forced into realising that the Greater Reich was a dangerous place for them. In the early years of National Socialism, men were far more likely to be arrested than women.[6] Most arrests in the pogrom were of Jewish men, not women. However, it soon became clear that gender was not a defence against brutality and murder.[7] Increasingly, families clamoured to get their daughters out of Germany and Austria. I therefore examine the three routes by which young women and girls could escape: via nursing, domestic service visas and through the Kindertransport. Finally, this chapter explores the refugees' early lives in Britain, as foster children, nurses and domestic servants, and the reaction of the British public to their presence. The narratives illustrate the ambivalent nature of Britain's response to their plight. Despite the determination of these girls and young women to face the ordeals in their new lives, the price of safety was often the loss of caste, as they shifted from servant-employing status to homes where they themselves were the servant.

Life for Jews before National Socialism

Kitty Schafer was born into a cultured middle-class home in Vienna in 1921: 'Anyhow, I had a wonderful time and don't forget at that time, one can't mention it anymore, but for the Jews, I was seventeen, and the time was great. You had every facility in Vienna, to go skiing, go sporting, I even went to a dancing school, believe it or not.'[8] In the inter-war period, Jews comprised about ten per cent of the population in Vienna; in Berlin it was only about one per cent. Either despite or because of the relatively high ratio of non-Jews to Jews, the Jewish population of Vienna needed to manage a climate of antisemitism that pervaded the city.⁹ Yet, for young girls like Kitty, life was happy and full of contentment. Most Jewish children attended secular schools and were well integrated into the local community. This was partly, according to Walter Laqueur, because liberal Jews believed that by attending the same schools as other children, they would be more readily assimilated into society.¹⁰

Antisemitism also existed in Weimar Germany, though at a vastly different level to the murderous regime under National Socialism. Jews had been granted equal rights in 1919, but potential forms of exclusion remained. As Kerry Wallach argues, the desire to 'pass' as German rather than Jewish was an integral part of life for Jews in Weimar Germany.¹¹ Most Jews in Germany belonged to the middle class, and attending the *Gymnasium* would enable their children to remain so.¹² It was only after Jewish children were dismissed from secular schools in 1933 that Jewish schools found favour, at which point they were not only essential, but also served to protect children against the growing violence.¹³

The young German and Central European women and girls whose narratives form this book grew up in predominantly cultured homes with all the opportunities that a solid middle-class upbringing could offer in the inter-war period. Josephine Bruegel's father was a general medical practitioner (GP). She attended a girls' grammar school in Teplice-Sanov, in Czechoslovakia. Bruegel's childhood was sporty, academic and cultured; she even read the *Manchester Guardian* at a reading club she joined in 1931.¹⁴ Eva Flatow grew up on the Baltic coast of Germany. She enjoyed school, music, hiking, swimming and spending time with her friends.¹⁵ Hortense Gordon's father was a country GP. She grew up in a large house with her parents and her younger sister. The family was wealthy enough to own a car and employ a nanny to care for the children.¹⁶ Gertrude and Lotte Dann had privileged and contented childhoods, with a much loved and extended family group.¹⁷ Trudie Moos's memoirs also reflect a happy childhood, especially when she visited her beloved Uncle Oscar. Oscar was a doctor and Trudie wanted to follow in his footsteps: 'He took me very seriously and my avid interest in his surgery and gadgets stimulated him to explain all sorts of medical things to me.'¹⁸

Gertrude Roberts's childhood was not so happy, with little love from her mother. The family were, however, proud Germans, and Roberts remembered surprising her teacher when she told her the family had lived in the country for four hundred years.[19] These privileged and mostly happy lives only reinforced the cultural, educational and social difficulties refugees experienced when they arrived in Britain to work as maids. As Jennifer Craig-Norton argues, the domestic work expected from them was arduous, and in houses heated by open fires, cleaning was a Sisyphean task. Most of them were wholly unsuited to the work, having come from sheltered and affluent homes where they employed their own servants. These challenges were compounded as the refugees were not used to being treated as socially inferior, were not used to the British class structure and had frequently received no training in British household management.[20] As I argue in this chapter, the aspect of their new lives which the refugees found hardest to bear were the way they were treated by their British employers. In German homes, the maid was treated almost as part of the family; in their new British homes, refugees soon realised that servants were often regarded as barely human.[21]

Many of the young girls who eventually escaped to Britain identified as having normal childhoods. However, some noted a quiet threat – the obstacles the Jews of the Weimar Republic faced that were not part of the lives of other Germans.[22] Ruth Price recalled the moment at school, when she was only about six years old, when the teacher made her feel she was no longer part of the 'community'. Now 'I belonged to the Jewish community.'[23] Erna Harding, who trained as a nurse in Germany in 1916, recalled growing up in Thuringia, near Leipzig, which was, she stated, a very antisemitic place, and where she was the only Jewish girl in her class. At one point the daughter of an army officer joined her class and she 'persuaded the other children not to talk to me any more'. Later, she realised, 'they just wanted to get me out of their circle. But I never told my parents because I was afraid they would send me to Switzerland and I didn't want to leave home.'[24] Just after the end of the First World War, Lotte Dann's mother warned her of antisemitism: 'Therefore, being Jewish, you have to be extra well-behaved and quiet and not put yourself forward.'[25] Trudie Moos remembered the growing foreboding in 1932, when she was about ten years old:

> During that whole year I had overheard my parents and their friends having very serious conversations about politics and the threat of Nazis or Communists gaining the upper hand in Germany. I knew there were a lot of dissatisfied and unemployed people, many were bitter and angry ... There were also whisperings of Jews being persecuted under a Nazi regime and I was well aware of being Jewish, though we weren't practicing [sic] Jews.[26]

This nascent antisemitism meant that once Hitler came to power, many Jews were habituated to being cast as 'other', so therefore did not respond with any sense of urgency to the increasing anti-Jewish programme of the regime. Initially the new laws were seen as merely an extension of what many had always encountered, and thus most did not even consider escape.

The developing horror

When Hitler came to power in 1933 there were about half a million Jews living in Germany; approximately one-third lived in Berlin.[27] In the early months, whilst the Jews were certainly aware of his party's antisemitic ideology, little actually changed for them.[28] Few considered emigrating or even sending money out of the country.[29] Many thought that Hitler would not last.[30] Harding recalled:

> I was in Berlin [when Hitler came to power]. I wanted to leave earlier, but my family was very German, and said, 'oh no, that won't last and we won't leave.' My mother passed away in '38 and then I said, 'I am going to leave' and they said, 'oh no, nothing will happen.' But I sent my boy [her son Peter] when he was ten and a half alone to England ... My sisters didn't help me, they said I wasn't in my right mind to leave.[31]

If some Jews did see reasons to emigrate, historian Doron Niederland maintains that it may not be appropriate to refer the refugees in the early 1930s as refugees at all; rather, they were Jews who chose to come to live in Britain.[32] David Cesarani argues that initially the numbers of émigrés were not high. Some even returned to Germany when they found the reality of living in a foreign country too difficult.³³ Those Jews who wanted to emigrate were hindered by their limited knowledge of potential countries of refuge, lack of contacts and an inability to speak the language.³⁴ It has been suggested that Germany was in such a 'mess' that even some Jews felt Hitler should be given a chance. According to historian Claire Hilton, one psychiatrist at the Maudsley Hospital in London considered returning to Germany after the Reichstag fire, because he felt that if so many of the population had voted for Hitler, 'he must be a great man'.³⁵ Fortunately the doctor was persuaded to stay in Britain. Roberts recalled, 'nobody realised quite what sort of a person [Hitler] was, or perhaps they didn't want to realise'.³⁶ There were arguments that if and when the National Socialists attained power, they would become more sensible and willing to compromise.³⁷ Whilst anti-Jewish laws were passed soon after the National Socialists gained control of Germany, they were not always implemented and members of the public sometimes ignored them. Even when Hitler started to make Jewish life difficult, local populations did not necessarily follow edicts of prohibition. In rural areas the local community continued to frequent Jewish shops.³⁸ For many Jews in the early months of National Socialism, the erratic nature of anti-Jewish legislation supported the view that under Hitler's regime, they would simply experience an extension to the ever-present underlying antisemitism.³⁹

Thus, despite the increasingly precarious nature of life under National Socialism, Hitler's *raison d'être* – to make Germany and later all its occupied territories *Judenfrei*, or Jew-free – was not as carefully premeditated as some have suggested.⁴⁰ In the early years of National Socialism, the treatment of Jews by those in authority was conflicting and inconsistent. In her oral history interview, Price remembered her father being arrested in 1937, but because one of the Gestapo agents knew him, they let him go.⁴¹ In 1934, Margaret Marflow's autobiography notes her two best friends '"had" to "bid me goodbye". Not because they had suddenly turned into Anti-Semites, but because friendship with me would have endangered their fathers' careers.'⁴² Yet, as late as August 1938, Marflow was able to travel reasonably freely for a holiday in the Bavarian Alps.⁴³ Susi Lewinsky, who later came to Britain on a nursing visa, recalled a holiday in a small country house near Hamburg in the summer of 1938. However, she admitted that they 'avoided big places ... We cooked for ourselves on a hearth.' It was at this time that Lewinsky and her friends started to plan their escape to Britain: 'England let you enter only for household help or for nurse training when you were old enough. We could go as a team.'[44] In her memoir, Lewinsky wrote of what she called the 'comic imagination' of the conversation, as they planned to emigrate to England to work and discussed what work they could, or more accurately could not, do. Arguably therefore, even as late as 1938, the young women of Germany were not necessarily fearful of their position and considered emigration as an amusing diversion rather than a bid for their lives.

When Lewinsky returned to Hamburg, she found her living arrangements had become more challenging. Her landlord did not ask her to leave her lodgings, but 'the situation became uncomfortable to be with non-Jewish people'.[45] She felt that the owner was relieved when she left of her own volition.[46] As Nazi ideology intensified its grip on Germany, many ordinary Germans were increasingly willing to take advantage of antisemitic legislation. German Jewish household income was on average three times that of the non-Jewish population.[47] At a time of great financial hardship, such disparities could easily create discontent. Saul Friedlander maintains that although most ordinary Germans did not advocate violence, they were nevertheless pleased to see the Jews go without and perhaps even face some humiliation.[48] Edith Menkes Wolloch's family home was forcibly sold: 'they bought it for almost no money'.[49] Dina Gold, whose mother, Aviva, escaped to England in about 1936, describes the forced sale of the Wolff family furrier business premises that her great-grandfather had built: 'The land and building was [sic] sold for RM 1.8 million ($725,800 at the time) ... There were a few additional small expenses as well, so that at the end of it all he [Dina's Uncle Fritz] was left with RM 1,629 (just under $400 in those days).'[50]

On 7 April 1933, the Law for the Restoration of the Professional Civil Service was enacted. The law excluded all Jews working in the civil service – including schoolteachers and university academics – from their positions. On 22 April, doctors and dentists who practised within the state sector were barred and by September that year, Jewish lawyers were also banned from practising.[51] By rendering these professional Jews unemployed and unemployable and forcing the reduction of their assets and capital, it was increasingly difficult for them to escape.[52] Simultaneously, measures were escalated to make their living in Germany impossible. Ervin Staub argues that the increasing acquiescence to the boycott of Jewish shops, breaking ties with Jewish friends and acquisition of Jewish jobs could not solely be attributed to fear of the regime. There was, he argues, a 'cultural lilt' to anti-Jewish feeling within the 'Aryan' Germans.[53] Campaigns against Jewish business enabled middle-class party members to denounce their Jewish competitors and create a more favourable economic climate for 'Aryan' business.[54] As early as 1940, writers and journalists Yvonne Kapp and Margaret Mynatt argued that one ramification of the policy was the removal of talented Jews and their replacement with mediocre 'Aryans'.[55] Importantly for Jews, the loss of social status associated with professional work had a greater negative impact on men.

For those Jewish women who had worked outside the home, opportunities for retraining were limited. They nevertheless managed to adapt to their reduction in status, finding employment and volunteer work with Jewish organisations.[56] The woman who had been a housewife shifted from being the mistress of servants in her home to being the one who undertook the domestic work.[57] Husbands, however, struggled to move from bank manager or scholar to working-class employment or no employment at all.[58] Many men experienced what Marion Kaplan argues was a 'social death'.[59] These alterations in status and resilience did not change the gendered hierarchy. Women who were supposed to safeguard the psychological and spiritual wellbeing of the family were entrusted to 'make things work'.[60] The constant struggle to keep the household running with ever-dwindling resources kept them busy. Their position as wives and mothers who needed to feed the family placed them in direct daily contact with non-Jews. Women were therefore often more aware of the growing antisemitism and critically witnessed the pressures on their children. Women frequently tried in vain to encourage their husbands to see the increasing dangers and escape. In refusing to listen to wives' desire to flee, many families stayed to certain death.[61]

A truncated education

'Aryanisation' of German education began in 1933, as many Jewish children were dismissed from their state schools.[62] As Hitler occupied other countries, the pattern was similar, with Jewish children excluded from state schools and forced into Jewish schools or having no schooling at all. Given the centrality of school to all children's lives, such moves caused great suffering.[63] Laqueur argued that this expulsion was not universal and that children of war veterans were permitted to stay on longer. He admitted he was one of the last Jews to graduate from a secular *Gymnasium* in 1938.[64] For those who did not leave immediately, secular schools were often a place in which children increasingly experienced anti-semitism and its associated physical and psychological violence, from both teachers and fellow pupils. Parents began to remove their children from secular schools in a bid to protect them. Those children who arrived in Britain as refugees would feel severely affected by this truncated education.

In her oral history, Elisabeth Katz recalled there were two Jewish teachers at her secular school. One taught German and she was very German in her outlook; Katz remembered that she preferred non-Jewish children to the Jewish ones. But this 'Aryan outlook' could not save her. In about 1933 or 1934, 'there came two men to the door of her classroom and they asked [her] ... to take her purse with her and she was never seen again ... My parents weren't willing to discuss it.'[65] Rosa Sacharin recalled one teacher who promised to protect the Jewish children in her class.[66] However, as more teachers either joined the Nazi Party or as Party members were given the jobs of dismissed Jewish teachers, the indoctrination of German children took hold. Sacharin remembered all the children being taken out to look at the sky on a winter's evening and the teacher said, 'Children, you see that big star up there? That is the Jew star and is responsible for all our troubles.'[67] Sacharin was forced to leave her school two years later when, in September 1935, the Nuremberg Laws decreed German teachers could not be expected to teach Jewish children. She then attended a Jewish school, but attested that her education was broken by the events.

Hortense Gordon was refused entry to the prestigious high school in her town because she was Jewish.⁶⁸ Ruth Price recalled in her oral history, 'I don't think I was exactly barred from going there but, as things were going, my parents decided that it would be much better if I went to Jewish school.'⁶⁹ Edith Bown was forced to leave her secular school as early as 1934. Her memoir recalled how she was increasingly 'hounded' in the playground, but the situation became unbearable when the teacher also started to bully her and slapped her in front of the whole class: 'I did not go to school the next day.'⁷⁰ Her mother had wanted her to start attending a Jewish school for some time, but her father had resisted, believing that his membership of the *Reichsbund jüdischer Frontsoldaten* would save him and the family.⁷¹ He eventually realised this optimism was misplaced and Bown was sent to a Jewish school, which she attended until November 1938. Heidi Cowen's education was curtailed after her brother was thrown off a bridge. Luckily he survived.⁷²

On 9 November 1938, a pogrom was unleashed on the Jews of Germany. Synagogues across Germany and Austria were burned, shops smashed and homes violated. Ninety-one Jews were killed and within just twenty-four hours more than 30,000 Jewish men between the ages of 16 and 60 (about one-quarter of all those living in Germany) were arrested and sent to Dachau, Sachsenhausen and Buchenwald concentration camps. The fathers of Gordon and Roberts were amongst those detained.⁷³ Although the greater fear was reserved for Jewish men, the pogrom made it clear to all Jews that their position was not secure, that Hitler was not going to disappear and that the only way to save their lives was to escape. At the same time, Britain and other countries tightened their borders. The Home Office expressed its concern at the potential influx of many Jews.⁷⁴ This anxiety had been increasing following the annexation of Austria (*Anschluss*) in March 1938, when the Home Office started to prepare itself for the incursion of Austrian Jews. The Government was aware that Austrian Jews would likely be rendered stateless by their new German overlords and thus would prove difficult to remove once on British soil. There was agreement that wholesale restriction was not to be countenanced. The Government did not want to adversely affect its international reputation, nor did it want to prevent the emigration of those Jews who would be useful to the country. The decision was thus to implement visa restrictions, which would enable those Jews who would further British interests to enter, whilst preventing those who could be a burden or a potential threat.[75]

Escape to Britain: the Kindertransport, nursing and domestic service visas

According to Peter Alter, British immigration policy was based 'first and foremost on its own economic and political interests'.[76] Nevertheless, across the liberal democracies of Europe and the United States, 'Kristallnacht was a dramatic turning point in the way Nazism was perceived.'[77] Yet, coming just two months after the Munich Agreement, the British Government was caught between the certainty of the sort of regime they were connected to and the determination not to antagonise the Nazi leadership.[78] As Tony Kushner argues, 'foreign policy continued regardless', and the Government continued to engage in dialogue with Hitler and his regime.[79]

Following the pogrom there was an immediate response from the public. The Prime Minister, Neville Chamberlain, spoke to the House of Commons on the importance of doing something to help the Jews. However, no consensus could be reached and no clear idea of how to manage the 'Jewish Problem' was presented.[80] Kushner continues that if the British public were initially outraged, their interest in the pogrom soon faded.[81] The British press, including the right-wing press but excluding Fascist publications, condemned the actions of Nazi Germany towards the Jews.[82] The British public were therefore well aware of the atrocities. But apart from the *Manchester Guardian*, which maintained a consistent stance throughout, the press excused the leaders of Nazi Germany for the brutal way they treated the Jews. With such contradictory messages, the British public's attitudes could have been nothing other than ambivalent.

There were, however, some for whom the knowledge of the pogrom engendered action and ensured that the British Government would galvanise to support refugees. Schemes offering block visas for children and those women willing to work as domestic servants were established.⁸³ Saving women and children was far less politically problematic than rescuing men of working age. However, even these government escape routes relied on voluntary organisations and committed individuals to facilitate immigration. The rescue work of Nicholas Winton, Doreen Warriner, Trevor Chadwick and Rabbi Solomon Schonfeld have been the subject of a variety of studies.⁸⁴ Yet, despite deserved accolades for some individuals, both the Kindertransport and domestic service visa schemes have been subject to considerable and well-earned criticisms.

The inclusion of nursing as a means of escape has not been subject to the same level of scrutiny. Nevertheless, as this book identifies, it offered a third practical opportunity for escape for some women. Nursing offered something more than domestic service. For those who were interested or already engaged in medical or nursing work, it enabled the continuation of service in the healthcare field. It was also rampant opportunism on the part of the British Government and nursing profession. As war became increasingly inevitable, it was clear that there would not be enough nurses to care for the nation's sick and injured, combatants and civilians alike. Refugees came from educated and cultured homes and could be useful to hospitals. Whether the profession's leaders considered that such cultured young women might find the nursing world intellectually stifling and physically exhausting can only be speculation. However, there is little doubt that the desperation to leave Nazi territories would make them willing workers. Much has been made in the liberal imagination that commends saving so many women and children via these escape routes. The Kindertransport has been heralded as the bastion of altruism on behalf of the British Government and populace. The reality for the children who were saved was more problematic, as it was for those young women who came as nurses and domestic servants.

The Kindertransport

Kushner argues that the Kindertransport has become 'the most remembered and celebrated refugee movement in British history'.⁸⁵ In January 2020, the *Guardian* newspaper published an article quoting the Labour Peer and Kindertransportee Lord Alfred Dubs's plea for the child refugees from Syria:

> When I arrived in Britain as an unaccompanied refugee child fleeing the Nazis, I never thought I would end up in the Lords. But this country not only allowed me a life and gave me sanctuary, it also gave me opportunity. I certainly never imagined that 81 years later, in the same country that gave homes to 10,000 lone refugee children like me, I'd be fighting for just a few hundred to be allowed to find their families here.[86]

Despite the undoubted concern for the current child refugee crisis and the gratitude Dubs clearly feels towards Britain for saving his life, this vision of the Kindertransport is rose-coloured at best. According to Claudia Curio, a historian of child refugees, whilst the admission of children was a useful 'cushion [to] the inhumanity of policies towards alien immigration', it also distracted from the lack of humanitarian action on the part of liberal democracies.[87] It was, nevertheless, inured with ambivalence toward Continental Jews. It is acknowledged that many children's lives were saved by the scheme. Susan Cohen cites that by August 1939, 9,354 predominately Jewish children had been rescued.[88] Only about eleven per cent of German Jewish children who stayed in Germany survived the war and two million were murdered.[89] The rescue therefore of 10,000 by Britain is important. The underlying premise was that children would be saved but without their parents. The children's journey to Britain was fraught with danger and anguish at leaving their families and friends. Jennifer Craig-Norton argues that the parents' plight was desperate, but one that has been overlooked in a bid to create a narrative of 'salvation, success and happiness' for the children who were saved.[90]

Edith Bown recalled the day that she and her brother, Gert (Gerald), left Germany.[91] As the taxi took them to the railway station, she read a letter from her mother. Kindertransport historians Rebekka Gopfert and Andrea Hammel argue that the children themselves were rarely involved in the decision to emigrate. It was common for the Kinder not to realise that their parents were not going with them until they arrived at the railway station and their parents said goodbye. The separation from families would haunt many Kinder throughout their lives. Like other children, Edith and Gerald would not have known then that they would never see their parents again. Significantly, Edith did not dwell on these memories in her memoirs or oral history.[92] Edith and Gerald joined the other children and the train eventually left Berlin. At Aachen the train stopped:

> It seemed as if the uniformed men, SA or SS, wanted to search us and all the older children with passports. We were to leave the train, and I was petrified. However, the ladies of the party [English Quaker women assigned to chaperone the children on their journey] kept the SS men or the SA men arguing, until with German punctuality the train started moving again.[93]

Being harassed by SS officers was a common occurrence for those who escaped. The Germans may not have wanted Jews in their country, but nor did they want to make it straightforward for them to escape. The large red 'J' stamped on the passports of emigrating Jews (see Figure 1.2) did little to encourage the ease of travel.[94]

Mia Ross recalled, 'Eventually we stopped at the Austro-German frontier. There were several SS men there. We all had to open our suitcases and we were asked lots of questions and our passports were examined to see if we had a permit for England and also permission to leave the country.'[95] Susi Loeffler was a young girl when Hitler invaded Czechoslovakia. In July 1939, she was sent to Britain on one of the last Kindertransports out of Prague:

> Hordes of children and parents were there. All quite upset. Our luggage was minutely examined. I had a little opal ring on my finger and a modest gold bracelet which was taken off me. I am not going to tell you about our good-byes, it is too painful. I repressed that memory for 30 years and then I got flashbacks all the time and got quite sick here in Sydney ... We came by boat over the English Channel. Lots of us, children. I was just very strained and didn't take anything in very much.[96]

As Loeffler's words illustrate, many Kinder carried this loss and guilt into adulthood. Far from being rescued, many of these children were damaged by their survivor guilt and the traumatic knowledge that parents, siblings, grandparents and cousins had perished.[97] Eva Minden's grandfather had taken British nationality

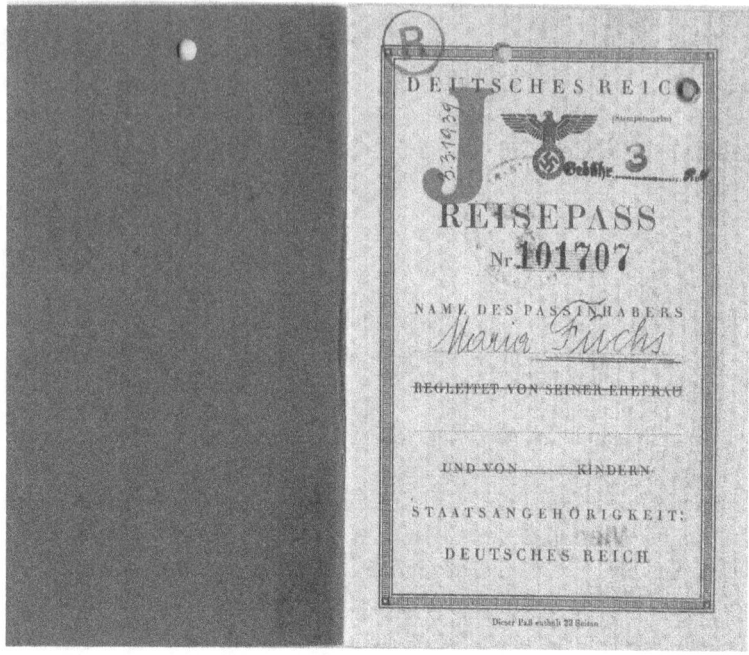

Figure 1.2 Maria Fuchs's (Mia Ross's) passport. Reproduced with kind permission of her sons, David and Paul Ross [fo. 60]

when he worked in Hull at the beginning of the twentieth century. Minden was fortunate therefore to have a British passport, as well as a German one. She was under strict instructions never to tell anyone of her dual nationality. However, being armed with a British passport, she would find access to that country easier. With the Nazi decree that all those with British nationality must register before 30 November 1938, her parents left Germany, leaving Minden and her sister Elizabeth to support their grandparents until it was safe for them to leave. The November pogrom meant that they needed to escape before they had fulfilled their duties, forcing the two sisters to travel to Amsterdam; their grandparents were murdered in the Holocaust. When the sisters reached the Dutch–German border, they were forced off the train by the Gestapo and were told to wait, which they did for hours. Their British passports saved them from missing the last train. In her memoir, Minden recalled her sister's indignation at the Gestapo: 'At last it was too much for Elizabeth. She said, "Do you examine all British subjects like this?"'[98] Eventually they were able to leave. They arrived in Amsterdam at midnight, relieved to find their father was there to meet them. Despite the apparent bravery of those evacuated on the Kindertransports, the departure and journey were harrowing events for these children. Being ripped from their parents and sent to a strange land, with a language they neither understood nor spoke, had a devastating effect on most of them. The vivid recollections of their departure and journeys to Britain speak to the continued influence of these memories, even eighty years later.

Heidi Cowen did not leave on the official Kindertransport. Unlike Minden, she had no sibling travelling with her and therefore travelled alone. The description of her escape reveals the terrifying nature of her journey:

> Yes. I had a very nasty experience. At the frontier I was taken out of the train and had to be stripped naked and everything was examined. And they made me miss my train, and I only had a twenty-four-hour permit to go through Belgium. And at sixteen by yourself that was pretty horrific. Anyway, I got dressed quickly, and somebody took pity on me, a woman, she said, 'there's a tram goes to Strasbourg, and if the train stops at Strasbourg, which there might well be [sic], you might catch your train again.' And I did that and caught the train in Strasbourg. But that was very stressful. At sixteen by yourself stripped naked, to start with, and then your suitcase opened and everything spilled on the floor – carefully packed, your only belongings.[99]

Beverley Chalmers, a historian of the Nazi abuses of women, describes 'forced nakedness' and sexualised degradation as part of the systematic humiliation and dehumanisation of Jews by the regime.[100] Cowen's experience was therefore by no means uncommon and her youth was no protection against such behaviour. Her description of the event was stoic. It is possible that within the oral history interview, she simply did not wish to dwell on the episode. The reasons Holocaust survivors do not 'tell' of certain experiences are varied, but include the words they find too unbearable to speak and events they simply cannot put into words for someone else.[101] Cowen turned instead to focus on her life in

Britain and her nursing work as the narratives that gave meaning to her being.[102] Tal Litvak Hirsch and colleagues argue that one of the most important tools for gaining a sense of personal coherence is the family.[103] In the interview Cowen moved quickly from the horror of her strip-search and potential inability to escape to her arrival in Britain, focusing on her good fortune at being met by her father's cousin. As with Rawraway's testimony at the beginning of the chapter, luck was central to the experience of flight from Nazism.

Most Kinder were not so lucky to have family or friends waiting for them on arrival. Rosa Sacharin left Berlin on 1 December 1938, aged 13, and arrived in Britain the next day. She left her mother in Germany, but her sister managed to escape on 1 September 1939, the date Germany invaded Poland. Sacharin's father had been arrested in 1935 and she never saw him again. In her oral history Sacharin recalled her arrival in Britain and placement at Dovercourt holiday camp, which 'was quite chaotic'. The organising committee appeared to be unsure of how to manage the children it had evacuated from Nazi Europe: 'it was winter time ... it wasn't really suitable, little hutlets, and there was no heating there, bitterly cold. We had ... I think I had one blanket, I kept my coat on and we all congregated in the dining room and just didn't know what was happening.' Sacharin remembered being asked to transmigrate to Australia, Ireland or Palestine, but refused, as she was fearful she would not see her mother again.[104]

The use of summer holiday camps such as Dovercourt enabled the authorities to provide shelter for the Kinder before they were taken to foster homes, but they were clearly not conducive to the needs of traumatised children. According to Veronica Gillespie, who worked with the Kindertransport, there was no heating in the sleeping accommodation during what was one of the harshest of winters.[105] The Kindertransport was not financed by the Government but by voluntary organisations, with a variety of underpinning rationales for action.[106] Whilst these organisations should be admired for attempting to rescue so many children from certain death, the schemes were haphazard. The Refugee Children's Movement, which oversaw the rescue and transport of the Kinder, was criticised for not respecting the children's religious and cultural backgrounds.¹⁰⁷ The reception camp at Dovercourt where Rosa Sacharin lived did not even have kosher food.¹⁰⁸ The lack of sympathy for children who had been ripped from their parents' homeland and sent to a country where they often barely spoke the language affected them deeply and for many years. For some, coercion to convert to Christianity removed the last vestiges of their links to their childhood, family and heritage.¹⁰⁹ A significant criticism of Nicholas Winton was that he cooperated with the Barbican Mission, a charity that offered to find homes for about one hundred Jewish children, so long as they would convert.¹¹⁰ Even when the children were placed in Jewish households the situation could be difficult, as there was a 'huge gulf that existed between British Jewry and those of the Continent'.¹¹¹ This gulf, according to Marion Berghahn, was due to the very different cultures between Anglo-Jewry, many of whom had arrived at the end of the nineteenth century from Eastern Europe, the so-called *Ostjuden*, and the newly arrived German and Austrian Jews. Anglo-Jewry considered the German Jews too assimilated and arrogant, whereas German Jews considered their British co-religionists too 'Jewish' and 'ghettoized'.¹¹²

One of the cruellest aspects of places like Dovercourt was the selection of refugees by potential foster families. Before March 1939, children were rescued and sent to the relative safety of reception camps, without their 'suitability' being assessed before they left Nazi territories.¹¹³ However, once in Britain, 'selection' of children occurred. Potential foster parents came to the camp and chose their refugees.¹¹⁴ Tragically, having been sent away by their parents, certain children were always left behind in these 'children's markets'.¹¹⁵ Younger girls, especially blonde ones, appealed to prospective carers, as did those without family connections but whose provenance was middle-class. Older boys were not popular.¹¹⁶ The younger and more Anglo-Saxon they looked, the easier they were to acculturate into 'Englishness', of which the loss of accent was a critical issue.¹¹⁷ As Curio argues, 'Few children could meet all these criteria.'¹¹⁸ Helen Jones, whose work focuses on British women's responses to the refugee crisis, maintains that in later life the Kinder remembered being treated as a 'sort of museum piece'. They recalled they were expected to be perennially grateful whilst having their accents laughed at and asked when they would return 'home'.[119] Anna Essinger, the German-born headmistress of a boarding school in Kent, successfully lobbied to change the selection process. Later transports had their foster parents allocated before they met the children.[120]

In the epilogue to her memoir, Edith Bown wrote, 'From the end of 1938 to the beginning of World War II in 1939, groups of shocked and exhausted children aged between four months and sixteen years arrived once or twice a week in London, usually at Liverpool Street station. From there they were boarded out around the British Isles.'[121] Edith and Gerald were sent to live in a hostel in Belfast vouched for by the Jewish community. On 26 June 1939, Bown's diary states, 'Well if I have to stay here, I shall go completely down the drain. Only work, dirty work. Nothing to learn.'[122] The couple who were allegedly caring for the children seemed to have little understanding of their situation: 'Mrs Hurwitz was here. She met us and asked us a few useless questions.'[123] Fortunately, Bown and her brother were sent to the Refugee Resettlement Farm in Millisle, Northern Ireland.[124] Both their recollections from this period in their young lives were positive. Gerald's written account for the *Belfast Jewish Chronicle* in 2005 stated, 'We had freedom, food, and a wonderful healthy life, in the beautiful Irish countryside. What more could you want?'[125] Edith Bown's recollections are equally as romantic and her writings suggest the proper care they received.[126] Whilst Gerald was able to stay at the farm for several years before being sent to school, Edith was sent out to work.

When Lee Fischer and her brother arrived in England in July 1939, they were sent to a family who ran a boarding house in Westgate-on-Sea. When war broke out two months later, the family moved to London and the maids left their positions. The gendered nature of 'refugeedom' meant that Fischer, aged only 14, had to become the maid.[127] Her brother, who was younger, was housed in the rather neglected annexe to the building and died from rheumatic fever shortly afterwards.[128] Rosa Sacharin describes how she was fostered by an elderly couple who had wanted an 18-year-old, 'but you will have to do'. The relationship was not good from the start: 'There was no warmth.'[129] The unmet need for attachment that Sacharin felt, separated from her family and friends, resonates across many narratives, with language and cultural differences exacerbating loneliness.[130] Fischer found things particularly difficult because of her poor English, as did Edith Bown.[131] Because Sacharin was only 13, she attended school during the day but was required to clean the house before school. In her memoir she recalled how she was originally given a nice bedroom but was soon moved into an attic room more suitable for a servant: 'I was lonely, spoke little and became withdrawn ... One day the older daughter, a married woman, took me shopping and said to me, "You German Jews deserve what was happening to you because you were not good Jews".'[132] These children's loneliness amongst people who appeared neither to understand nor care is particularly hard to absorb. Berghahn highlights the nature of the 'Germanness' of the German and Austrian Jew. The cultural differences were a significant challenge when both adult and child refugees attempted to assimilate into Britain.[133]

Although much of the literature describes the hardships that these children had to manage, the narratives of some young refugees do identify kindliness and even love in some foster homes and schools.[134] Leonore Lowton's own family perished in the Holocaust, but her Welsh foster family accepted her as one of their own: 'And, well, I was just always treated as one of the nieces and they just accepted me.'[135] They even respected her Jewish heritage.[136] Susi Loeffler felt she was very lucky to be given a home with a Miss Hurst, a single woman in Tunbridge Wells: 'She was a sweet lady. She had been a music teacher and played the violin in the local orchestra. I got to hear all the great artists, refugees from the continent ... I was simply ecstatic to hear Ida Haendel.' Loeffler did start to attend school, but admitted her English was not good enough. Once the Kinder reached 16 years old, they were expected to seek employment. Loeffler continued, 'After a few months I felt I no longer could impose on Miss Hurst. So, I decided to stand on my own feet.' Despite her poor command of the language, she found work as a cadet nurse in a cottage hospital.[137] Craig-Norton argues that most refugees were forced to leave school at the age of 15 or 16 and enter useful employment.[138] The Minutes of the Executive Committee of the Domestic Bureau on 19 May 1939 demonstrate that the matter of girls' employment was discussed at length:

Letters were read from the Council for German Jewry and the Christian Council for Refugees, accepting the ultimate responsibility for these girls, and authorising the Domestic Bureau to bring them over on the conditions laid down by the Home Office ... The Chairman [sic] reported that she was in touch with the Children's Committee concerning the domestic permits for girls originally brought over under the children's scheme, who wished to enter domestic employment on reaching the age of 16.[139]

Transmigration had been one of the conditions of the support for 10,000 children to escape to Britain, but the war made this impossible.[140] Thus, the requirement to maintain themselves became essential for the Government and the Central Office for Refugees, who would otherwise need to support them financially. Although Loeffler was able to gain employment as a cadet nurse as soon as she was old enough, for most the default occupation was domestic service. In this they joined the 20,000 predominantly female Jewish refugees who escaped Nazi territories on domestic service visas.

Domestic service

The decision to enable 10,000 children to enter Britain was largely an appeasement to criticisms of the Government's lack of support for Jewish refugees. The provision of domestic service visas was a concession to the middle-class women of Britain, who could no longer find household staff. The proliferation of middle-class households in the nineteenth century created the need for an army of domestic servants to clean, polish and feed the homes of the nation.[141] Even the humblest of middle-class homes brought girls in from rural areas to be what historian Sue Bruley calls 'live-in drudge[s]'.[142] The work was unpopular, with long hours, close supervision and lack of privacy. For most servants in the typical one- or two-servant household, the life was also lonely.[143]

The offer of domestic work as a method of escape from Nazi territories was founded in what Craig-Norton calls 'coldly pragmatic' decisions rather than humanitarian concern for the plight of Jewish women.[144] British middle-class housewives could not find sufficient working-class women to clean their homes. The recruitment of refugees was organised through the Domestic Bureau of the Council for German Jewry, which was established in 1938 and located alongside the Nursing and Midwifery Department at Bloomsbury House in London.[145] The Bureau also regulated the treatment of refugees in private households. It considered the work it supported to be 'one of the largest pieces of constructive work for the refugee'. Its work involved 'removing large numbers of women from intolerable conditions and giving them the opportunity of earning their living'.[146]

One in three refugees who came to Britain came as domestic servants.[147] At a time when middle-class women in Britain were experiencing what was known as the 'servant crisis' and Jewish women were desperate to escape Nazi persecution, the Government offered domestic service as the prima facie option.[148] There is little doubt that these women were exploited and that the decision to allow them to escape to Britain was self-serving. Kushner goes further and quotes one refugee as maintaining that they may have been given refuge, but this did not equate to any real security.[149] A more positive outlook is offered by women's historian Anne Summers, who argues that we cannot ignore that their lives were spared.[150] In July 1939, the Home Office threatened to stop issuing domestic service visas if the number reached saturation point.[151] The escape of 20,000 women who arrived on these visas before hostilities commenced was therefore a positive outcome. Furthermore, as the war progressed most were able to leave domestic service and take up more worthwhile work. Nevertheless, this did not remove the months and sometimes years of misery and humiliation working in other people's houses. The literature is replete with stories of the appalling treatment of refugee domestics. In some instances, they were forced to sleep and eat with the dogs, even being required to eat the dogs' food.[152] Sexual advances by the men in the house were not uncommon.[153] According to Louise London, refugees were literally 'chained' to domestic service.[154]

Gertrude Dann came to Britain on a domestic service visa and was employed by a family far less cultured, wealthy or educated than her own. One evening after she and her sister had eaten leftover chicken from their employers' dinner, Dann recalled that the mistress of the house told them, 'Will you remember that you will never, and I repeat NEVER, have in the kitchen what we have in the dining room. You can have cocoa or semolina or cheese.'[155] Later in her memoir she remembered her wealthy Aunt Minna visiting in her chauffeur-driven car. at which point Dann's employer conceded she was different from her previous maids. Dann recalled, 'Aunt Minna was very pleased that the purpose of her visit was fulfilled.'[156] However, whilst Dann's recollection of this event has comedic value, the reality of the superior class of the refugee to the employing family led to considerable difficulties. In her semi-autobiographical novel, Lore Segal summed up the problem eloquently as she described her parents' situation as 'married couple' domestic servants to a Mr and Mrs Willoughby:

> And so the Willoughbys had put my parents in their place; the refugees belonged to the class of people who eat in the kitchen, sleep on cheap mattresses ... – which goes to show that people have, after all, an innate sense of justice and cannot with equanimity be served by their fellows when these too closely resemble themselves.[157]

The Domestic Bureau's edict that 'good conditions include also warm, comfortable accommodation in the house and adequate wholesome food' were followed in some employing households, but not all.[158] Yet the refugees themselves were chastened to remember that 'they are received into English households through friendliness and good will and it behoves them to be a credit to their people and to their religion as the public are apt to judge all from one'.[159] The implication was clear: the British were suspicious of Continental Jews and it was the responsibility of the refugees to ensure they did nothing to fuel this antipathy. Cilly Haar, aged 17, left Germany and arrived in Britain some time in 1939. She spent three days on a kibbutz and then went to a family:

> And so, it came that I went to an English family outside Luton. There I spent two very happy years. They treated me like a daughter, you didn't even know at the time there was a war on. I learned to cook, I learned how to display an English table flower arranging [sic]. They taught me how to speak English. I believe that those early impressions of my life made me a positive person because there were lots of people who were not as lucky as me.[160]

The requirement for refugees to be grateful to Britain for their rescue means that many of the testimonies portray a happier picture of these early months than were actually experienced. Haar's opening lines about her time in England are full of promise and kindness. Only later in the interview does she admit to aspects of her life which highlighted that she was neither a guest nor a foster daughter but a paid servant.[161] Similarly, her memoir notes, 'The only thing I really hated was wearing a uniform and cap. I felt so labelled, but that's what they wished me to wear, so I had to do it.'[162] Gordon escaped to England on a domestic service visa in July 1939 and arrived in 'Southampton, I think. Then I was picked up by my employer and taken to their home where I was introduced to the kitchen, which was, after all, my domain, and the scullery and the other staff. I was more or less the senior.'[163] Two months later the other maids left to engage in war work and Gordon stayed on for another two years. She admitted that it was hard work: 'I started at half-past five in the morning because otherwise the boiler would have gone out.'[164] Despite this she was treated reasonably well and considered the work to be good preparation for her nurse training.

Lisbeth Hockey also escaped to Britain on a domestic service visa. Hockey was not strictly Jewish but 'non-Aryan'. She had been unaware of any Jewish heritage growing up, but following the *Anschluss*, her Jewish ancestry became important and her need to leave Austria paramount. Being 'non-Aryan' she was helped by the Quakers, who supported the escape of many who did not come under the jurisdiction of Jewish organisations. Hockey found a position as governess to the children of the Wedgwood family and was sent to their home in Devon: 'they were such lovely people and took great care of me'.[165] Susi Linton's initial experience as a domestic servant was also a positive one. Miss Parry, who acted as a liaison for Linton, visited her when she first arrived. Linton was staying at the Catholic Teachers' College in Liverpool, which had offered to take Jewish refugees to help ease them into British life: 'So she said, "There is an English clergyman from a vicarage, who particularly asked for a Jewish girl, to do domestic work, to be an au-pair" ... So I thought, what my father said, "be with Jewish people". But then I thought, "This is a good man, he asked for a Jewish girl"... They, from day one, they were absolutely wonderful. They couldn't do enough for me.'[166]

Sadly, following the fall of France to the Nazis in the spring of 1940, the Government instituted a raft of new regulations for refugees.[167] Linton was unable to stay in Liverpool – a port city. Despite the vicar vouching for her at the tribunal, she was forced to take a job inland and chose Manchester as it had a large Jewish community. The Refugee Committee found her a job with a wealthy family: 'It was a nightmare from day one ... "Clean the steps, get breakfast ready and start the washing in the garage." That's the way they talked to me, there was no personal contact, no sympathy, nothing, nothing.' Linton left after eight weeks and found another job, but it was no better: 'They would let the food go bad rather than give me anything to eat.'[168] Linton was saved by the war: 'We were allowed to do wartime jobs ... So I was the first who went back to the Refugee Committee, "Can I train as a nurse?" Which I always – which I might have done even in Germany. And they said, "Unfortunately, it will not be possible". Because in those days you had to pay for the training, couldn't do it.' Several weeks later, when Linton was invited back to the office and offered nursery-nurse training, she took the opportunity.[169]

In the booklet 'Domestic Bureau: Some suggestions for employers and employees', the Bureau acknowledged the possibility of poor treatment, which it cited as a rationale for leaving without notice.[170] However it failed to acknowledge openly, at least not in any of the documents located for this study, the poor conditions under which many refugee servants were forced to work and live. There was even a level of blame imposed on those refugees who changed employment shortly after arrival, which was usually because of poor treatment.[171] Even if the Bureau had been able to acknowledge and act upon the appalling treatment of some refugee servants, it had no jurisdiction over those refugee servants brought to Britain as Kinder and forced to work as domestic help.[172]

The Domestic Bureau attempted to organise social workers to monitor young girls who worked as servants, but this was a largely unsuccessful endeavour, especially once hostilities began and travel was curtailed.[173] Following the death of her brother, Lee Fischer was taken to Manchester by her cousin, who lived there: 'In short ... when I was 16, I became a maid in another family and I stayed there for two years being mother's helper. And

I did a lot of things like cleaning vegetables and stuff and doing laundry.' According to her oral history interview, Fischer accepted this because her parents had told her 'to be grateful that we're in England and not to worry and just do what we were told'.[174] When Mia Ross left her school in Tottenham, she was sent to a family in a small village outside Saffron Walden. She was expected to build the fires, cook and clean and remove the dead mice from the kitchen: 'Life was not too pleasant as I had to do lots of jobs I was not used to and I missed the company of my friends and the family I had been staying with in Saffron Walden.' Her existence was made worse by the hostility of the woman of the house, who 'found many faults with my work'.[175] Ross discovered that this animus was the result of the woman's pregnancy and she thus tried to please her. But she acknowledged that this was not easy. Like Ross, Roberts was sent to domestic service jobs as soon as she left school. The Refugee Committee sent her to one household, but she admits they clearly did not check the family's credentials:

> I remember once she threatened me with a carving knife. I mean I don't know how I behaved, all I knew is I was scrubbing stairs, I was unhappy, I was crying, I was getting distraught letters from my parents, I was writing to them and all I wanted at that time was to try and communicate with my parents, find out where they were, tell them what I was doing because I had become ... Oh no, no, I was an enemy alien, what was I doing in her country, you know, she was suspicious like a lot of people were at that time.[176]

As the narratives above attest, the view of the Domestic Bureau that these young girls 'wished to enter domestic employment' was inaccurate. I have not found one personal testimony from a child refugee stating that she was glad to be offered domestic service work. They took the positions because they had no alternative. Given the supportive and loving homes from which most of these young girls came, even without the moments of physical violence Roberts described, this would have been a highly challenging period in their lives. Tragically, given the inability of the Refugee Committee to provide financial support to refugees, it appears the vetting procedures for prospective employers were not as diligent as they should have been, compounding the girls' misery. Historical scholarship on refugees who came on domestic service visas and the Kindertransport may only be quite recent, but there is a reasonable body of literature that has focused on these two refugee groups. Those who came on nursing visas have, however, been largely missing from the historical canon. It is acknowledged that the number was never even close to the 20,000 who came on domestic service visas. However, nursing was the only other sphere of work that enabled the British Government to take a more generous approach to the immigration of adult Jews.[177]

Nursing visas

The decision to enable women refugees to come to Britain on nursing visas was based on similar opportunism as the invitation to those coming as domestic servants. Middle-class hospital matrons wanted to staff their hospitals, just as middle-class wives wanted to staff their homes. Nursing was nominally considered a profession and therefore higher in the social strata than service. But it was hard work, with long hours and petty discipline, conditions which made it difficult to recruit British women and girls into the profession. The nursing elite had long wished for the profession to enlist educated, middle-class women into its ranks, but its attempts had not been effective. The opportunity to bring educated, cultured refugees into nursing was a potential answer to the class issue. Their religion and Continental backgrounds, not to mention their refugee status, marked them as different and to many somewhat infra dig.[178]

Margot Hodge was a student nurse at the Jewish Hospital in Berlin. In her memoir she recalled that she was relatively safe in the hospital, but it was clear that if she was going to survive, she needed to leave Germany.[179] She wrote for help to the Jewish refugee agency in London. As she had family friends in Leeds in the north of England, she was given a visa to move to that city and train at St James's Hospital. She recalled that the matron of the hospital in Berlin was not pleased when she resigned, either despite or perhaps because of the growing dangers for Jews in Germany. The matron made Hodge work her month's notice.[180] She arrived in England on 4 July 1939. Elisabeth Katz was a student nurse at the Jewish Hospital in Frankfurt during the November pogrom. Unlike Hodge, although the patients felt safe inside the hospital walls, she did not. In her oral history she recalled, 'And there, I have never seen so many people, they looked for shelter. They were piled in corridors. Every bed taken. They all came in because they knew if they were in a hospital, they were safe.'[181]

The horror Katz experienced was not reserved for the plight of the patients. At a time when the physicians in a hospital were considered close to God, she had to watch whilst they committed suicide: 'And there were several of the physicians who jumped out of the windows as the Gestapo came through the door. There were others who had cyanide ready. It was an absolutely ghastly experience. I can see it before me, but I can't really put it into words.' It was this experience that compelled Katz to leave Frankfurt for England: 'I just applied OK and I was lucky ... I think all the nurses did. England wanted student nurses.'[182] The fact that Katz and Hodge had worked as nurses in Germany and were therefore already reasonably experienced would have undoubtedly supported their applications. In her oral history Katz remembered, '[Bloomsbury House] worked to get people out and get people processed and get them to England as an immigrant, either as a student nurse, or you get out as a housekeeper ... so you applied and waited.' Katz was accepted at St Luke's Hospital in Bradford, West Yorkshire and she flew to England early in 1939.[183] German nursing qualifications were not recognised by the General Nursing Council, so despite Katz's and Hodge's considerable nursing experience in Germany, both were required to start their nurse training from the beginning.[184] Given that Hodge could barely speak English, starting as a junior probationer was probably useful. However, the decision was also opportunistic for the hospitals. They could employ competent nurses for the full training period, which meant paying lower salaries if they did not take their previous training into account.

Josephine Bruegel was a medical student at the German University in Prague. In October 1938, the university demanded certification of Bruegel's 'Aryan' heritage, and in its absence, she was barred from re-registering for the last semester of her studies. Although this was before the German invasion of Czechoslovakia, the German University was under Nazi rule. Fortunately, the Dean was a friend of her family and as she was so close to qualifying, gave her special dispensation to continue. In her memoirs, Bruegel admitted that although at the time she did not fear for her life in Prague, she nevertheless decided that she ought to leave and made plans to emigrate the United States.[185] She received the required affidavits through her boyfriend, but he decided to emigrate with his mother instead, leaving Bruegel behind. By the end of 1938, the situation for the Jews in Czechoslovakia was becoming more perilous.

Medicine may have been an acceptable and popular career choice in Central Europe, but women were largely kept out of the profession in Britain.[186] The lack of money only added to the challenges of gaining access to Britain as a woman doctor. Bruegel was recommended to the Quakers for consideration to enter England on a nursing visa:

> Sometime in January 1939 I was called for interview by a representative of the Quakers, to see if I was the right sort of person to come to England to be a nurse. They were extremely polite and just asked about my interest in nursing and my knowledge of languages. Having got my exit permit I went to Masaryk station and boarded a train on 30th March 1939. This would take me to England via Holland. I remember packing my fur coat and taking a typewriter, my university documents and my recipe book, but not much else. My mother came to see me off. With the egotism of the young, it did not occur to me to consider how she felt. She was very fit, not yet sixty, and not an old woman in outlook. I did not think of it as a long-term thing, nor that she was alone. I took it that she was surrounded by friends and that she would not leave, that her life would be restricted, but not threatened by the Germans. But, had I known this was the last time I would see her.[187]

The main work of the Quakers was with those who were classed as 'non-Aryan', 'since those of Jewish faith were able to obtain assistance from their own Community'.[188] Nevertheless, although Quakers mainly helped 'non-Aryans', they did also support Jews like Bruegel. Throughout the 1930s, a number of Quaker women and men lived and worked in Germany and Austria to help those in peril from the Nazis.[189] Despite Britain and Germany not being at war at the time, their position was not without danger. According to Laurence Darton's account, from the very beginning of Hitler's ascension to power, the Quakers sought ways to help the Jewish population. Darton himself visited the British Embassy asking if he could help Germany's Jews: 'The next morning at an early hour my whole family suddenly found itself under Gestapo arrest.'[190] Darton and his family were released, but it is clear Darton had subjected them all to significant risk.

Bruegel was fortunate to escape to Britain only two months after her initial interview with the Quakers, before she experienced any severe episodes of antisemitism. Furthermore, whilst many on her train through Germany were strip-searched, she was not, and she arrived in Holland unscathed.[191] Susi Lewinsky's memoirs describe a far more protracted and frightening time as she tried to leave Germany. Lewinsky recalls that all Jews were required to submit their passport. On the day she delivered hers, 'All Jews had to pick up an identification card with a photo of the left profile with the left ear uncovered; to our names were added Sara, or Israel. We had to carry it with us all the time.'[192] Lewinsky reflected how she and her friends had joked during their summer holiday earlier that year about the possibility of escaping as nurses or housemaids. These were, she acknowledged, now the only options for emigration. She was helped by a Dr Samson to find a connection in London to support her application to enter Britain on a nursing visa: 'It was a nerve-wrackin [sic] existence. These waves of terror kept us alert. Periodically the manhunts were on ... We spent much time in the streets.'[193] In February 1939, Lewinsky received her preliminary notice of her acceptance for nursing in Britain. Yet even now the desperation did not end. She endeavoured to sell what she could and decide what she could take with her, given the ever-changing laws on emigration for Jews: 'My visa arrived in March. I planned tentatively to leave at the beginning of April. The police, some other authorities had to be informed ... and above all, the Gestapo had to send an officer to check the contents of my baggage.'[194] Finally, on 9 April, Lewinsky was ready to board the boat to England, but once again there were bags to be checked by the Gestapo: 'Only then were we free to board the ship to England. A few persons had to stay behind because they caused suspicion. What was their fate?' On arrival in Britain, she sent her parents the following letter:

If only I could comprehend that I am really here in London. Never did I imagine to feel so relieved to be out of Germany. I hope it's not a dream. My boatride [sic] was a beautiful experience under a blue and sunny sky with very agreeable people. And after all the running around of the last days. One could not be certain up to the last moments if all the necessary papers were obtained. I was so petrified that war would break out and I was in a hurry to book my trip for the shortest way to get away. I did not expect the Gestapo again before boarding the boat.[195]

Lewinsky started her nurse training in mid-April 1939 at the Dreadnaught Hospital in Greenwich.

Conclusion

Before the accession of Hitler, Jews in Germany, Austria and Czechoslovakia did experience a certain amount of antisemitism, but their largely middle-class lives enabled a mostly happy and successful existence. From 1933 onwards, these lives changed in progressively more hostile and dangerous ways. The loss of professional careers, university places and schooling left many with little option but to escape. Yet emigration is a profoundly challenging event, and many chose not to go. The pogrom in November 1938 brought into stark relief the threat to life. The arrests of men and boys nourished the belief that women and girls would be saved from Nazi brutality, yet there was a developing sense that all Jews were in danger. It had been considered dangerous for daughters to travel alone. Furthermore, gendered expectations kept some of them at home to support elderly family members. Parents now urged them to leave. As increasing numbers of Jews desperately tried to escape, the liberal democracies tightened their border controls. Nevertheless, as this chapter identifies, for children and women, three escape routes were created. Coming on nursing or domestic service visas or the Kindertransport ensured as safe an entry onto British soil as possible. But this does not mean that once here refugees were accepted entirely. As Marion Berghahn argues, Britain was a country of transit and not settlement.[196]

Children as young as the 13-year-old Rosa Sacharin had even been asked, almost on arrival, if they would immediately transmigrate. Despite this expectation, those who arrived on nursing visas came on the understanding that they would be able to qualify first and transmigrate after. The knowledge that they would be able to stay in Britain for the full three or four years of their training may have given them a sense of security because, like many Jewish refugees, their decisions were imbued with opportunism. While the refugees were student nurses, they would staff the nation's hospitals and be paid a paltry sum. Once qualified and therefore more expensive members of staff, they would be expected to leave not only the hospital but also the country. However, on 3 September 1939, Britain declared war on Germany, and all possibility of transmigration ceased. The women and girls who had arrived on the Kindertransport, or on nursing and domestic service visas, would remain in Britain until at least 1945. Their experiences during the war will be explored in the next chapter.

Notes

1 Miraculously, the Jewish Hospital in Berlin remained open throughout the war. The reason for allowing it to continue with a retinue of Jewish medical and nursing staff was partly because it offered the only place where half-Jews and those married to 'Aryans' could receive treatment. For further details see 'Traces of war: The Jewish Hospital in Berlin' (2020). https://www.tracesofwar.com/articles/5561/Jewish-hospital-in-Berlin-during-the-Nazi-period.htm [accessed 19 August 2022].
2 It has not been possible to verify her employment at St Thomas's Hospital. Given the lack of reciprocity of registration between Germany and Britain, it may be that she was able to work as a nursery nurse.
3 See advice from Council for Refugees with Horsburgh plea. Central Office for Refugees, 'Circular No. 100. B: Nursing and medical auxiliaries, 1. Hospital nursing (6 June 1941). Report on the work of the Aliens War Service Department 1939–1944: Volume 1. HO 213/2093/3, National Archives.
4 Lola Hahn-Warburg, testimonial for Ruth Rawraway, 26 January 1939. Personal archive. Lola Hahn-Warburg was a refugee who arrived in Britain and was to lead the Refugee Children's Movement

in London. Recent research from Paul Weindling points to her 'selection' processes for Viennese Jewish children. According to Weindling, 'Hahn-Warburg saw the issue as if being worthy of a place on a Kindertransport was equivalent to emigration to Palestine, where physically and mentally high-quality youths were required' (p. 19). Paul Weindling, 'The Kindertransport from Vienna: The children who came and those left behind', *Jewish Historical Studies* 51, 1 (2020): 16–32. https://doi.org/10.14324/111.444.jhs.2020v51.003 [accessed 27 September 2023]. According to Jennifer Craig-Norton, from 1939, social work assessments were required to see if the family had any history of 'psychological breakdown' and in March 1939, children of Polish decent were excluded. Jennifer Craig-Norton, *The Kindertransport: Contesting Memory* (Bloomington: Indiana University Press, 2019), 244. See also Sybil Oldfield, '"It is usually she": The role of British women in the rescue and care of the Kindertransport Kinder', *Shofar: An Interdisciplinary Journal of Jewish Studies, Special Issue: Kindertransporte 1938/39 – Rescue and Integration* 23, 1 (2004): 57–70; Rose Holmes, 'The politics of compassion: The Refugee Children's Movement and caring for the Kinder', *Jewish Historical Studies* 51, 1 (2020): 51–67. https://doi.org/10.14324/111.444.jhs.20 20v51.005 [accessed 27 September 2023].

5 Declaration of British Nationality and Status of Aliens Act, 1914. Home Office certificate No. A7 2.6751, Ruth Anneliese Simon (14 June 1947). Personal archive.
6 Dalia Ofer and Lenore J. Weitzman, 'Introduction: The role of gender in the Holocaust', in Dalia Ofer and Lenore J. Weitzman (eds), *Women in the Holocaust* (New Haven, CT: Yale University Press, 1998), 6.
7 David Cesarani, *Final Solution: The Fate of the Jews, 1933–1949* (London: Pan Macmillan, Kindle edition, 2017), 243.
8 Kitty Schafer (Kaufmann), oral history interview by Jane Brooks on 30 August 2017. Personal archive.
9 Kerry Wallach, *Passing Illusions: Jewish Visibility in Weimar Germany* (Ann Arbor: University of Michigan Press, 2017), 14.
10 Walter Laqueur, *Generation Exodus: The Fate of Young Jewish Refugees from Nazi Germany* (London: I. B. Tauris, 2004), 2.
11 Wallach, *Passing Illusions*, 4.
12 Till van Rahden, 'Jews and the ambivalences of civil society in Germany, 1800–1933: Assessment and reassessment', *Journal of Modern History* 77 (2005): 1026.
13 Marion Berghahn, *Continental Britons: German-Jewish Refugees from Nazi Germany* (Oxford: Berg, 1988), 53.

14 Josephine Bruegel, 'Reminiscences', 3. Oral history interview by Sylva Simsova between 1998 and 2001. OSP 2122, Wiener Holocaust Library, London.
15 Yarm School Assembly, A talk on the theme of 'Great Lives', 2 June 2014. A talk given by Eva Flatow's son, Dr David Gordon.
16 Hortense Gordon, oral history interview by Jane Brooks at her home in London on 27 October 2017. Personal archive.
17 Gertrude Dann, 'Memoir', Leo Baeck Institute (LBI) Memoir Collection (ME978). Leo Baeck Institute Oral History Archive, Berlin and New York.
18 Gertrud (Trudie) Moos, 'I Remember: My Life Story' (printed 1995), 12. A biographical database of European Medical Refugees in Great Britain, 1930s–1950s, Oxford Brookes University, Oxford.
19 Gertrude Roberts, oral history interview by Alan Dein on 23 January 1982. Audio 184. Oral History Collection, Jewish Museum, London.
20 Laqueur, *Generation Exodus*, 201.
21 Jennifer Craig-Norton, 'Refugees at the margins: Jewish domestics in Britain, 1938–45', *Shofar: An Interdisciplinary Journal of Jewish Studies* 37, 3 (2019): 302.
22 Benjamin Ziemann, 'Weimar was Weimar: Politics, culture and the employment of the German Republic', *German History* 28, 4 (2010), 562. https://doi.org/10.1093/gerhis/ghq114 [accessed 27 September 2023].
23 Ruth Price (Schulvater), oral history interview by Helen Lloyd at her home in Crowle on 29 July 2004. Interview 68, Refugee Voices: Association of Jewish Refugees (AJR) Audio-Visual Testimony Archive, British Library, London.
24 Erna Harding, oral history video interview by Peter Ryan in Walnut Creek on 11 April 2011. Gift of Jewish and Children's Services of San Francisco, the Peninsula, Marin and Sonoma Counties. United States Holocaust Memorial Museum (USHMM), Washington, DC.
25 Lotte Dann-Treves, 'Memoir'. Leo Baeck Institute Berlin Collection (ME979), Leo Baeck Institute, Berlin and New York.
26 Moos, 'I Remember', 23.
27 Laqueur, *Generation Exodus*, 1.
28 Cesarani, *Final Solution*, 43.
29 Laqueur, *Generation Exodus*, 12.
30 Berghahn, *Continental Britons*, 58.
31 Harding, oral history video interview.
32 Doron Niederland, 'Areas of departure from Nazi Germany and the social structure of the emigrants', in Werner E. Mosse, Julius

Carlebach, Gerhard Hirschfield, Aubrey Newman, Arnold Pauker and Peter Pulzer (eds), *Second Chance: Two Centuries of German-Speaking Jews in the United Kingdom* (Tübingen: J. C. B. Mohr, 1991), 57.

33 Cesarani, *Final Solution*, 116.
34 Bill Williams, *Jews and other Foreigners: Manchester and the Rescue of the Victims of European Fascism, 1933–40* (Manchester: Manchester University Press, 2011), 1.
35 Claire Hilton, 'A Jewish contribution to British psychiatry: Edward Mapother, Aubrey Lewis and their Jewish refugee colleagues at the Bethlem and Maudsley Hospital and Institute of Psychiatry, 1933–66', *Jewish Historical Journal* 41 (2007): 213.
36 Roberts, oral history interview.
37 Cesarani, *Final Solution*, 70.
38 Saul Friedlander, *Nazi Germany and the Jews: Volume I, The Years of Persecution, 1933–1939* (London: Phoenix, 1997), 21.
39 Ervin Staub, *The Roots of Evil: The Origins of Genocide and Other Group Violence* (Cambridge: Cambridge University Press, 1989), 100.
40 Cesarani, *Final Solution*.
41 Price, oral history interview.
42 Margaret Marflow, 'For my Grandchildren' (2001), 41. A biographical database of European Medical Refugees in Great Britain, 1930s–1950s, Oxford Brookes University, Oxford.
43 Marflow, 'For my Grandchildren', 45.
44 Susi Lewinsky, 'Memoirs, 1911–1940'. Leo Baeck Institute Memoir Collection (ME1628): A32/6. Leo Baeck Institute, Berlin and New York.
45 Lewinsky, 'Memoirs, 1911–1940', 79.
46 Lewinsky, 'Memoirs, 1911–1940', 79.
47 Cesarani, *Final Solution*, 44.
48 Friedlander, *Nazi Germany and the Jews*, 324.
49 Edith Menkes Wolloch, oral history interview at her home on 21 March 2006. Interview 2297, Austrian Heritage Collection (AHC) Oral History Archive, Leo Baeck Institute, Berlin and New York. https://digipres.cjh.org/delivery/DeliveryManagerServlet?dps_pid=IE2981299 [accessed 1 October 2023].
50 Dina Gold, *Stolen Legacy: Nazi Theft and the Quest for Justice at Krausenstrasse 17/18, Berlin* (Chicago: American Bar Association Publishing, 2016), 63. Dina's uncle Fritz was sent to Auschwitz on 1 March 1943, where he was murdered.

51 Martin Gilbert, *Kristallnacht: Prelude to Destruction* (London: Harper Perennial, 2006), 120–1. See also USHMM, Holocaust Encyclopedia, 'Law for the Restoration of the Civil Service.' The Law initially excluded those who had been in post since 1 August 1914, First-World-War veterans and those who fathers or sons had been killed in that conflict. https://encyclopedia.ushmm.org/content/en/timeline-event/holocaust/1933–1938/law-for-the-restoration-of-the-professional-civil-service.

52 Frank Caestecker and Bob Moore (eds), *Refugees from Nazi Europe and the Liberal European States* (New York: Berghahn Books, 2010), 211.

53 Staub, *Roots of Evil*, 118. It is not the intention of this book to undertake a detailed analysis of the part the German population played in the Holocaust. There is a wealth of literature which analyses this most difficult of questions. See for example, David Cesarani (ed.), *The Final Solution: Origins and Implementation* (London: Routledge, 1994); Friedlander, *Nazi Germany and the Jews*; Donald Bloxham and Tony Kushner (eds), *The Holocaust: Critical Historical Approaches* (Manchester: Manchester University Press, 2005); Christian Wiese and Paul Betts (eds), *Years of Persecution, Years of Extermination: Saul Friedlander and the Future of Holocaust Studies* (London: Continuum, 2010). It should also be that acknowledged that antisemitism was endemic throughout the liberal democracies as well, including Britain. This nascent antisemitism will be identified throughout this book.

54 Frank Bajohr, *'Aryanisation' in Hamburg: The Economic Exclusion of Jews and the Confiscation of their Property in Nazi Germany* (New York: Berghahn Books, 2002), 22.

55 Yvonne Kapp and Margaret Mynatt, *British Policy and the Refugees, 1939–1941* (London: Frank Cass, 1997), 14.

56 Judith Tydor Baumel, *Double Jeopardy: Gender and the Holocaust* (London: Vallentine Mitchell, 1998), 6.

57 Marion Kaplan, 'Prologue: Jewish women in Nazi Germany', in Sibylle Quack (ed.), *Between Sorrow and Strength: Women Refugees of the Nazi Period* (Cambridge: Cambridge University Press, 1995).

58 Dalia Ofer and Leonore J. Weitzman, 'Introduction: The role of gender in the Holocaust', in Dalia Ofer and Leonore J. Weitzman (eds), *Women in the Holocaust* (New Haven, CT: Yale University Press, 1998), 4.

59 Marion Kaplan, *Between Dignity and Despair: Jewish Life in Nazi Germany* (New York: Oxford University Press, 1998), 5.

60 Ofer and Weitzman, 'Introduction', 3.
61 Kaplan, 'Prologue: Jewish women in Nazi Germany', 37.
62 Berghahn, *Continental Britons*, 53.
63 Deborah Dwork, *Children with a Star: Jewish Youth in Nazi Europe* (New Haven, CT: Yale University Press, 1991),15.
64 Laqueur, *Generation Exodus*, 4–5.
65 Elizabeth Katz (Rosenthal), oral history video interview by Sandra Bendayan on 4 August 1994. Gift of Jewish and Children's Services of San Francisco, the Peninsula, Marin and Sonoma Counties. USHMM, Washington, DC.
66 Rosa Sacharin (Goldschal), oral history interview by Barbara Mortimer on 28 April 2010. Interview T407, Oral History Collection, Royal College of Nursing (RCN), Edinburgh.
67 Sacharin, oral history interview.
68 Hortense Gordon, oral history interview by Sharon Rapaport in London on 3 July 2004. Interview 65, Refugee Voices: AJR Audio-Visual Testimony Archive, British Library, London.
69 Price, oral history interview.
70 Edith Bown (Jacobowitz), 'Memories and reflections: A refugee's story' (1938). RCN Archives, Edinburgh, 8.
71 The *Reichsbund jüdischer Frontsoldaten* (Reich Federation of Jewish Front-Line Soldiers) was founded in February 1919. As an organisation of German Jewish soldiers, it worked to demonstrate loyalty to Germany and to ensure that the sacrifice of Jewish soldiers in the trenches of the First World War was not forgotten. Cesarani, *Final Solution*, 53.
72 Heidi Cowen (pseudonym) and Ruth Shire, oral history interview by Jane Brooks at Ruth Shire's home in the West Midlands on 13 February 2018. Personal archive.
73 Gordon, oral history interview 2004; Roberts, oral history interview.
74 Bernard Wasserstein, *Britain and the Jews of Europe, 1939–1945* (London: Clarendon Press, 1979), 11.
75 Gemma Romain, 'The *Anschluss*: The British response to the refugee crisis', *Journal of Holocaust Education* 8, 3 (1999): 87–102.
76 Peter Alter, 'Refugees from Nazism and cultural transfer to Britain', *Immigrants and Minorities* 30, 2/3 (2012): 193.
77 Gilbert, *Kristallnacht*, 16.
78 Tony Kushner, *The Holocaust and the Liberal Imagination: A Social and Cultural History* (Oxford: Blackwell, 1994), 48.
79 Kushner, *Holocaust and the Liberal Imagination*, 50.
80 Susan Cohen, *Rescue the Perishing: Eleanor Rathbone and the Refugees* (London: Vallentine Mitchell, 2010), 113.

81 Kushner, *Holocaust and the Liberal Imagination*, 51.
82 Andrew Sharf, 'Noah Barou Memorial Lecture: "Nazi racialism and the British Press, 1933–1945"', delivered at University College London (London: World Jewish Congress, 16 December 1963).
83 Louise London, 'British immigration controls procedures and Jewish refugees, 1933–1939', in Werner E. Mosse, Julius Carlebach, Gerhard Hirschfield, Aubrey Newman, Arnold Pauker and Peter Pulzer (eds), *Second Chance: Two Centuries of German-Speaking Jews in the United Kingdom* (Tübingen: J. C. B. Mohr, 1991), 506.
84 See for example, Cohen, *Rescue the Perishing*; Craig-Norton, *Kindertransport*.
85 Tony Kushner, *Journeys from the Abyss: The Holocaust and Forced Migration from the 1880s to the Present* (Liverpool: Liverpool University Press, 2017), 42.
86 Alf Dubs, 'We simply can't turn our backs on vulnerable refugee children', *Guardian* (10 January 2020), www.theguardian.com/commentisfree/2020/jan/10/refugee-children-lone-reunite-rights-dublin-regulation [accessed 8 March 2021].
87 Claudia Curio, 'Were unaccompanied child refugees a privileged class of refugees in the liberal states of Europe?', in Frank Caestecker and Bob Moore (eds), *Refugees from Nazi Europe and the Liberal European States* (New York: Berghahn Books, 2010), 183.
88 Cohen, *Rescue the Perishing*, 113.
89 Dwork, *Children with a Star*, xxiii. See also Ruth Barnett, 'The acculturation of the Kindertransport children: Intergenerational dialogue on the Kindertransport experience', *Shofar: An Interdisciplinary Journal of Jewish Studies* 23, 1 (2004): 100–8.
90 Craig-Norton, *Kindertransport*, 239, 240.
91 At some point – and it is not clear when – Gert Jacobowitz became Gerald Jayson. As the Anglicised version is the name under which he published his recollections of Millisle, that is the name that will be used throughout the book.
92 Rebekka Gopfert and Andrea Hammel, 'Kindertransport: History and memory', *Shofar: An Interdisciplinary Journal of Jewish Studies* 23, 1 (2004), 25. Gopfert and Hammel continue that Kinder reunions did not start to occur until about the 1980s, when most those who managed to survive the camps were dead: 'One can see here a coming out of the shadow of the Auschwitz survivors. Many Kinder were for the first time enabled to articulate for themselves and society that also they had survived traumatic experiences about which they grieve and must, to this day come to terms' (25).

93 Bown, 'Memories and reflections', 19.
94 Frank Caestecker and Bob Moore, 'From *Kristallnacht* to war, November 1938–August 1939', in Frank Caestecker and Bob Moore (eds), *Refugees from Nazi Europe and the Liberal European States* (New York: Berghahn Books, 2010), 277.
95 Mia Ross (Maria Fuchs), 'War memories', 2.
96 Susi Loeffler, 'The Family Löffler: Part V – 1939: Escape of Susi' (unpublished ms, 2017), 8. Susi emigrated to Australia in the 1950s and lived there until her death in 2018.
97 Benz and Hammel, 'Emigration as rescue and trauma', 4.
98 Eva Minden, *How it all Started with the Shoes: Memoirs of a Career in Nursing from 1934–1951* (Baltimore, MD: Novice Publishers, 2021), 28.
99 Cowen, oral history interview.
100 Beverley Chalmers, 'Jewish women's sexual behaviour and sexualized abuse during the Nazi era', *Canadian Journal of Human Sexuality* 24, 2 (2015): 189; see also Ofer and Weitzman, 'Introduction', 7.
101 Henry Greenspan, 'The unsaid, the incommunicable, the unbearable, and the irretrievable', *Oral History Review* 41, 2 (2014): 229–43.
102 Mahua Sarkar, 'Between craft and method: Meaning and inter-subjectivity in oral history analysis', *Journal of Historical Sociology* 25, 4 (2012): 578.
103 Tal Litvak Hirsch, Alon Lazar and Orna Braun-Lewensohn, 'Sense of coherence during female Holocaust survivors' formative years', *Journal of Loss and Trauma* 21, 5 (2016): 361.
104 Sacharin, oral history interview.
105 Veronica Gillespie, 'Working with the "Kindertransports"', in Sybil Oldfield (ed.), *This Working-Day: Women's Lives and Culture(s) in Britain, 1914–1945* (London: Taylor & Francis, 1994), 127.
106 Curio, 'Were unaccompanied child refugees a privileged class?'
107 Cesarani, *Final Solution: The Fate of the Jews*, 282.
108 Cesarani, *Final Solution: The Fate of the Jews*, 282.
109 Gopfert and Hammel. 'Kindertransport: History and memory', 23.
110 Craig-Norton, *Kindertransport*, 78.
111 Kushner, *Holocaust and the Liberal Imagination*, 240.
112 Berghahn, *Continental Britons*, 232–3.
113 Curio, 'Were unaccompanied child refugees a privileged class?', 175.
114 Oldfield, '"It is usually she"', 62.
115 Rosa M. Sacharin, *The Unwanted Jew: A Struggle for Acceptance* (Tullibody: Diadem Books, 2014), 49.
116 Gopfert and Hammel, 'Kindertransport: History and memory', 23.

117 Marion Berghahn, 'Women émigrés in England', in Sibylle Quack (ed.), *Between Sorrow and Strength: Women Refugees of the Nazi Period* (Cambridge: Cambridge University Press, 1995), 75–6; Craig-Norton, *Kindertransport*, 113.
118 Curio, 'Were unaccompanied child refugees a privileged class?', 175.
119 Helen Jones, 'National, community and personal priorities: British women's responses to refugees from the Nazis, from the mid-1930s to early 1940s', *Women's History Review* 21, 1 (2012): 143.
120 Oldfield, '"It is usually she"', 62. Anna Essinger was German-born and educated in the United States. She returned to Germany after the First World War and established a progressive school near Ulm, where she had been born. When Hitler came to power, she managed to relocate the school to Bunce Court in Kent.
121 Edith Bown, 'Fur das Kind: 2008 Liverpool Street Station', in 'Memories and Reflections'.
122 Bown, 'Memories and reflections' (26 June 1939), 26.
123 Bown, 'Memories and reflections' (22 June 1939), 26.
124 Millisle had originally been a training farm for young European Jews to learn agricultural skills. From 1939, when it was clear that Jews were not welcome in several parts of Europe, it was changed into a refugee camp for children and young people. It was finally dismantled in 1947. Gerald Jayson (Jacobowitz), 'The farm', written for the *Belfast Jewish Chronicle* (September 2005). Millisle Farm 1760, Wiener Holocaust Library, London.
125 Jayson, 'The farm', 4.
126 Bown, 'Memories and reflections: Copy of a BBC talk in 1962', 34.
127 Lee Fischer (Liesl Einstein), oral history interview by Jane Brooks on 12 October 2017. Personal archive.
128 Fischer, oral history interview.
129 Sacharin, *Unwanted Jew*, 51.
130 Laqueur refers to the trauma of separation and loss of all that was familiar, family, friends and environment. Laqueur, *Generation Exodus*, 291
131 Fischer, oral history interview; Bown, '"Dear Uncle": in Memories and reflections' (10 November 1939), 35.
132 Sacharin, *Unwanted Jew*, 53.
133 Berghahn, *Continental Britons*, 205.
134 Curio, 'Were unaccompanied child refugees a privileged class?'; Jennifer Craig-Norton, 'Contesting the Kindertransport as a "model" refugee response', *European Judaism* 50, 2 (2017): 25; Craig-Norton, *Kindertransport*. For the full range of first-hand accounts of the Kinder, see Karen Gershon (ed.), *We Came as Children: A Collective*

Autobiography of Refugees (London: Papermac, 1989); Bertha Leverton and Shmuel Lowensohn, *I Came Alone: The Stories of the Kindertransports* (Sussex: Book Guild, 1990).
135 Leonore Lowton (pseudonym), oral history interview at her home in the Midlands by Jane Brooks on 12 February 2018. Personal archive.
136 Judy Tydor Baumel-Schwartz maintains that this contrasted with the situation in the United States, in which Kinder were kept in religiously suitable homes. However, she acknowledges that because Britain was affected by the war in a way that the United States never was and needed to evacuate children from British parents as well as refugees, it meant that refugees were often resettled as part of the child evacuation scheme. Judy Tydor Baumel-Schwartz, 'The rescue of Jewish girls and teenage women to England and the USA during the Holocaust: A gendered perspective', *Jewish History* 26 (2012): 223–45. For a useful analysis of the comparative experiences of Kinder and British evacuees see Edward Timms, 'The ordeals of Kinder and evacuees in comparative perspective', *Yearbook of the Research Centre for German and Austrian Exile Studies* 13 (2012): 125–40.
137 Loeffler, 'Family Löffler: Part V – 1939', 10. Ida Haendel was in fact younger than Susi. Haendel was born in Poland in 1928, she made her London concert début in 1937 playing Beethoven's Violin Concerto at the Royal Albert Hall under the direction of Sir Henry Wood. In order to evade child labour laws, she was billed as being older than her real age, which may account for the confusion.
138 Craig-Norton, *Kindertransport*, 46.
139 Minutes of the Executive Committee of the Domestic Bureau of the Central Office for Refugees (19 May 1939), 2. Domestic Bureau Executive Minutes, 11 January 1939–17 January 1941 and Correspondence 1939–1941. ACC/2793/01/01/07, London Metropolitan Archives (LMA).
140 A draft letter to E. N. Cooper at the Home Office from the German Jewish Aid Committee raised the anxieties of the Committee as to the number of refugees arriving in Britain and their ability to support them. The Committee therefore recommended that 'Our efforts must, in the first instance, be concentrated on the younger generation, by giving them an opportunity of training and retraining, with a view to emigrating the vast majority of them overseas.' German Jewish Aid Committee to E. N. Cooper (14 September 1938), 2. ACC/2793/04/05/01, LMA.

141 Shani D'Cruze, 'Women and the family', in June Purvis (ed.), *Women's History Britain, 1850–1945* (London: UCL Press, 1995).
142 Sue Bruley, *Women in Britain since 1900* (Basingstoke: Palgrave, 1999), 8.
143 Lucy Delap, *Knowing their Place: Domestic Service in Twentieth-Century Britain* (Oxford: Oxford University Press, 2011), 48.
144 Craig-Norton, 'Refugees at the margins', 298.
145 Rose Holmes, 'Love, labour, loss: Women, refugees and the servant crisis in Britain, 1933–1939', *Women's History Review* 27, 2 (2017): 291.
146 Domestic Bureau, 'Memorandum to the Council for German Jewry', 2. ACC/2793/5/DB/1, LMA.
147 Angela Davies, '"Belonging and unbelonging": Jewish refugee and survivor women in 1950s Britain', *Women's History Review* 26, 1 (2016): 131. http://dx.doi.org/10.1080/09612025.2015.1123028 [accessed 25 September 2023].
148 Jennifer Craig-Norton, 'Servitude, displacement and trauma: Jewish refugee domestics in Britain, 1938–45', in Paula A. Michaels and Christina Twomey (eds), *Gender and Trauma since 1900* (London: Bloomsbury, 2021).
149 Tony Kushner, 'Asylum or servitude? Refugee domestics in Britain, 1933–1945', *Bulletin of the Society for the Study of Labour History* 53, 3 (1988): 25.
150 Anne Summers, *Christian and Jewish Women in Britain, 1880–1940: Living with Difference* (London: Palgrave Macmillan, 2017), 184.
151 Letter from H. Z. Oates to 'Madam', Home Office, 31 July 1939, 2. ACC/2793/04/05/01, LMA.
152 Kushner, 'Asylum or servitude?', 22; Berghahn, *Continental Britons*, 120; Berghahn, 'Women émigrés in England', 78. When refugees refer to eating the dogs' food, they were eating the same leftovers from their employers' meals as the dogs ate. They were not eating what we would now refer to as 'dog food', that is, food specifically created for dogs.
153 Berghahn, 'Women émigrés in England', 78.
154 Louise London, *Whitehall and the Jews, 1933–1948: British Immigration Policy, Jewish Refugees and the Holocaust* (Cambridge: Cambridge University Press, 2000), 71.
155 Dann, 'Memoir', 12.
156 Dann, 'Memoir', 7.
157 Lore Segal, *Other People's Houses: A Novel* (London: Sort of Books, 2018), 132–3. While most refugee domestic servants were women,

some married couples were able to escape together and find work as 'married couple domestics'. In this instance Segal's mother worked in the house and her father was employed first as the butler, but was soon demoted to the gardener (p. 127).

158 Central Office for Refugees Domestic Bureau, 'Domestic Bureau: Some Suggestions for Employers and Employees' (London: Central Office for Refugees Domestic Bureau, c. 1938), 6. ACC/2793/5/DB/1, LMA.
159 Central Office for Refugees Domestic Bureau, 'Domestic Bureau', 7.
160 Cilly Haar (Brauer), oral history interview by Jane Brooks at her home in London on 4 September 2017. Personal archive. The reference to living on a kibbutz is interesting. I have not found any other references to this type of living arrangement for refugees in all the texts consulted for this book. It is possible it was simply a place of initial refuge from where refugees were sent for employment.
161 Haar, oral history interview.
162 Cilly Haar, *Then and Now: The Memories of Cilly Haar, nee Brauer*, 17. There are no publications details with this memoir; it was given to me by the author at the time of our oral history interview.
163 Gordon, oral history interview, 2017.
164 Gordon, oral history interview, 2004.
165 Lisbeth Hockey, oral history interview at her home (interviewer not specified) in Edinburgh on 27 December 1987, 8. Interview T26. Oral History Collection, RCN, Edinburgh.
166 Susi Linton, oral history interview by Rosalyn Livshin on 19 October 2004, 15. Interview 78, Refugee Voices: Association of Jewish Refugees (AJR) Audio-Visual Testimony Archive, British Library, London.
167 Rachel Pistol, '"Heavy is the responsibility for all the lives that might have been saved in the pre-war years": British perceptions of refugees, 1933–1940', *European Judaism* 40, 2 (2017): 45.
168 Linton, oral history interview, 19.
169 Linton, oral history interview, 20. It is unclear why the Refugee Committee told her she could not train as a nurse because one had to pay for the training. This was untrue; the fact that student or probationer nurses did not pay for their training was one of the reasons why it was possible for other refugees to take up the profession.
170 Central Office for Refugees: Domestic Bureau, 'Domestic Bureau', 5.
171 Letter from H. Z. Oates to 'Madam', 2.
172 Holmes, 'Love, labour, loss', 301.

173 Executive Council of the Domestic Bureau, 'Minutes', 23 June 1939, ACC/2793/5/DB/1, LMA.
174 Fischer, oral history interview.
175 Mia Ross (Maria Fuchs), 'War memories', 11.
176 Roberts, oral history interview.
177 Kushner, 'Asylum or servitude?', 20.
178 Historian of refugees and humanitarianism Peter Gatrell argues that to be a refugee is to have one's attributes of social distinction eroded to a point of 'pure deprivation'. Peter Gatrell, *The Making of the Modern Refugee* (Oxford: Oxford University Press, 2015), 49.
179 Margot (Pogorzelski) Hodge, 'My Life, 1920–1943', 2004. 633. Library and Archives, Rubenstein Institute, USHMM, Washington, DC, 46b.
180 Hodge, 'My Life, 1920–1943', 48.
181 Katz, oral history video interview.
182 Katz, oral history video interview. Katz was in fact one of thirty-three nurses from the Jewish Hospital in Frankfurt who managed to escape to Britain. My thanks to Eva Marie Ulmer Otto for sending me these nurses' names and brief biographical details. In her interview Katz admitted that for years she could not even fly into Frankfurt, which is a major airport hub in Germany, and that she never again visited the city. Katz does not explain why only physicians had cyanide pills and not the nurses. It is possible that nurses were considered too inconsequential to be targeted by the Gestapo.
183 Katz, oral history video interview.
184 Paul Weindling, 'Medical refugees and the modernisation of British medicine, 1930–1960', *Social History of Medicine* 22, 3 (2009): 499.
185 Josephine Bruegel, 'Memoirs', 26. Wiener Holocaust Library, London. https://wiener.soutron.net/Portal/Default/en-GB/RecordView/Index/23314 [accessed 27 September 2023].
186 Weindling, 'Medical refugees and the modernisation of British medicine', 499.
187 Bruegel, 'Memoirs', 28 (original ellipses).
188 Lawrence Darton, 'An account of the work of the Friends Committee for refugees and aliens, first known as the Germany Emergency Committee of the Society of Friends, 1933–1950.' Issued by the Friends Committee for Refugees and Aliens, 1954. Friends Meeting House Library, Euston Road, London, 4.
189 Jones, 'National, community and personal priorities', 124.
190 Laurence Darton, 'An account of the work of the Friends Committee for refugees and aliens'.
191 Bruegel, 'Reminiscences', 29.

192 Susi Lewinsky, 'Memoirs, 1911–1940'. Leo Baeck Institute Memoir Collection (ME1628): A32/6, Leo Baeck Institute, Berlin and New York.
193 Lewinsky, 'Memoirs, 1911–1940', 81.
194 Lewinsky, 'Memoirs, 1911–1940', 84.
195 Lewinsky, 'Memoirs, 1911–1940', 86.
196 Berghahn, *Continental Britons*, 77.

2

The nursing world

I went for the interview and since I had not enough schooling, I had to write an essay, and apparently that essay helped me to get into nursing. And I started nursing in March 1943 ... and that was the same year my parents were deported to Auschwitz. So basically, I was on my own. I was never a teenager. I grew up very fast.[1]

This quotation from Lee Fischer's oral history interview identifies the kaleidoscope of emotions she experienced as a young Jewish refugee embarking upon her nursing career. Fischer came from a middle-class background and was hoping to study medicine. Her ambitions were thwarted by the rise of National Socialism and her education was truncated. Her decision to enter nursing was linked to her former ambition and the death of her brother shortly after arriving in Britain.[2] Her work as a domestic servant had been arduous and lonely; nursing was seen as a positive alternative. Fischer learnt of her parents' deportation the year she started nursing, though she did not say whether she knew the fate that awaited them. She did not have sufficient schooling to enter nurse training, but the matron of Booth Hall Children's Hospital in North Manchester was prepared to take her. It is unclear if her willingness to accept Fischer as a probationer nurse was out of sympathy or the desperate need for nursing staff during a time of war.[3] Being on the outskirts of Manchester would have made Booth Hall a less popular training hospital than those in the centre, which might have increased Fischer's chances. Furthermore, a nurse furnished with only her children's nursing registration would not have been considered fully trained.[4] By 1943, however, there is little doubt that the need for nurses on the home front – including those trained to care for children – was critical.[5]

This chapter focuses on the nursing world into which the refugees were recruited. It begins with an analysis of the situation of nursing and the nursing profession in the 1930s through a review of a series of commissions and reports. Several of these commissions were established by those outside nursing, although they tended to have some nursing input. Nevertheless, this input was usually from London hospital matrons, who were invariably from very different social and educational backgrounds than most of their nursing staff. I then turn to the specific issue of recruiting refugees and the organisations involved in the drive to bring them into the nursing profession. This is followed by an examination of the attitudes of the nursing press and ordinary nurses towards their refugee colleagues. To put the nurses' experience in context, I consider in some detail how the medical profession responded to refugee doctors. As I argue, those antagonistic to the employment of Jewish nurses hardly needed to look beyond reporting by the National Socialist regime in the nursing press and the anti-refugee mood of the medical profession to find evidence for their prejudices.

This chapter then considers the experiences of refugees in accessing hospital training. Drawing on personal testimonies from a number of oral histories and written narratives, I demonstrate the difficulties that many faced in locating a hospital that would accept them. Several of the refugees' attempts to gain places at London teaching hospitals were thwarted because voluntary hospitals barred Jews and 'foreigners'. As I identify, such antipathy on the part of the voluntary hospitals meant that the municipal hospital system was able to recruit young women from far more educated and cultured backgrounds than was usual. Some of these refugee nurses turned to the Socialist Medical Association (SMA), closely linked to the municipal hospital system, and especially the London County Council (LCC) hospitals. It was those hospitals within the LCC system and two hospitals in the East End of London, the London Hospital, Whitechapel and the Jewish Hospital, which offered some kindly and supportive respite from the many challenges these young women faced. The responses of the two East End hospitals, particularly, bring into stark relief the influence of the refugees' Jewish heritage on decisions as to whether to admit them as nurses. The response of the LCC demonstrates an acknowledgement of the talents these young women could bring to less prestigious establishments. In the final section, I consider individual refugees' experiences of interview and admission into nurse training schools.

The state and status of nursing

On 11 October 1930, Dr Esther Carling, the medical superintendent at the Berkshire and Buckingham tuberculosis sanatorium, wrote a letter to the *Lancet*: 'The medical profession seems curiously asleep in the face of an approaching crisis. More and more the doctor depends on the nurse; less and less will he find her.' Educated young women and their parents, she continued, preferred that they stay on at school and study teaching, business or social work, although 'nursing is a great work and can make use of the best that any human being has to offer'. The manner in which nurses were trained did not attract intelligent women and thus, 'we are letting it slip as an opportunity for our well-educated girls'.[6] Letters from nurses themselves flowed into the *Lancet* following Carling's letter. One published anonymously was particularly clear in its analysis of the problem:

> The modern educated girl is going to be nobody's 'handmaiden', and the medical profession having exploited the handmaiden idea of the nursing profession, the servile attitude of the nurse has resulted in a loss of social status, which the girl whose brothers are often doctors is not prepared to accept. Medical science would be practically wasted unless there was a profession such as ours prepared to assist in its application. What is that service worth to the medical profession and the community? It has never been properly acknowledged by the former or paid by the latter, and when it is the finest women in the country who fill its ranks.[7]

Publicly voiced concerns relating to nurse recruitment and retention from within and outside the profession could not be ignored. On 5 November 1930, the *Lancet* announced its decision to hold a Commission of Inquiry. The Lancet Commission published its 'Final Report' about the nursing recruitment and retention crisis in 1932.[8] The 'Final Report' highlighted petty rules, harsh discipline and poor financial remuneration. Nursing leaders wanted to recruit educated, middle-class girls but had always struggled to access this cohort of potential recruits in any meaningful numbers. If the Commission's ultimate desire was to alter the 'conditions of service in the nursing profession ... to attract a far larger proportion of those girls who ... will stay at school until they are 18', their mission was unsuccessful.[9]

Many of the accusations were valid. However, the Commission failed to acknowledge the involvement of the medical profession, who wished to maintain absolute authority on the wards, and hospital administrators, who wished to keep the costs of running hospitals to a minimum. Indeed, the early panel members of the Commission included only two nurses – both hospital matrons – alongside five medical men.[10] It is most likely that the cause of nursing's unpopularity lay in multiple places, including those in charge of nursing, those in charge of hospitals and the work itself. Attrition rates remained excessively high throughout the decade. In the introduction to the 'Final Report', it is noted: 'We have confined our attention as far as possible to proposals which would involve adaptation rather than fundamental change in the system on which [the] nursing services of this country are at present carried.'[11] Following the publication of the 'Final Report', the *Daily Telegraph* informed its readers, 'Unless a remedy can be found, we shall soon be faced with a grave shortage of trained nurses.'[12]

According to nursing historian Anne Marie Rafferty, the downturn in the economic climate did offer some improvements in the recruitment of British women. This upsurge enabled the College of Nursing to impose restrictions on the employment of foreign probationers, including Jewish refugees.[13] The improvements in the recruitment of British nurses did not last, and in 1937 the Interdepartmental Committee on Nursing Services was established by the Ministry of Health Board of Education, under the chairmanship of Lord Athlone.[14] The Committee's remit was to review the reasons for nursing shortages. It concluded that there were many young women interested in the profession but that the requirement for more and more nurses outstripped recruitment.[15] Advances in medical science were placing greater burdens on the hospital system, which required ever-increasing numbers of skilled nursing staff. It recommended that nurses' hours be reduced to a 96-hour fortnight, with better remuneration and superannuation provision. The voluntary hospitals, even the famous ones in London, could ill afford such improvements.[16] The lack of real change meant that in 1938, the Association of Nurses reported that 38 per cent of probationer nurses left in the first year and only 50 per cent ever qualified.[17] Fortunately for hospital finances, the war intervened, preventing the implementation of the Committee's recommendations.

The Royal College of Nursing was disappointed that the Athlone recommendations were abandoned because of the war. Thus, in 1941 they implemented a Reconstruction Committee, with Lord Horder as its chairman.[18] Its published report condemned nurse training as the perpetuation of 'unintelligent repetitive work', which was, the report argued, 'one of the greatest dangers of youth to-day'.[19] As the war progressed, the nurse staffing crisis worsened. In 1943, Sheila Bevington, a lecturer in industrial psychology at the London School of Economics, published *Nursing Life and Discipline*. Comprising over five hundred interviews with all grades of nursing staff, her research highlighted the by-now familiar criticisms of the nursing world. Bevington, however, went further than merely offering the usual condemnations of the system, using her industrial psychology training to illustrate the root causes of the difficulties. She described developing understandings of how to manage mistakes: 'When a mistake is made, the authority in charge *investigates the cause,* instead of simply *observing the symptom* and *rebuking the offender.*' The overworked and harassed ward sister was unlikely to have the time for such measured responses. Bevington insisted that young women would be entering nursing with modern ideas; if they found a more draconian approach to discipline, 'many of the more intelligent and high-spirited (the best material from which to fashion future Matrons) may well quit nursing in search of a more progressive attitude elsewhere'.[20] Unlike the Lancet Commission's 'Final Report', Bevington did not place the blame on hospital matrons; rather, she argued, 'the conservative nursing traditions of Doctors, Governors, and Sisters often seriously handicap [reforming matrons'] efforts'.[21]

As the crisis of war ended in 1945, the situation still had not improved. Gladys Carter, a Canadian nurse and economist and Evelyn Pearce, author of *A General Text Book of Nursing*, regretted that nurse training was still mired in strict timetabling, menial and repetitious work and learning by rote.[22] Young women, as Bevington had argued, who would not subjugate themselves to the regime, abandoned training.[23] Thus, throughout the 1930s and during the war itself, the nursing profession continued in its struggle to recruit and retain women in its ranks. In order to bolster its numbers, the profession turned to less traditional cohorts of girls and young women.[24]

Recruiting refugees

By 1938 the College of Nursing reconsidered its refusal to accept the services of foreign women into nursing. In part this was due to growing sympathies towards Jewish refugees from Nazi Europe, but there was also growing concern about severe nursing shortages as the country moved closer to war.[25] Not all British nurses supported the recruitment of refugees into their profession.[26] The issue once again exposed the paradoxical situation of British nursing: there were not enough young women willing to enter nurse training; yet across the nursing elite and the wider profession, some opposed the recruitment of women who did not fit the imagined ideal of a British nurse. The lack of recruits meant that the work was harsher and discipline tighter for those who stayed. A high turnover of junior nurses meant that ward sisters needed to maintain strict obedience to guarantee both an effective environment for the sick to heal and the moral universe they believed was necessary to ensure suitable recruits into the profession.[27] Ultimately such an environment would make the conditions less amenable to young women, especially those from educated backgrounds.

During the 1930s, a number of voluntary organisations were established to care for and support refugees from Nazi Germany. One of these organisations, the German Jewish Aid Committee, identified nursing and domestic service as two potentially useful escape routes for Jewish women, and thus established a Nursing Committee. As historian John Stewart maintains, overlapping causes and a proliferation of organisations led to the implementation of the Central Co-Ordinating Committee for Refugees.[28] This organisation moved into Bloomsbury House in London and thereafter became known by that name. In 1938, the Committee received a request from the Home Office to establish two subcommittees, the Domestic Service Bureau and the Nursing and Midwifery Committee, also known as the Nursing and Midwifery Department (hereafter the Department).[29] The 1939 Annual Report of the Council for Jewish Refugees reflected on the Department's superseding work that had 'previously been done by private persons on a small scale'. The report concluded that following the establishment of the Department, 'a continuous flow of applicants was admitted, after individual examination by the Home Office, till the outbreak of war'.[30]

Several refugees whose narratives comprise this book identify the Department as critical to their escape, arrival or employment opportunities in Britain. Marion Berghahn argues that not all refugees were keen to be dependent on the Refugee Committee and found its presence in their lives in Britain a humiliation. Those who managed without its support, she continues, were pleased to be able to succeed independently.[31] Despite occasional misgivings, the Department and Bloomsbury House became an important support mechanism for many.

In a letter from the Merseyside Coordinating Committee written on 2 March 1939, Elizabeth Parry informed Susi Linton that if for any reason she needed to leave Germany before 1 May, Bloomsbury House would find her accommodation. Thus, when Linton arrived in Britain on 16 April 1939, she lodged at the Catholic Teachers' Training College in Liverpool. After two weeks acclimatising to British life, she reported to Bloomsbury House as directed for her domestic service placement.[32] Bloomsbury House itself offered some short-term accommodation, as well as help with finding employment. When Josephine Bruegel first arrived in April 1939 from Czechoslovakia, she was able to stay there until her first job caring for a small child began.[33] Kitty Schafer's uncle, who was already living in London, applied for Kitty to come to Britain via Bloomsbury House so she could get a visa. It is not clear if she came through the Nursing and Midwifery Department or the Domestic Bureau. Her oral history acknowledged both visa options and that she had always wanted to be a nurse. Schafer recalled that all the decisions relating to her escape to Britain were taken by her uncle: 'I knew nothing, because don't forget at that time I was in Vienna. I knew nothing. It was left to my uncle, who was there [in London], to find out all the things that are necessary, where to apply.' By the time she arrived in Britain in 1939, her father had also settled in England and she lived with him until she commenced at East Croydon Hospital.[34] Margaret Marflow's memoir described the worrying time for her parents as they waited for visas for Margaret and her brother. Whilst waiting, Marflow's father's sister and her husband committed suicide, compounding the family crisis. It was, Marflow maintained, Bloomsbury House that managed to bring her and her brother to England.[35] Trudie Moos also found Bloomsbury House to be a lifeline, as it was through the Department that an interview for nursery-nurse training was organised.[36] Elisabeth Katz recalled that Bloomsbury House was where the Jewish organisations were located: 'they worked to get people out and get people processed'. It was through the Department that she received her nursing visa and was offered the position at St Luke's Hospital in Bradford, Yorkshire.[37]

The Department was particularly important in placing refugees in hospital nurse-training schools recognised by the General Nursing Council. The Home Office were determined to maintain direct contact with the Department, thus guaranteeing that its organisation was in line with government policies.[38] They therefore requested that Miss G. V. Hillyers, matron of St Thomas's Hospital in London, take over as chairman [sic], Miss E. M. Pye, president of the Midwives' Institute as its vice-chairman and Miss Frey, the daughter of an exiled Austrian doctor, as its secretary, to ensure its smooth running.[39] Having such high-profile members of the two professions leading the Department lent a certain authority, but it did not mean that the refugees were welcomed into all hospitals. The London teaching hospitals, including St Thomas's, demonstrated a particular ambivalence to recruiting from this cohort of young women.

Nursing and the refugees

Lisbeth Hockey, Annie Altschul, Josephine Bruegel, Edith Bown, Lee Fischer and Rosa Sacharin were all intelligent young women with promising options before Hitler came to power. Hockey and Bruegel were medical students; Altschul studied mathematics at the University of Vienna. Although Sacharin, Bown and Fischer were not old enough to reach university before escaping Nazism, all were ambitious. Bown and Fischer wanted to study medicine. Unusually for girls in Britain who entered the nursing profession at that time, Sacharin stayed at school, passed her Higher Leaving Certificate and was awarded prizes in English, geography and commercial subjects.[40] However, apart from teaching and social work, few professions in Britain accepted women with grace.

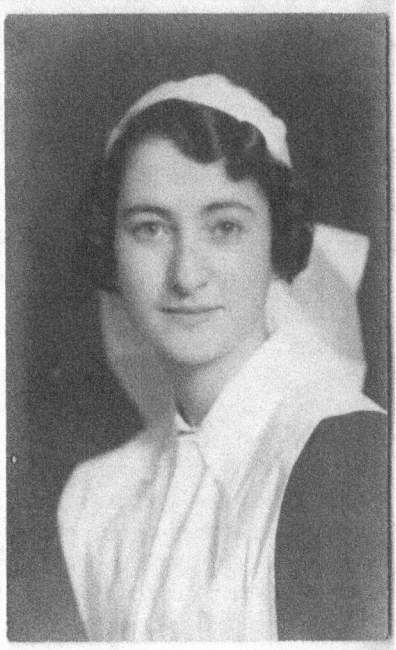

Figure 2.1 Aviva Gold in her Princess Margaret Rose Hospital uniform, date unknown. Reproduced with kind permission of her daughter, Dina Gold [fo. 110]

Most refugee girls were encouraged into domestic service or nursery nursing.[41] Hospital nursing was considered the most suitable option for the more academic refugees 'to pursue their advanced educational goals'.[42] Aviva Gold was encouraged into nursing by an old friend of her mother's – Dr Martha Turk, who was keen that all child refugees should access some sort of training: '[Turk] saw it as a way to gain professional training I could use anywhere in the world. She arranged for me to train at the Princess Margaret Rose Hospital in Edinburgh. I wasn't at all unhappy there, though it was very hard work.'[43]

The crisis in recruitment and retention of nurses made the willingness to accept Jewish refugees both sensible and humane. In late 1938, Mr Stephany, a member of the Central British Fund for World Jewish Relief, observed in 'Notes for the Home Secretary's speech', 'A number, also, of well-educated girls and young women are being placed in training for hospital nursing, and meet a definite need of our hospitals, which was not satisfied by English girls.'[44] As war loomed ever closer, British nurses clamoured to join up for military service, keen for adventure and to escape the stifling atmosphere of civilian hospitals.[45] The nursing elite and Government were only too aware of the impending staffing disaster. As chair of the Department, Hillyers published an open letter in the *Nursing Times*, requesting that hospitals and nurses in Britain consider the recruitment of refugees. As the journal was associated with the College of Nursing, the *Nursing Times* would have reached many nurses across the country:

> All candidates will be officially interviewed abroad in the first place and will be required to furnish certificates of birth and good health, in addition to answering a very detailed questionnaire. The completed dossiers of all candidates recommended as suitable for training will be forwarded to the nursing sub-committee, who will make the final selection and obtain vacancies for them in recognised training schools in England and Wales. These candidates will then be allowed to come to this country to take their full nursing training, with the object of fitting them to take posts abroad ... Publicity was given to the scheme by circularizing the matrons of training schools recognized by the General Nursing Council, who were asked to place the matter before their hospital committees for their sympathetic consideration.

We feel the need is imperative, and we ask all leaders of the nursing profession to assist in extending a helping hand to those who are in great distress at the present time.[46]

The edict was clear. Once qualified, these nurses were expected to transmigrate, but they would at least be given the opportunity of training. What is not stated is that in return they would offer hospitals cheap labour – essential to the nation, given the recruitment crisis. Nevertheless, despite this opportunism, Hillyers's sympathy is apparent. On 10 December 1938, the *Nursing Mirror and Midwives' Journal* (hereafter *Nursing Mirror*) published a shortened version of the decision outlining the entry requirements for training: 'They must be over nineteen, unmarried, and must have reached the necessary standard of education as laid down by the General Nursing Council.'[47] As mentioned above, Lee Fischer's acceptance at Booth Hall Hospital was predicated on her writing an essay. It appears therefore that the regulations laid down in 1938 could easily be waived as the necessity for nurses increased during the war.

British nurses wrote to both the *Nursing Times* and *Nursing Mirror* offering their support. On 26 November 1938, a 'Sister' wrote begging her fellow nurses to help:

> None of us can open our daily papers and remain unmoved at the desperate predicament of the German Jews. Can we not – those of our profession – do something to aid this human suffering. Many of these poor wretched creatures are well-educated young women, girls brought up in refinement, now flung helplessly into a chaotic world without mercy or pity.
>
> The doors of some of our hospital training schools have already been opened to a few of them, but the number is as yet quite inadequate. If such a scheme [to support these young women to enter nursing] could be launched, I, for one, would be pleased to accept responsibility for the welfare of one of these girls, to take her into my flat, to fit her out with uniform and books prior to her entrance into some approved hospital training school, and give her a home for off-days and holidays.[48]

No such scheme was launched and the lack of a 'home' for days off and holidays remained a problem for refugee nurses.[49]

Appeals to nurses to help, however, continued in the nursing press, on one occasion even acknowledging the value of meeting people from different backgrounds. On 31 August 1940, M. H. Campbell addressed a letter to the matrons of the nation's hospitals in *Nursing Mirror*:

> So make room for an alien nurse if you can, take more than one if that is possible, and you will find that not only have you added a hard worker and an intelligent nurse to your staff, but that through contact with a fellow human being with a different background, your own life and that of your other nurses has gained in wideness of outlook and variety of interest.[50]

It is unclear if a call on behalf of embracing difference would have appealed to many in Britain, given the general suspicion of 'foreigners', but Campbell's plea on grounds of developing a 'wider outlook' shows that some were open to new ideas and broader understandings.[51] In general, requests for help were grounded in sympathy for those in adversity, rather than the benefits of meeting and working with people from outside the small island of Britain. In Pye's appeal on behalf of those training as midwives, the reflection of victimhood is all too apparent. On 10 June 1939 she wrote to *Nursing Mirror*:

> No one can come into contact with these victims of a social upheaval without great sympathy for their tragic stories and admiration for their courage and determination in starting a new life, stripped of all they possess save character and education, and the work of helping them is of deep human interest ... Helpers are wanted to give regular time to interviewing and giving information to enquirers.[52]

The 1939 Report of the Central Council for Jewish Refugees identified that 'The Midwives Sub-Committee enabled a number of women doctors to take up midwifery training.'[53] On 12 August 1939, Pye wrote again to *Nursing Mirror*: 'I should be most grateful if you would allow me to make known an urgent need for text books on midwifery, for the use of medical women refugees who have received permission to enter as pupil midwives in this country.'[54] The opportunity for medical women to retrain as midwives was highly gendered and not questioned either by the male-dominated Central Council for Jewish Refugees or the nursing and midwifery professions. The demand to escape Nazi Germany and Austria was such that women doctors were prepared to take this option for escape and work.

In a letter to *Nursing Mirror* on 11 February 1939, M. C. S. asked, 'May a Jewish woman M.D. of Vienna, who is a gynaecologist, take her C.M.B. [Central Midwives' Board exam] without general training? Where does one apply for special dispensation?'[55] The answer confirmed the ambivalence towards refugees and the opportunism of hospitals to benefit from the expertise of these medically trained women without paying for it: 'Midwifery training is open to people not generally trained, but it usually takes two years instead of one for non-State Registered Nurses.'[56] No dispensation was offered, but the address of the Nursing and Midwifery Department was provided for applicants.

There is some evidence that those who were supported by the British Federation of University Women and were sent to hospitals in Scotland had their medical degrees taken into account and were able to complete their midwifery training more quickly.[57] Even so, as Anne von Villiez argues, for a female doctor to take a position as a nurse or midwife was a 'step backwards'.[58] Sylva Simsova, who interviewed Bruegel, suggests that Bruegel was not happy working as a nurse in Bognor Regis and argues that this is because she wanted to be a doctor.[59] However, in her memoir Bruegel admitted that she 'seriously considered nursing' when she was deciding on her career, 'but nurse training had not been properly established in ... Czechoslovakia at that time ... Had my father been alive I would have taken up nursing in England. I enquired, but I did not want to leave my mother.'[60] Bruegel criticised the hierarchical structure of nursing, specifically at the convalescent hospital in Bognor, but she had been happy in her previous nursing jobs.[61] Although she was keen to return to medicine as soon as this was made possible, she did not appear to view nursing as a poor alternative. Despite valid criticisms of the scheme, the involvement of elite midwives like Pye enabled female refugee doctors to at least find work in a profession associated with medicine, which was not an option for their male colleagues. Thus, whilst gendered attitudes towards women doctors stopped the British medical profession from welcoming Continental female practitioners into its midst, gender was critical in enabling these women to escape. Nursing and midwifery were suitable professions for a woman, and women doctors desperate to flee Nazi Europe were ideal recruits.

Not all nurses were keen to have Jewish refugees in their profession. Nurses, like the population as a whole, were susceptible to the same fears of 'foreign invasion' and anxious about their income in a time of high unemployment.[62] Britain might not have been as systemically antisemitic as some countries, but that does not mean that antisemitism was absent. That said, it not surprising that many were fearful of an influx of refugees at a time of economic crisis.[63] Tony Kushner argues that in the 1930s many Britons were suspicious of Jews because they were Jews.[64] Nevertheless, British women were generally more supportive of Jewish refugees than British men. Helen Jones argues that on a local level, British women engaged philanthropically with Jewish refugees, 'often in opposition to the dominant patriotic discourse'.[65] This female activism and support were not, however, universal.

Any antipathy towards refugees might have been bolstered by ongoing engagement with those within the National Socialist regime, as reported in the nursing press. In July 1935, the *Nursing Times* reported on two nurses touring the Rhine.[66] In December, College member G. M. Y. stated her desire to see 'what the Germans are really like' and her decision to visit Frau Oberin Hubler of the Bad Homburg *Mutterhaus*:[67] 'It was all I could do not to burst out laughing at the way everyone who came into the [rail] carriage said "Heil Hitler" to everyone else. But later I found myself unconsciously returning the greeting.'[68] In *Travellers in the Third Reich*, Julia Boyd maintains that in the early years of the regime, tourists could retain some moral compass and make the salute, but later, when the true brutality of the regime became all too apparent, their discomfiture increased.[69] A cartoon in the Christmas issue in the same year (see Figure 2.2) demonstrates the College of Nursing's uncertainty of attitude between Fascist Germany and Communist Russia: 'Those who join the College study tours cannot escape some political implications.'[70]

Throughout the 1930s, the nursing press not only reported on members of the College who visited Germany but also on Nazi accolades for British nurses. On 15 January 1938, *Nursing Mirror*

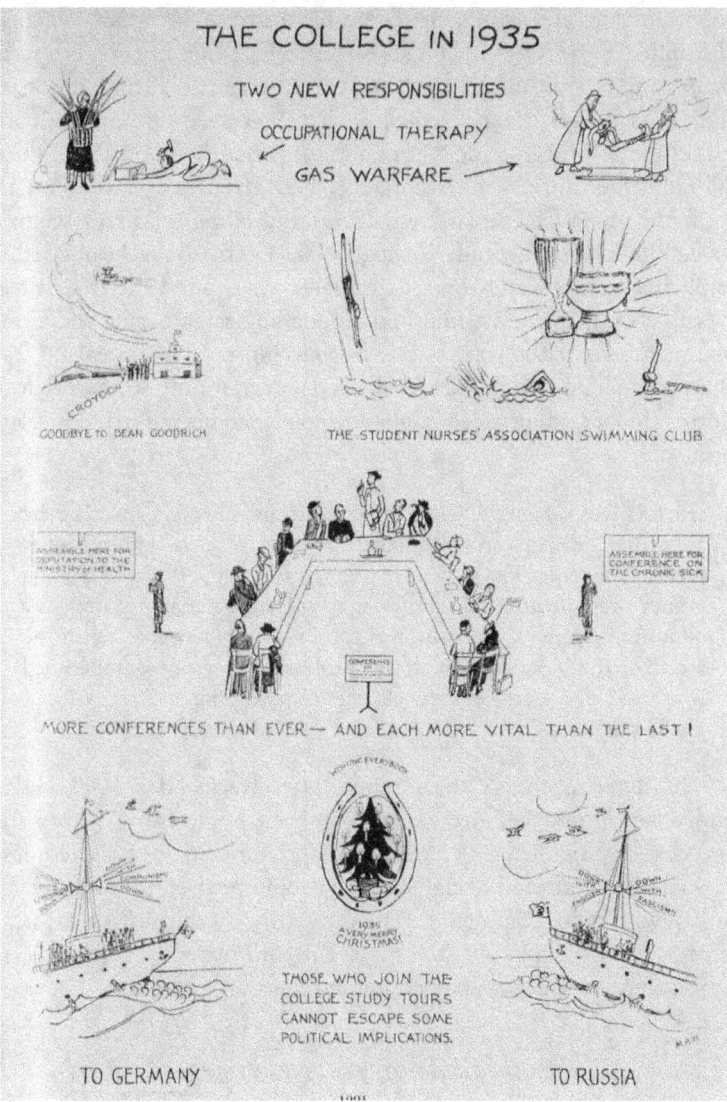

Figure 2.2 Cartoon showing the push and pull between Communist Russia and Nazi Germany, *Nursing Times*, Christmas edition, 1935. Published with permission of Gale and Royal College of Nursing, https://link.gale.com/apps/doc/OPRIIE463744181/WMNS?u=rcnur&sid=bookmark-WMNS&xid=47265fc4 [fo. 116]

reported that Herr Hilgenfeld, the head of the National Socialist charitable organisation, 'lays stress on the fact that nursing is a vital profession'.[71] In August of that year, the same journal reported that Miss Ellis, formerly a theatre sister, received an honour from Hitler himself for nursing German sailors after the bombing of their ship. Furthermore, King George VI had given her permission to wear the medal.[72] The *Nursing Times* and *Nursing Mirror* seemed to demur in their attitude towards Nazi Germany; only one letter explicitly antagonistic towards refugees was found in either. It is possible that, given assumptions about nurses as caring individuals, members of the profession were circumspect in appearing less than compassionate in the public arena, even if only to their fellow nurses. In December 1938, a nurse who signed herself 'Anglo-Scott' argued:

> Doctors are safeguarding themselves against an alien invasion by admitting only a certain number of medical men and potential medical students. The same menace may eventually threaten nursing homes ... Some hospitals are trying to solve the nursing shortage by admitting refugees, but how will the British probationer relish the fact that the key positions in our profession may one day be filled by aliens? There are very few chances of promotion as it is, without giving the highest posts to Jewesses. Humanity begins at home.[73]

This letter received a sharp rebuttal two weeks later. L. H. Lewis ended her letter, 'Might I simply remind "Anglo-Scott", "but for the Grace of God ...".'[74] Nevertheless, the nursing press's acquiescence to the National Socialist regime could be used to reinforce an anti-Jewish refugee polemic. The antipathy by the British medical profession to refugees in their midst further buttressed some nurses' ambivalence to Jewish women joining their profession.

The medical profession and refugees

In 1933, Lord Dawson of Penn, President of the Royal College of Surgeons, infamously told the British Government that the number of refugee doctors 'who could usefully be absorbed or teach us anything could be counted on the fingers of one hand'.[75] Unfortunately for the refugees, Lord Dawson was not alone in holding such anti-German and anti-Jewish views. The British Medical Association and the Medical Practitioners Union held similar anti-immigrant views. Throughout the 1930s both organisations worked to stymie the acceptance of refugees into British medicine.[76] On 4 July 1938, representatives of the British Medical Association, the Royal Colleges of Physicians and Surgeons, the University of London and the Society of Apothecaries met with Sir Samuel Hoare, the Home Secretary and Lord Winterton, the Chancellor of [the] Duchy. The purpose of the meeting at the Home Office was to discuss the possibility of work for Jewish medical refugees. The decision was taken 'that it would only be possible to admit a limited number, that any such admissions must be the subject of careful selection, and that a committee representing the medical profession should be set up to assist in the selection'.[77]

Individual doctors were no less vociferous in their antipathy and far less guarded in the professional press than their nursing colleagues. On 2 April 1938, a Dr Goodwin wrote to the *Lancet* cautioning against the recruitment of refugee doctors from Continental Europe who would have 'a decided advantage over our own recently qualified men and women in that they are men of previous experience in practice'[78] – a statement that precluded the possibility of female doctors from the Continent arriving for work, despite ranks of women in medicine in Germany and Austria. Two weeks later a wholehearted response was published:

> I should like to express most heartily my agreement with the common-sense protest made by Mr. Goodwin and Dr. Endean against the policy of encouraging Jewish émigrés from Middle Europe to practise in this country. The medical profession is now very overcrowded and often for one vacant appointment there may be as many as thirty candidates, all of whom may be excellent men who would fill the job admirably ... and be of benefit to the profession as a whole. It might be pertinent to inquire whether other professions are suggesting the same policy, and whether lawyers, engineers, civil servants, and so forth in this country are welcoming fresh competition in the shape of Jewish refugees from Middle Europe; or is ours the only profession encouraging this misplaced philanthropy?[79]

Even those supportive of medical refugees acknowledged that their chances of employment were low. An article in the *Lancet* in 1934 requested that British medical colleagues offer financial support to refugees: 'There is no question of the employment of more foreign medical practitioners in Britain, and this is recognised by the Fund.'[80] Louise London's critical analysis of the anti-refugee stance by the medical and dental professions identifies the limited concern for the refugees themselves and the professions' absolute determination to maintain the status quo.[81] Vivian Lipman, a historian of Judaism in Britain, notes the recommendation that Continental dentists call themselves 'Mr' and not 'Dr', and that they should remember not to criticise dental work performed by British dentists – something that might have been a challenge, given the number of unqualified practitioners in the country at the time.[82]

Karola Decker's work on medical refugees places the Home Office and the medical establishment at the centre of the lack of support. The medical profession, she argues, made it increasingly difficult for German and later Austrian medical practitioners to practise or even requalify in Britain.[83] The Home Office 'adopted a selective, if not manipulative, approach to the refugee problem, and decisions were based on its judgment of the individual case. This approach worked in favor of the rich and famous and allowed for cherry picking in the spheres of science.'[84] The exception to this was the welcome afforded to a number of Jewish refugee psychiatrists at the Maudsley Hospital, where they were able to reach consultant level. Other teaching hospitals in London might have employed eminent psychiatrists, but they remained in relatively junior positions.[85] Paul Weindling argues that this analysis can be contested when viewed against the access the ordinary refugee practitioner had to medical work. Instead, he suggests, the narrative is more nuanced, with the need to view European refugee doctors as bringing the opposing forces of British medicine into stark relief.[86] Continental doctors were more likely to be research-led, whereas the British medical profession was dominated by elite honorary physicians and surgeons, whose traditional space was private practice.[87] Notwithstanding Weindling's more positive analysis of the situation for medical refugees, most historians point to control of numbers at best, and downright antipathy at worst.[88] The only open letter written by British medics in support of refugee doctors was found in the *Nursing Times*, not the medical press. As these doctors were members of the Peace Campaign, it is likely that they did not speak for many of their professional colleagues. Furthermore, they did not ask for the British medical profession to support Austrian Jewish doctors to work in Britain; instead, they asked the profession and the public in all countries to 'stand by members'.[89]

If the nursing profession looked to medicine to strengthen its resolve against welcoming refugees, the Government thought differently.[90] Given the nursing shortages, it was probably correct to question the anti-refugee stance of the General Nursing Council and the College of Nursing.[91] However, there were elements of gender and class bias as well. According to Stewart, the Government appears to have accepted the medical profession's concerns about jobs for qualified practitioners but easily dismissed the nursing profession's similar worries.[92] Nevertheless, despite an apparent willingness to support the recruitment of nurses (but not doctors), the *a priori* stance of both the professions and government was one of suspicion towards refugees. Even after refugees were enabled to return to work after the period of mass dismissals in 1940, a quota for them was maintained.[93] Thus, hospitals reluctant to employ refugees needed only to look to the British Government and the professional organisations to reinforce any anti-refugee polices, official or unofficial, that they wished to sanction.

Accessing hospital training

Voluntary hospitals and refugee nurses

Several of the refugees whose narratives form this study described wishing to train at London teaching hospitals and finding their access barred. Hortense Gordon stated, 'Because we weren't allowed to go into voluntary hospitals and once I finished my children's qualifications I applied to go to UCH or General, whatever they were called, Royal Free now, wouldn't take me because I was a foreigner.'[94] Trudie Moos was advised by Miss Crowe, the matron at her nursery-nurse training institution, to apply to the London Hospital, perhaps because she was aware they were sympathetic towards Jews.[95] However, Moos was attracted to King's College

Hospital in London, where her cousin Carla was a radiography student, and she submitted her application in 1941. The matron at King's refused her on the grounds of her being 'foreign'. Moos was, however, successful in her application to the Royal Free Hospital in London. Her choice of the Royal Free was fortunate, as the matron, Miss Elizabeth Cockayne, had also accepted another refugee for nurse training and thoughtfully placed them in the same set.[96]

Marianne Parkes wrote in her memoir, 'the London hospitals would not accept me because of my questionable status as a "friendly enemy alien"'.[97] It is not known how many hospitals she applied to, but it appears that she was refused by more than one. She eventually trained at Sutton and Cheam Hospital in Surrey, where she suggested that the senior staff 'seemed to have the impression that I started the war for my own amusement. Work-wise that was often difficult.'[98] This attitude fits what Sonya O. Rose maintains were long-held stereotypes of Jews as self-serving, cowardly and only interested in personal gain.[99] Such beliefs were understandably distressing to the young refugees and difficult to sustain, given their willingness to work as hospital nurses. Charlotte Kratz admitted that in Germany nursing was not deemed an appropriate profession for educated young women.[100] It was not therefore a career she considered when she arrived in Britain. However, she became ill with appendicitis in 1941 and following surgery at St Mary's Hospital, Paddington, she was evacuated to Park Prewitt Hospital in Basingstoke. Park Prewitt was part of the St Thomas's sector hospitals and whilst there she was cared for by St Thomas's Hospital nurses. She admitted later:

> I thought, well yes, perhaps I would become a nurse after all as this was as good a job as any. I had to go to St Thomas's because by then I'd learnt it was the place to go to. But Thomas's was pretty selective in those days and pretty choosy. It took me two years to get them to accept me ... they didn't think I was the sort of person they normally had. But I eventually managed to find a friend of my aunt's and uncle's, who in turn was friendly with the senior almoner at St Thomas's, and she told them that perhaps I might be the right person after all.[101]

Kushner argues that there were a number of places in which Jews were not welcome in Britain, even Anglo-Jews. These included public schools, universities and clubs.[102] Within institutions themselves, antisemitism could make Jews unwelcome. Polish medical students at the University of Edinburgh made refugee students sit at different tables, as they had back in Poland.[103] It is not clear if the university did anything to prevent such ostracism. As Yvonne Kapp and Margaret Mynatt argued, Jewish refugees were allowed to work and study but only if their British counterparts accepted them, and not all did.[104] The London teaching hospitals tried to impose restrictions similar to those of other anti-Jewish establishments. To support their anti-refugee policy, they needed only to follow the line of many in government. Susan Cohen cited the belief of Sir John Anderson, the Home Secretary, in 1940, that an increased influx of refugees from Nazi Europe would increase antisemitism.[105] Some thought that sending refugees across the country would help stem antisemitism in the capital.

According to Peter Alter, those refugees who were willing to move to depressed areas like the North-East were accepted over those who wished to remain in London. In April 1939, the Board of Deputies of British Jews promoted the preference for refugees to be located across the country.[106] Colin Holmes is clear in his exposition of the problem: 'the number and concentration of immigrants exercised an important influence over the development of hostility in the local population and even beyond'.[107] Because antisemitism tended to be worse in areas that had fewer refugees, the dispersal of refugees across the country might therefore have been counterproductive.[108] Furthermore, it increased the isolation of vulnerable young people who had fled the horrors of Nazism only to find themselves alone in often hostile places.

An isolating experience

Edith Bown realised that she did not have enough education to go to university, but had promised herself 'to do either history or medicine when I was young'.[109] Once her situation in Northern Ireland was settled and she had reached the age of 18, she started to see nursing as a good opportunity. Her diary entry for 27 June 1941 stated, 'I have written to four hospitals and have had one refusal. Three letters went to England and one to Belfast. Mrs Kohner and I have ordered *The Nursing Times*.'[110] In her oral history she admitted, 'nobody would have a Jew and an enemy alien'.[111] On 18 January 1942, she had still not received an offer of a place: 'anyway, I hope soon to get into a hospital'.[112] She added this note in 1990: 'I started at the Ards District Hospital in September 1942.'[113] It had taken Bown over a year to find a hospital training school that would accept her. She acknowledged that Newtonards Hospital 'wasn't the sort of hospital people applied to. No Protestant would apply there. There was one Protestant nurse there, the others were Catholics. They were at each others [sic] throats the whole time while I was there.'[114]

Even for those who did not describe hostility, being sent far from family and newly found friends could add to the distress of these young women who were already suffering from the loss of all that was familiar, including language and culture. Mia Ross was 16½ when she left Austria in March 1939. She admitted that people were kind, but she struggled with the English language, which initially made life and developing friendships difficult for her.[115] On completing her school-leaving exams in 1940, when still only 17 years old, Ross became a domestic servant. Like most of the refugees whose work as domestic servants was explored in the previous chapter, Ross did not particularly like the work. However, she was fortunate that her ex-headmistress continued to take an interest in her and searched for a nurse-training position. In her memoir Ross admitted it could not have been easy to find a training hospital for her: 'There were quite a number of hospitals out of bounds either near the coast or near munitions factories or in other places where even friendly aliens were not allowed.' In the end Ross was accepted as a student nurse at the Keighley and District Victoria Hospital in West Yorkshire. As a domestic servant with the family near Saffron Walden, Ross wrote how she missed the company of those friends she had made since arriving in Britain. Having been relocated to Keighley, she was now over two hundred miles away from the friends she had met only two years previously. Ross described being circumspect about becoming a nurse: 'I started training as a nurse in the hospital in March 1941. I must say I was pleased to have finished my work as a domestic, but I had quite mixed feelings about my future as a hospital nurse. Being a "friendly alien" during war time left you with a very limited choice of jobs or career.'116

A supportive world

Despite the difficulties that many refugees experienced, there were those willing to support them. The matron at Booth Hall accepted Fischer without sufficient education and Ross's headmistress maintained their relationship after Ross had left school. But even those who found supportive environments struggled with the language and cultural differences between Germany and England. Kitty Schafer attended her interview with her father because she could not speak sufficient English. Having been accepted as a probationer nurse, Schafer recalled the kindness of her patients as they tried to teach her English:

> I loved the patients, you know why? Because they all had a bet, who could teach me English better, or rather quicker? So, whenever I came to their bed, 'remember Nurse Kaufmann, this is a glass, repeat after me, this is a glass, this is, this is, this is' ... I soon learnt. And I thought it was wonderful, oh, I thought it was absolutely terrific.[117]

However, the joy of learning the language could not make up for the cultural difficulties. Schafer acknowledged that the Viennese were emotional people: 'the English people, as you know, did not like to show their emotions, so we couldn't quite get on so well together. But I tried to learn, and I did learn.'[118]

Rosa Sacharin wrote in her memoir that she was 'apprehensive and had a rather negative attitude' about becoming a nurse.[119] Her oral history recalled that Miss Clarkson, the matron of York Hill Hospital, Glasgow, was warned by the wife of the minister who 'rescued' Sacharin from domestic service that she 'wasn't very keen to go into nursing'. Sacharin admitted that she didn't know why she felt like that, but 'it's something I'd never experienced, it wasn't part of my history, I mean if you have been in hospital or if you have somebody in the family who was nursing or something like that, then you internalise that in a sense ... and to me this is ... what is that? What do I do there?' Despite the negative feelings, Sacharin went to her interview, but as it ended, she asked the matron, 'how long would I have to stay before I could leave? And she smiled and said, "Well, Miss Goldschal, if we don't like you, or you don't like us, then you can leave after three months", and I was accepted. I started nursing on 3rd August 1943 and I hated it.' After three months, Sacharin wrote her letter of resignation. Clarkson decided that instead of accepting it, she would send Sacharin to a children's convalescent home in the country. Sacharin recalled, 'it was a much freer and easier atmosphere ... And I grew up.'[120]

Charlotte Hoxter arrived in Britain in 1933 or 1934. Like several other refugee nurses, she had originally wanted to enter the medical profession. As this was not possible, after a series of caring jobs, she decided to train as a nurse. Hoxter applied to the London Jewish Hospital, which had been founded in 1919.[121] The Jewish Hospital was clearly a safe space for Jewish refugees to train as nurses. However, an article in the *Jewish Chronicle* in the 1940s decried the lack of enthusiasm of Jewish girls and young women to access its nurse-training school: 'For the refugee trainees in England, or the majority of them at any rate, have become nurses only after the bitterness of Nazi persecution has given them a rude awakening.'[122] In his thesis on the Jewish Hospital, Howard Rein maintains that the lack of interest shown by Jewish women to enter the hospital as nurses was in large part due to the lack of facilities there.[123] A major fundraising campaign had been undertaken in 1935 for a purpose-built Nurses' Home. An article in the *Jewish Chronicle* identified the optimism with which this was viewed, referring to the 'important development in its history ... when the ceremony of laying the foundation-stone of the long overdue and urgently needed Nurses' Home was performed by the Marchioness of Reading'.[124]

The new Nurses' Home was eventually opened in 1939.[125] It was bombed during the Blitz only a year later.[126] However, the lack of amenities did not adversely affect Hoxter's love of nursing and on qualification she undertook midwifery training at the British Hospital for Mothers and Babies in Woolwich. This was a most fortunate decision on her part. The father of Miss Gregory, the matron, was Dean of St Paul's and a friend of the Archbishop of Canterbury. It was through the Archbishop that Hoxter's parents were brought out of Germany to safety in Britain.[127] Lisbeth Hockey applied to the London Hospital Whitechapel because it had its own swimming pool.[128] Miss Littleboy, the matron, agreed she would accept Hockey as a probationer nurse if she learnt sufficient English in three months: 'So I learnt English in three months and I was very proud of myself, you know, because, I really worked hard at it, and eventually got accepted at The London.'[129] The London Hospital's close relationship with the East End Jewish community was likely a critical factor in their acceptance of Hockey.

Even in the very early years of the twentieth century, the London Hospital, Whitechapel had accommodated Jewish religious practices and accepted Jewish staff.[130] The hospital had cared for the East End Jewish community since its inception in 1741, and according to historian Gerry Black, most requests by the Jewish community were accepted by the hospital. Appointments included 'a Jewish almoner, Jewish members on the House Committee of the hospital and on its Board of Governors, and even a separate mortuary and ice chambers for deceased'.[131] Of the London teaching hospitals, the London Hospital and the Royal Free were the most welcoming to refugees. It was, however, the hospitals of the London County Council (LCC) and, to some extent, their neighbours in the Middlesex and Surrey County Councils which led the way in supporting refugees to become nurses.

Alice Fink started her training as a children's nurse at the Jewish Hospital in Berlin in 1937.[132] She qualified as a nursery nurse on 31 March 1938 and was due to commence her general nurse training in October that year. Fortunately for Fink, she had a cousin in England who managed to find her a place in London to train as a general nurse. Fink escaped Germany on a nursing visa and began her training at the Miller Hospital in Greenwich on 14 November 1938, only five days after the November pogrom, during which her father was arrested.[133] Fink had some English lessons before she left for Britain, though she admitted that as they were from a German woman, they were not entirely helpful. Most of the nurses at the Miller Hospital were working-class girls with strong accents, making her ability to understand their English a challenge, 'But, the matron and the sisters who handled these things at the hospital were very considerate.' The matron even ensured that Fink was placed on the children's ward because she knew Fink had worked with children and thought that it would make things easier for her.

Fink recalled that the home sister was called Sister Darling, 'and that is exactly what she was. She was so concerned for my integration.' Sister Darling even made sure that one of the other girls who was Fink's size lent her a long dress for the Christmas ball: 'they were very good to me'.[134] The Miller Hospital was part of the LCC hospital system, which according to Paul Weindling was particularly favourable towards refugee nurses and doctors.[135] At least eight of the nurses whose testimony comprise this book trained at LCC hospitals. As an organisation it willingly accepted refugees in numbers not experienced in other establishments, taking two refugees as probationer nurses at each of its 37 training schools.[136]

In 1929, the Local Government Act sought to improve the nation's health by dissolving the Poor Law and placing hospital provision under local authority rule. Councils were enabled to 'appropriate' hospitals that had been under Poor Law provision.[137] According to Stewart, if this appropriation was slow in some parts of the country, London worked 'vigorously to exploit [the power] with the result that in the 1930s [the LCC] was the largest single provider of hospital beds in Britain, and possibly the world'.[138] Its health provision included 141 hospitals, including maternity, general and mental health hospitals, employing over 26,000 staff, of which 8,000 were female nurses.[139] Of the mental health hospitals, the Maudsley is particularly important in the story of Jewish refugees as it operated on an open policy, bringing a number of Jewish psychiatrists to work in it.[140] Annie Altschul trained as a mental health nurse at Mill Hill Hospital, which had been requisitioned for the Emergency Medical Service by the Maudsley.[141]

Approximately forty per cent of all public general hospital beds in England and Wales came under the LCC.[142] But the LCC hospitals, with their history in the Poor Law, suffered the stigma of being somewhat infra dig next to the London teaching hospitals. Therefore the employment of educated Jewish refugees was likely to have been seen as a coup for hospitals that did not usually recruit from the middle classes. Although Epsom Hospital, where Altschul completed her general nurse training, was part of Surrey rather than the London County Council, her view that 'the hospital had never met anyone with any intelligence before'[143] might also have been true for some of the smaller LCC hospitals in poorer boroughs.

Once war was declared, Josephine Bruegel was evacuated from the Princess Elizabeth Children's Hospital, a voluntary hospital in the East End where she commenced her nurse training, to Whipps Cross Hospital in Leytonstone. She maintained that Whipps Cross was 'better equipped' than the Princess Elizabeth.[144] Nevertheless, she continued, 'The nurses were not as well-educated as in the voluntary hospital.' Most were from working-class backgrounds.[145] Nurses themselves were aware of the two-tier system and the reality that theirs were regarded as 'second class nurse training schools'.[146] Despite the difficulties that their second-class status afforded municipal hospitals, the sheer size of the LCC enabled those nurses who trained within it a broad range of nursing experience. It also enabled appointments to be made to the LCC itself and not individual hospitals, something that created wider opportunities of further training, promotion and the transfer of pensions.[147] Furthermore, the LCC had the backing of the Socialist Medical Association (SMA).

The SMA was established in 1930. Its founding president, Surgeon Somerset Hastings, was, according to John Stewart, a powerful ally of the LCC. Many of the leading SMA figures were key participants in London's Labour movement.[148] The SMA wanted to end the voluntary hospital system, which it saw as divisive, and lobbied instead for a municipal system that was free for all, rich and poor, and one that supported the health of the capital.[149] As Frank Honigsbaum argued, the SMA did more than any other medical organisation to support Jewish refugees from Nazism.[150] This policy worked to the SMA's advantage, as it was partly because of refugees that it enhanced its membership and therefore its influence in the 1940s.[151] Significantly for the story of refugee nurses in Britain, the SMA recruited nurses as well as doctors into its midst, including refugees.[152] The secretary of the London branch wrote to the London Labour Party calling for the LCC to take as many doctors and nurses as was possible.[153] Charles Brook, a London general medical practitioner, London County Councillor and founding member of the SMA, appealed for non-British nurses to be employed by LCC hospitals, citing the shortage of nurses. Those refugees with appropriate qualifications and English language, he argued, could be of great value to the city's health needs.[154]

Ruth Shire and Heidi Cowen trained at Staines Emergency Hospital, within the provision of the LCC's neighbour, Middlesex County Council. Both were members of the SMA. In her oral history Shire recalled:

> And we were extremely lucky because the matron of our hospital was a very modern woman. She had been married. I'm not sure if she was a widow. But she had all the modern ideas. And she was in touch with doctors who were all very keen on the idea of the SMA, which was then started, the Social [sic] Medical Association. And so, the whole atmosphere of the hospital was one of looking ahead and treating the nurses as people who wanted to do vocational work, as well as learning. Very keen on education.[155]

The SMA medical staff worked with the matron, Miss Lang, in the education of the nursing staff, spending considerable time lecturing them on the hoped-for benefits of a national health service.[156] According to Shire, Lang was particularly keen on refugee nurses, taking about ten in total. Shire maintained that Lang 'was very clever because she realised that the girls, the refugee girls, all had a fairly decent primary education – and they were all young of course – and a certain amount of secondary part. So she had a lot of refugees.'[157] Cowen agreed that the matron was supportive of Jewish refugee nurses, though contested the number. According to Cowen, Lang accepted thirty, which she acknowledged was 'unusual in those days'.[158]

For matrons such as Lang, the matron of the Miller Hospital and Littleboy at the London, the decision to take Jewish refugees into their hospital training programmes was undoubtedly a pragmatic one, particularly for the smaller, less prestigious hospitals. Recruiting nurses with culture and education was not easy. However, in many instances these matrons appear to have gone beyond the normal recruitment drives to make their refugee nurses' new lives in Britain easier. Shire recalls Lang giving extra ration cards to her refugee nurses so that they could prepare Passover meals:

> I then went to the matron and we suggested to her could we do the food for the patients who were Jewish. And she said yes. And she gave us some coupons, because you must have coupons during the time, and we could buy our food with these coupons; so bread

and so on. And we did it for almost a week, which was the right time, and she let us carry on with this – probably not too exactly. But it showed her enlightenment, not ours.[159]

Conclusion

Nursing was both a pragmatic work option for female Jewish refugees and rampant opportunism on the part of the Government and the nursing profession. Not all the refugees whose narratives comprise this book were keen to avail themselves of the opportunity to enter nurse training. The very limited work choices for refugees meant that nursing was certainly a better option than the alternatives, particularly domestic service. Nevertheless, there were those like Sacharin and Ross, who were at best unsure about nursing as a career. However, most appear to have viewed nursing as a genuine prospect for independence and a worthwhile career. As the war progressed and refugees were entitled to join either the Auxiliary Territorial Service (ATS) or munitions factories, nursing appears to have remained an acceptable prospect.[160]

The Government and profession may have presented nursing as a useful career choice for refugees, but that did not necessarily correspond to hospitals opening their doors. Several of the refugees who sought places at the famous London teaching hospitals struggled to gain acceptance to them. The refusal of voluntary hospital training schools to accept refugees was to the benefit to the hospitals of the LCC and less prestigious training schools around the country. However, not even all these hospitals, often desperate for recruits, treated the refugees well, and many struggled to gain places in even the most remote areas of Britain. Furthermore, once the refugee had gained her place, the security of the hospital training school was not necessarily assured. For some, accolades from the matron and senior staff were a welcome experience after the chaos of their lives under National Socialism. For others, antisemitic and anti-German feelings were never far from the surface. The mass dismissals in the spring of 1940 were to test the most resilient of these young women.

Notes

1 Lee Fischer (Liesl Einstein), oral history interview by Jane Brooks on 12 October 2017. Personal archive.
2 Fischer's brother became ill some time after arriving in Britain, but no doctor was called to see him. Eventually he was brought into the main house from the annexe, where he lived with the other boys, so his sister could care for him. She noticed his urine was the colour of coffee and took a specimen to the doctor close by. Fischer's brother was immediately taken to hospital in an ambulance and diagnosed with rheumatic fever. Sadly, he was already in multi-organ failure and he died soon after, on his sister's fifteenth birthday.
3 Those nurses in training in the middle years of the twentieth century were still sometimes called 'probationers' and sometimes the more modern 'student nurses'. Both terms are used in the book.
4 Children's nurses were registered under a supplementary register, as were male nurses and psychiatric nurses. Robert Dingwall, Anne Marie Rafferty and Charles Webster, *An Introduction to the Social History of Nursing* (London: Routledge, 1988), 91.
5 Conscription for single women and childless widows between the ages of 20 and 40 was established in December 1941. Later in the war this was extended to those between 19 and 43 years old. Penny Summerfield, *Reconstructing Women's Wartime Lives: Discourse and Subjectivity in Oral Histories of the Second World War* (Manchester: Manchester University Press, 1998), 45; National Archives, 'Focus on women in uniform; Women in World War II – Introduction', www.nationalarchives.gov.uk/womeninuniform/wwii_intro.htm [accessed 29 June 2021].
6 Esther Carling, 'Recruitment for nursing. To the Editor of the Lancet', *Lancet* (11 October 1930): 826.
7 Anonymous, 'The position of nursing: Past and present', *Lancet* (15 November 1930): 1092.
8 For a detailed discussion of 'The Final Report', its ramifications and the limited response to it, see for example, Monica E. Baly, *Nursing and Social Change* (London: Routledge, 1995); Anne Marie Rafferty, *The Politics of Nursing Knowledge* (London: Routledge, 1996).
9 Lancet Commission, 'The Final Report on Nursing' (London: Lancet Commission, 1932), 56.
10 Anonymous, 'Position of nursing', 1090–3.
11 Lancet Commission, 'Final Report', 11.

12 Anonymous, 'A shortage of nurses', *Daily Telegraph* (19 February 1932).
13 Rafferty, *Politics of Nursing Knowledge*, 153. The College was not alone in its antipathy towards foreign nurses. Sir Francis Freemantle's discussion of the Athlone Committee findings was recorded by *Hansard*. He maintained: 'One of the obvious suggestions for dealing with the problem has been the use of foreign women nurses from abroad. The addition of foreigners of either sex has to be limited, I fear, by certain other considerations, but the Home Office have not been averse to considering whether they can stretch a point in favour of those who can do useful service in the nursing world.' *House of Commons debut, 'Nursing services', vol. 346 (18 April 1939), 205*. https://api.parliament.uk/historic-hansard/commons/1939/apr/18/nursing-services [accessed 7 June 2023].
14 Lord Athlone was the cousin of King George V.
15 Anne Bradshaw, *The Nurse Apprentice, 1860–1977* (London: Routledge 2001), 90.
16 Dingwall et al., *Introduction to the Social History of Nursing*, 103.
17 Susan McGann, Anne Crowther and Rona Dougall, *A History of the Royal College of Nursing, 1916–90: A Voice for Nurses* (Manchester: Manchester University Press, 2009), 97.
18 Rafferty, *Politics of Nursing Knowledge*, 169. The College of Nursing received its Royal Charter in 1939, becoming the Royal College of Nursing.
19 Royal College of Nursing, Chairman: Lord Horder, 'Nursing Reconstruction Committee: Section II, education and training' (London: Royal College of Nursing, 1943), 11.
20 Sheila M. Bevington, *Nursing Life and Discipline: A Study Based on over Five Hundred Interviews* (London: H. K. Lewis, 1943), 4 (original emphasis).
21 Bevington, *Nursing Life and Discipline*, 1. There is a caveat to this. In the introduction to the study, Bevington admitted that she was more likely to have been given access by the more reforming matrons than the less progressive. This will have undoubtedly affected the responses she received (p. 3).
22 Gladys B. Carter and Evelyn C. Pearce, 'Reconsideration of nursing: Its fundamentals, purpose and place in the community, 4: Training of nurses in hospital', *Nursing Mirror and Midwives' Journal* (16 February 1946): 331–2.
23 Dingwall et al., *Introduction to the Social History of Nursing*, 118.

24 Jane Brooks, 'From "unwanted Jew" to "a brighter professional future": Kinder girls and the nursing profession in wartime Britain', *Jewish Historical Studies: Transactions of the Jewish Historical Society of England* 51 (2019): 68–85.
25 McGann et al., *History of the Royal College of Nursing*, 105.
26 Paul Weindling, 'Refugee nurses in Great Britain, 1933–1945: From a place of safety to a new homeland, in Susan Grant (ed.), *Russian and Soviet Healthcare from an International Perspective* (London: Palgrave Macmillan, 2017), 244.
27 For a full and detailed discussion on the creation of the moral nurse and the training of character, see particularly Rafferty, *Politics of Nursing Knowledge*, Chapter 2: 'The character of training and training of character', 23–41.
28 John Stewart, 'Angels or aliens? Refugee nurses in Britain 1938–1942', *Medical History* 47 (2003): 154.
29 For the sake of consistency, the name used for this organisation throughout the book will be the Nursing and Midwifery Department, unless specifically stated otherwise. The nomenclature of this organisation is not consistent in the archives or oral history data. In the 1939 Annual Report for the Central Council for Jewish Refugees, the section dealing with the organisation is subheaded 'Nursing and Midwifery Department', but then discusses the work of the 'Committee'. Central Council for Jewish Refugees, 'Annual Report of the Council for 1939', 14. ACC/2793/S/A/84, London Metropolitan Archives (LMA). In her letter to the *Nursing Times* outlining the work of the Department, Hillyers refers to herself as the 'Chairman, nursing sub-committee of the Co-Ordinating Committee for Refugees'. G. V. Hillyers, 'Refugee nurses', *Nursing Times* (10 December 1938): 1310.
30 Central Council for Jewish Refugees, 'Annual Report of the Council for 1939', 14.
31 Marion Berghahn, *Continental Britons: German-Jewish Refugees from Nazi Germany* (Oxford: Berg, 1988), 118.
32 Susi Linton, oral history interview by Rosalyn Livshin on 19 October 2004, 16. Interview 78, Refugee Voices: Association of Jewish Refugees (AJR) Audio-Visual Testimony Archive, British Library, London. Linton does not say what role Parry had within the Merseyside Coordinating Committee, only that she had signed the letter.
33 Josephine Bruegel, 'Reminiscences': oral history interview by Sylva Simsova between 1998 and 2001. OSP 2122, Wiener Holocaust Library, London.

34 Kitty Schafer (Kaufmann), oral history interview by Jane Brooks on 30 August 2017. Personal archive.
35 Margaret Marflow, 'For my Grandchildren' (2001), 50–1. A biographical database of European Medical Refugees in Great Britain, 1930s–1950s, Oxford Brookes University, Oxford.
36 Gertrud (Trudie) Moos, 'I Remember: My Life Story' (printed 1995), 36. A biographical database of European Medical Refugees in Great Britain, 1930s–1950s, Oxford Brookes University, Oxford.
37 Elisabeth Katz (Rosenthal), oral history video interview with Sandra Bendayan on 4 August 1994. Gift of Jewish and Children's Services of San Francisco, the Peninsula, Marin and Sonoma Counties, United States Holocaust Memorial Museum (USHMM), Washington, DC.
38 Hillyers, 'Refugee nurses', 1310.
39 Stewart, 'Angels or aliens?', 155.
40 Rosa Sacharin (Goldschal), *The Unwanted Jew: A Struggle for Acceptance* (Tullibody: Diadem Books, 2014), 67.
41 Jennifer Craig-Norton, *The Kindertransport: Contesting Memory* (Bloomington: Indiana University Press, 2019), 159.
42 Craig-Norton, *Kindertransport*, 158.
43 Aviva Gold (Wolff) quoted in Dina Gold, *Stolen Legacy: Nazi Theft and the Quest for Justice at Krausenstrasse 17/18, Berlin* (Chicago: American Bar Association Publishing, 2016), 75.
44 Mr Stephany, 'Central British Fund for World Jewish Relief: Notes for the Home Secretary's speech' (*c.* late 1938), 3. Acc/2793/04/05/01, LMA.
45 For a full and detailed discussion of British nurses' rapid volunteering for military service, see for example, Penny Starns, *Nurses at War: Women on the Frontline, 1939–45* (Stroud: Sutton Publishing, 2000); Jane Brooks, *Negotiating Nursing: British Army Sisters and Soldiers in the Second World War* (Manchester, Manchester University Press, 2018).
46 Hillyers, 'Refugee nurses', 1310.
47 Anonymous, 'Helping the refugee nurse', *Nursing Mirror and Midwives' Journal* (10 December 1938): 357.
48 Sister, 'For the sake of humanity', *Nursing Mirror and Midwives' Journal* (26 November 1938): 305.
49 In her oral history interview Lee Fischer recalled being invited to English girls' homes as she had nowhere else to go on her days off. Ruth Shire reflected on the practical issues related to refugee nurses not having a home away from the hospitals. Fischer, oral history

interview; Ruth Shire, oral history interview by Jane Brooks at her home in the West Midlands on 13 February 2018, 7. Personal archive.
50 M. H. Campbell, 'Guests of our nation', *Nursing Mirror and Midwives' Journal* (31 August 1940): 516.
51 For a useful discussion of the suspicion many in Britain felt towards 'foreigners', see for example, Colin Holmes, *A Tolerant Country?: Immigrants, Refugees and Minorities in Britain* (London: Faber & Faber, 1991).
52 E. M. Pye, 'Midwifery training of refugees', *Nursing Mirror and Midwives' Journal* (10 June 1939): 380.
53 Central Council for Jewish Refugees, 'Annual Report of the Council for 1939', 14.
54 E. M. Pye, 'Text books for refugees', *Nursing Mirror and Midwives' Journal* (12 August 1939): 680.
55 M. C. S., 'Refugee and training', *Nursing Mirror and Midwives' Journal* (11 February 1939): 695.
56 Anonymous, 'Reply to M. C. S.', *Nursing Mirror and Midwives' Journal* (11 February 1939): 695.
57 Susan Cohen, '"Crossing borders": Academic refugee women, education and the British Federation of University Women during the Nazi era', *History of Education* 39, 2 (2010): 175–82.
58 Anne von Villiez, 'The emigration of women doctors from Germany under National Socialism', *Social History of Medicine* 22, 3 (2009): 564. Some of the refugees clearly did feel this was a step backwards, but not all. Hockey was highly critical of the theoretical training she was given at the London Hospital, decrying the honorary medical staff who provided the teaching as offering 'diluted medicine'. Lisbeth Hockey, oral history interview at her home (interviewer not specified) in Edinburgh on 27 December 1987. Interview T26, Oral History Collection, RCN, Edinburgh. Alternatively, Lee Fischer was clear: 'I felt that as a nurse I could be more helpful to the patient instead of a doctor, who goes in and out, and only sees the patient for a few minutes. I was able to be longer the patient and take care of them.' Fischer, oral history interview.
59 Sylva Simsova, 'Who were the pre-Second World War refugees from Czechoslovakia?', in Charmian Brinson and Marian Malet (eds), *Exile in and from Czechoslovakia during the 1930s and 1940s*. Yearbook of the Research Centre for German and Austrian Exile Studies: Volume II (Leiden: Brill, 2009), 90.
60 Josephine Bruegel, 'Memoirs', 21. Wiener Holocaust Library, London. https://wiener.soutron.net/Portal/Default/en-GB/RecordView/Index/23314 [accessed September 2023].

61 Bruegel, 'Reminiscences', 10.
62 Rachel Pistol, '"Heavy is the responsibility for all the lives that might have been saved in the pre-war years": British perceptions of refugees 1933–1940', *European Judaism* 50, 2 (2017): 42.
63 Berghahn, *Continental Britons*, 43.
64 Tony Kushner, *The Persistence of Prejudice: Antisemitism in British Society During the Second World War* (Manchester: Manchester University Press, 1989), 11. It should be noted that by the middle years of the war the Mass-Observation project noted a fall in anti-Jewish sentiment across the country to about 13 per cent. Tony Kushner, *The Holocaust and the Liberal Imagination: A Social and Cultural History* (Oxford: Blackwell, 1994), 187.
65 Helen Jones, 'National, community and personal priorities: British women's responses to refugees from the Nazis, from the mid-1930s to early 1940s', *Women's History Review* 21, 1 (2012): 121.
66 Anonymous, 'Awake or dreaming?: The impressions of the German tour, June 1935', *Nursing Times* (13 July 1935): 684–6.
67 The *Mutterhaus* or 'motherhouse' system was established in Germany in the nineteenth century and was the pre-eminent system of organising nursing work and the nurses themselves. The Motherhouse provided a community in which the Deaconesses, as they were called, could live and from where they would provide nursing and humanitarian aid to the community around them. See Evelyn R. Benson, 'Nursing in Germany: A historical study of Jewish presence', *Nursing History Review* 3 (1995): 190.
68 G. M. Y., 'I: Christmastide with Frau Oberin Hubler', *Nursing Times* (21 December 1935): 1237.
69 Julia Boyd, *Travellers in the Third Reich: The Rise of Fascism Through the Eyes of Everyday People* (London: Elliott & Thompson, Kindle edition, 2017), 164–5.
70 Anonymous, 'Cartoon – The College in 1935: Two new responsibilities – Occupational therapy and gas warfare', *Nursing Times* (21 December 1935): 1221. https://link.gale.com/apps/doc/OPRIIE463744181/WMNS?u=rcnur&sid=bookmark-WMNS&xid=47265fc4 [accessed 28 September 2023]. Julia Boyd suggests that throughout the early to mid-1930s travellers held an almost morbid interest in Russia and Germany, visiting both in order to confirm rather than defy their expectations of the two regimes. Boyd, *Travellers in the Third Reich*, 11.
71 Anonymous, 'Germany's shortage', *Nursing Mirror and Midwives' Journal* (15 January 1938): 362.

72 Anonymous, 'Nurse's German honour', *Nursing Mirror and Midwives' Journal* (20 August 1938): 478.
73 Anglo-Scott, 'Humanity begins at home', *Nursing Mirror and Midwives' Journal* (24 December 1938): 446.
74 L. H. Lewis, 'Refugee nurses', *Nursing Mirror and Midwives' Journal* (7 January 1939): 513 (ellipses in the original).
75 Lord Dawson of Penn, cited in Kushner, *Holocaust and the Liberal Imagination*, 83; Paul Weindling, 'Medical refugees and the modernisation of British medicine, 1930–1960', *Social History of Medicine* 22, 3 (2009): 490.
76 Kushner, *Holocaust and the Liberal Imagination*, 83.
77 Anonymous, 'Refugee doctors from Austria', *British Medical Journal* (9 July 1938): 79.
78 Aubrey Goodwin, '"Our colleagues in Austria": To the Editor of The Lancet', *Lancet* (2 April 1938): 808. In his argument, Goodwin states, 'To the latter is added the distinction of being "continental" practitioners, in the eyes of the British public a mark of distinction that places them at once in a higher category than ourselves.' It thus appears that whilst there were many in the medical profession who agreed with Dawson that refugee doctors should not be supported to work in Britain, there was some discrepancy as to their professional worth in the eyes of the public.
79 A. C. Lysaght, '"Our Colleagues in Austria": To the Editor of The Lancet', *Lancet* (16 April 1938); 914–15.
80 Anonymous, 'Refugee scientists', *Lancet* (21 April 1934): 860.
81 Louise London, *Whitehall and the Jews, 1933–1948: British Immigration Policy, Jewish Refugees and the Holocaust* (Cambridge: Cambridge University Press, 2000), 42.
82 Vivian D. Lipman, 'Anglo-Jewish attitudes to the refugees from Central Europe 1933–1939', in Werner E. Mosse, Julius Carlebach, Gerhard Hirschfield, Aubrey Newman, Arnold Pauker and Peter Pulzer (eds), *Second Chance: Two Centuries of German-Speaking Jews in the United Kingdom* (Tübingen: J. C. B. Mohr, 1991), 528.
83 Karola Decker, 'Divisions and diversity: The complexities of medical refuge in Britain, 1933–1948', *Bulletin of the History of Medicine* 77, 4 (2003): 852.
84 Decker, 'Divisions and diversity', 851.
85 Claire Hilton, 'A Jewish contribution to British psychiatry: Edward Mapother, Aubrey Lewis and their Jewish refugee colleagues at the Bethlem and Maudsley Hospital and Institute of Psychiatry, 1933–66', *Jewish Historical Journal* 41 (2007): 215.

The nursing world   121

86 Weindling, 'Medical refugees and the modernisation of British medicine', 490. Paul Weindling, 'The impact of German medical scientists on British medicine: A case study of Oxford, 1933–45', in Mitchell G. Ash and Alfons Sollner (eds), *Forced Migration and Scientific Change: Émigré German-speaking Scientists and Scholars after 1933* (Cambridge: Cambridge University Press, 1996), 87.

87 Weindling, 'Medical refugees and the modernisation of British medicine', 490.

88 See for example, Holmes, *Tolerant Country?*, 31; Walter Laqueur, *Generation Exodus: The Fate of Young Jewish Refugees from Nazi Germany* (London: I. B. Tauris, 2004), 200; Susan Cohen, *Rescue the Perishing: Eleanor Rathbone and the Refugees* (London: Vallentine Mitchell, 2015), 155.

89 W. Russell Brain, W. McAdam Eccles, Arthur Ellis, Richard W. B. Ellis, David Forsyth, R. D. Gillespie, Donald Hunter, Arthur Hurst, Robert Hutchison, Horder, Alan Moncrieff, J. P. Monkhouse, E. P. Poulton, H. E. Roaf, John A. Ryle, Adrian Stephen, C. P. Wilson and W. H. Wynn (Medical Peace Campaign), 'The medical profession in Austria', *Nursing Times* (26 March 1938): 338.

90 Paul Weindling cites a letter from A. V. Hill, physiologist, Nobel prize-winner and MP for Cambridge University, in which Hill maintains that civil servants were scared of the medical profession and the profession itself had little interest for anything except its own members. Weindling, 'Impact of German medical scientists on British medicine', 87. The Government's attitude to nursing, a female profession, had always been different. If the Government allowed the medical profession to regulate itself with limited interference, this was not true of its engagement with nursing, having imposed a number of restrictions on its ability to self-govern. For details on the involvement of the Government on the regulation of nurses, see Baly, *Nursing and Social Change*; Rafferty, *Politics of Nursing Knowledge*.

91 For a useful discussion on the use of non-British nationals in the NHS, see for example, Roberta Bivins, 'Picturing race in the British National Health Service, 1948–1988', *Twentieth Century British History* 28, 1 (2017): 83–109. Here Bivins reflects on a 1965 article in *The Times*, in which it was argued that whilst people of colour faced 'unpleasant racism' in industry, the same could not be said for those in the NHS, where they were not 'obviously competing for jobs' (p. 97).

92 Stewart, 'Angels or aliens?', 153.

93 Anonymous, 'Aliens may nurse again', *Nursing Mirror and Midwives' Journal* (9 November 1940): 121.

94 Hortense Gordon, oral history interview by Jane Brooks at her home in London on 27 October 2017. Personal archive. There is a lack of clarity as to which hospital Gordon applied. UCH (University College Hospital) is quite different from the Royal Free. She ultimately ended up training at St Stephen's Hospital in Fulham. This is further complicated by the acknowledgment that Moos did train at the Royal Free and that Miss Cockayne, the matron, was sympathetic to refugees. It is likely therefore that Gordon was mistaken and applied to UCH not the Royal Free.

95 Moos, 'I Remember', 45.

96 Moos, 'I Remember', 45. Hospital training schools took several 'sets' or intakes per year of student or probationer nurses. This cohort of students would progress through their training together and usually formed strong bonds.

97 Marianne Parkes, 'The Past and Other Pastimes' (no date), 8. A biographical database of European Medical Refugees in Great Britain, 1930s–1950s, Oxford Brookes University, Oxford.

98 Parkes, 'Past and Other Pastimes', 8.

99 Sonya O. Rose, *Which People's War?: National Identity and Citizenship in Wartime Britain 1939–1945* (Oxford: Oxford University Press, 2003), 96.

100 Charlotte Kratz, oral history interview at her home in Eastbourne on 16 September 1988. Interview T37, Oral History Collection, RCN, Edinburgh. The attitude towards nursing by the Germans and at this juncture, Nazi Germans, is usefully summarised by Ellen Ben-Sefer and Linda Shields in their analysis of the nursing school in the Warsaw Ghetto. They raise the question as to why the nursing school was allowed to continue, when the medical school and all other forms of learning were not. They suggest that nursing was considered a vocation and not a profession and therefore not a threat to the suppression of intellectual life of the Jews. It also may have been the gender makeup of nursing; women were less of a threat to the regime. Finally, they suggest that given the levels of typhus, tuberculosis and other infectious diseases which could spread beyond the ghetto, having nurses who could work to prevent such spread was advantageous. Arguably, therefore, Ben-Sefer and Shields point to nursing being understood as useful but not academic. Ellen Ben-Sefer and Linda Shields, 'Courage under adversity: Luba Bielicka-Blum (1906–1973) and the nursing school of the Warsaw Ghetto', *Health and History: Journal of the Australian and New Zealand Society for the History of Medicine* 18, 2 (2016): 31.

101 Kratz, oral history interview.
102 Kushner, *Persistence of Prejudice*, 10.
103 Bernard Wasserstein, *Britain and the Jews of Europe, 1939–1945* (Oxford: Clarendon Press, 1979), 117.
104 Yvonne Kapp and Margaret Mynatt, *British Policy and the Refugees, 1939–1941* (London: Frank Cass, 1997), 29.
105 Cohen, *Rescue the Perishing*, 136.
106 Peter Alter, 'Refugees from Nazism and cultural transfer to Britain', *Immigrants and Minorities* 30, 2/3 (2012): 190–210.
107 Holmes, *Tolerant Country*, 83.
108 Jones, 'National, community and personal priorities', 136.
109 Edith Bown (Jacobowitz), oral history interview by Barbara Mortimer in Maidstone on 24 May 2008. Interview T379, Oral History Collection, RCN, Edinburgh.
110 Edith Bown (Jacobowitz), 'Memories and reflections: A refugee's story' (1938). RCN Archives, Edinburgh, 55.
111 Bown, oral history interview.
112 Bown, 'Memories and reflections', 56.
113 Bown, 'Memories and reflections', 56.
114 Bown, oral history interview.
115 Mia Ross (Maria Fuchs), 'War memories', 4.
116 Ross, 'War memories', 11–13.
117 Schafer, oral history interview.
118 Schafer, oral history interview.
119 Sacharin, *Unwanted Jew*, 68.
120 Rosa Sacharin (Goldschal), oral history interview by Barbara Mortimer on 28 April 2010. Interview T407, Oral History Collection, RCN, Edinburgh.
121 Information about Charlotte Hoxter was given via email and telephone. My thanks to Hoxter's daughter for giving her time to tell me about her mother.
122 Anonymous, 'Home section: Part time training is suggested to popularise the nursing profession', *Jewish Chronicle* (c. late 1940s): 14. Military collection: War nurses' file, Jewish Museum of London.
123 Howard Irving Rein, 'A Comparative Study of the London German and the London Jewish Hospitals', PhD thesis, University of Southampton, 2016.
124 Anonymous, 'The London Jewish Hospital: New home for nurses. Lady Reading lays foundation-stone', *Jewish Chronicle* (22 July 1938): 29.

125 Rein, 'Comparative Study of the London German and the London Jewish Hospitals', 249.
126 Rein, 'Comparative Study of the London German and the London Jewish Hospitals', 253.
127 Charlotte Leopold Hoxter, 'How my parents Dr. Robert Hoxter and Luise Hoxter received their immigration permit to England'.
128 Hockey, oral history interview, 1987.
129 Hockey, oral history interview, 1987. Miss Gertrude May Littleboy was matron at the London Hospital from 1931 to 1941. There is a suggestion that she was part of 'the old regime' and was not keen to take on the mantle after Miss Monk, who was later President of the RCN. My thanks to Sarah Rogers for the information on Littleboy. Personal correspondence, 4 May 2020.
130 Anne Summers, *Christian and Jewish Women in Britain, 1880–1940: Living with Difference* (London: Palgrave Macmillan, 2017), 42.
131 Gerry Black, 'The struggle to establish the London Jewish Hospital: Lord Rothschild versus the barber', *Jewish Historical Studies* 32 (1990–92): 338. The London maintained firm links with the Jewish Hospital, as the admission of that hospital's bombed-out nurses discussed above attests. Significantly it appears that they created nurse-training links too. Esta Lefton maintained in her oral history that she trained at both the London Jewish Hospital and the London Hospital in 1946. Esta Lefton, oral history interview by Susan McGann in North London on 16 February 2004. Interview T253, Oral History Collection, RCN, Edinburgh.
132 Alice Fink (Redlich), oral history interview by Lyn E. Smith in November 1997. Interview 1775, Sound Archive, Imperial War Museum, London.
133 Fink's father was released a week after his arrest, by which time Fink had already started her nurse training.
134 Fink, oral history interview.
135 Paul Weindling, 'Medical refugees and the modernisation of British medicine', 505.
136 Cohen, 'Crossing borders', 178.
137 Becky Taylor, John Stewart and Martin Powell, 'Central and local government and the provision of municipal medicine, 1919–39', *English Historical Review* 122, 496 (2007): 401.
138 John Stewart, 'The finest municipal hospital service in the world'?: Contemporary perceptions of the London County Council's hospital provision, 1929–39', *Urban History* 32, 2 (2005): 329. See also Esyllt Jones, 'Nothing too good for the people: Local labour and London's

interwar health centre movement', *Social History of Medicine* 25, 1 (2011): 84–102.
139 Stephanie Kirby, 'A splendid scope for professional practice: Leading the London County Council Nursing Service, 1929–1948', *Nursing History Review* 14 (2006): 31–57.
140 Aleksandra Loewenau, 'Between resentment and aid: German and Austrian psychiatrist and neurologist refugees in Great Britain since 1933', *Journal of the History of the Neurosciences* 25, 3 (2016): 359.
141 Annie Altschul, oral history interview by Jane Brooks at her home in Edinburgh on 7 August 2001. Personal archive; Steve Tilley, 'Three nurses: Stories of refugee nurses in Scotland', *Scottish Review* (March 2018); Anonymous, 'Lost hospitals of London: Mill Hill Emergency Hospital', (no date). https://ezitis.myzen.co.uk/millhill.html [accessed 27 March 2020].
142 Nick Hayes, 'Did we really want a National Health Service? Hospitals, patients and public opinions before 1948', *English Historical Review* 127, 526 (2012): 631.
143 Altschul, oral history interview.
144 Bruegel, 'Reminiscences', 9.
145 Bruegel, 'Reminiscences', 11.
146 Kirby, 'Splendid scope for professional practice', 42.
147 Kirby, 'Splendid scope for professional practice', 39.
148 John Stewart, '"For a healthy London": The Socialist Medical Association and the London County Council in the 1930s', *Medical History* 42 (1997): 417–36.
149 Stewart, '"For a healthy London"', 420.
150 Frank Honigsbaum, *The Division of British Medicine: A History of the Separation of General Practice from Hospital Care* (London: Kogan Page, 1979), 260.
151 Stewart, 'Angels or aliens?', 154.
152 Kirby, 'Splendid scope for professional practice', 35.
153 John Stewart, *The Battle for Health: A Political History of the Socialist Medical Association* (London: Routledge Revivals, 2018), 106.
154 Stewart, 'Angels or aliens?', 154. There was even a call for refugee doctors to be given posts as nurses. Stewart, *Battle for Health*, 106.
155 Shire, oral history interview.
156 Zoe Josephs, *Survivors: Jewish Refugees in Birmingham, 1933–1945* (Birmingham: Meridian Books, 1988): 128.
157 Shire, oral history interview.

158 Heidi Cowen (pseudonym) and Ruth Shire, oral history interview by Jane Brooks at Shire's home in the West Midlands on 13 February 2018. Personal archive.
159 Shire and Cowen, oral history interview.
160 These were the choices that Sacharin herself noted in her oral history. Sacharin, oral history interview.

3

War nurse

Kitty Schafer was happy training to be a nurse in Croydon. However, she was not even able to complete her first year because in June 1940, she was dismissed:

> The bombshell, a letter came, 'your contract has been terminated, you cannot stay in the hospital anymore', because Croydon had an airport. I don't know what they thought I would do at the airport. But still, so, being stupid, naïve or whatever you like to call it, I took everything personally. I couldn't understand what they did to me, when I was good and being praised by matron, of all people, and so I had to leave. So, well, I did have to leave. I went back to London and stayed with my father, and the Blitz started, and we spent our time in the shelter, et cetera. Then one day, and I couldn't get a job or course in the area the selections were very, very hard, but at least I wasn't interned. And one day a letter came, we need nurses who would like to come back. And I said, 'I would love to, but provided I could go back to my matron, and to the hospital.' 'No. You cannot.' They gave me other alternatives. So I told them, 'if I'm not good enough to go to my matron, I don't want it anyway'.[1]

As this quote demonstrates, being turned away from the one place that offered some normality and security after all the horrors of persecution and escape was challenging for refugee nurses. This chapter thus explores the considerable hardships that the war years imposed on these young women. It examines refugees' wartime work as they negotiated dismissal, internment and reinstatement within the gendered expectations of women's place during the conflict. It begins with the 'phoney war' and the early war work of the refugees. This is followed by an analysis of the repercussions from the fall of France, the dismissal of alien nurses from hospitals across the country and the internment of some of them. As I argue, even those who were not enthusiastic about nursing found the period destabilising, as it plunged them back into a world of uncertainty after the relative calm of hospital training. I consider the scapegoating of Jews in Britain and the impact of public antisemitism on refugee nurses. Finally, the chapter explores the relaxation of employment regulations for refugees and the influx into nursing of those who had arrived on domestic service visas and the Kindertransport.

The 'phoney war' and enemy alien status

When war was declared on 3 September 1939, the population of Britain expected bombs and immediate danger to life. According to military historian Brian Bond, within minutes of the announcement that Britain was at war, the air-raid sirens created 'pandemonium in Whitehall'.[2] The panic that ensued sent the public 'scurrying for inadequate shelter'.[3] All the sirens were false alarms.

The Allied Forces and civilians were prepared for war, but nothing happened for the first ten months. This period soon became known as the 'phoney war'. It was a time of war without war. Civil defence systems were organised and civilians were employed to work within the Air Raid Precautions (ARP), but there was little for them to do. The Civil Nursing Reserve had been organised in 1938 as an 'essential component of the wartime emergency services'.[4] Nurses and their assistants might initially have been keen to contribute to the war effort, but the Reserve soon started to disband. Many of the women – only about a quarter of whom were registered nurses – were 'bored by the lack of work and sought alternative employment'.[5] With war geographically removed from Britain and in the absence of aerial bombardment, life for most of the population changed little in those early months.[6] Joel Morley, a historian of morale during both world wars, even refers to the phoney war by the less well-known name, the 'Bore War'. His research on Mass-Observation data identifies the anti-climax felt by Britons and their increasing lack of engagement in and apathy for the war effort.[7]

The declaration of war changed the status of Jewish refugees in Britain.[8] Those who had fled the Greater Reich were no longer refugees to be pitied, but enemy aliens; 'for the average Englishman we were after all Germans'.[9] Sheer Ganor, a historian of German Jewry, maintains that British authorities assumed all refugees were faithful to their homeland and therefore not to be trusted.[10] According to refugee historian Colin Holmes, the Government ordered 'an immediate review' of all Germans and Austrians living in Britain. Having already collected details of aliens, all the Government needed to do was to categorise them into designations based on their potential danger to the country.[11] Category A persons were interned and Category B were left at liberty, but had certain restrictions placed on them. Category C were 'persons certified as "refugees from Nazi oppression" and freed from restrictions other than those applied to friendly aliens'.[12] None of the refugees whose stories comprise this book were placed in the A category. Both Elisabeth Katz and Margot Hodge were designated as Category B. There does not appear to be any reason why they should have been categorised as more potentially dangerous than other nursing refugees. Hodge's memoir does suggest a link to northern cities: 'I found out years later, that in the north, particularly in the Bradford and Leeds areas, there had been a number of infiltrations into textile mills and colleges by undesirables, who pretended to study, but were in fact suspect.'[13] It was even recognised at the time that the designations were frequently arbitrary and dependent to some extent on the official considering the case.[14] Even those placed in Category C could not be assured of fair treatment from the British public.

According to Tony Kushner, over 8,000 women domestics were sacked within the first two weeks of war.[15] One reason for this mass dismissal was the dislocation caused by the war, as 'mistresses had either been evacuated or had lost their income'.[16] The other reason was starker: the British did not want to employ Germans in their homes.[17] The rationale for this was gendered, nationalistic and class-based. Jewish refugee domestics were 'foreign, female and inhabited that dangerous world below stairs'.[18] Nevertheless, women refugees were generally viewed with less suspicion than their male compatriots. In her monograph on women in the Special Operations

Executive, Juliette Pattinson argues that women were popular for courier roles because they could pass controls more easily than men.[19] Women were less likely to be suspected of nefarious activity. This very gendered notion of women's obedience was critical to the more lenient treatment proffered to female refugees.

When war was declared, those refugees working as hospital nurses were able to continue their employment. The majority were working in and around London, including Annie Altschul in Ealing, Lisbeth Hockey at the London Hospital, Whitechapel (see Figure 3.1), Edith Menkes Wolloch at the Women's Hospital in Marylebone and Annaliese Pearl in Hackney. Others had been sent to the Midlands and as far north as Yorkshire. Eva Flatow was working at Northampton General Hospital, Margot Hodge at St James's Hospital in Leeds and Elizabeth Katz at St Luke's in Bradford.

With the advent of war, the clearest signs to the refugees of their change in status were the imposition of a five-mile radius, the prohibition on cycling and the requirement to register as an 'enemy alien'.[20] Marion Berghahn also highlights the curfew that was imposed.[21] The refugees' narratives do not dwell on these physical restrictions. Their work as nurses was heavily prescribed and there was little time for leisure pursuits. Nevertheless, the new designation of 'enemy alien' did have a psychological impact on them. In her memoir Trudie Moos recalled the pain at being labelled an 'enemy alien', as 'nobody could have been more grateful to England than we were'.[22] Alice Fink noted the shock of the label but acknowledged the very real fear of invasion.[23] Both Moos and Marflow recalled the personal distress they experienced when being considered German by the English.[24] The 1951 United Nations Convention on the Refugee states that the term 'alienage' refers to 'a person who is outside the country of his [sic] nationality, or if he has no nationality the country of his former habitual residence'.[25] It is the very nature of 'being outside' one's own country, that is, alienated from it, that enables people to gain refugee status.[26] Whilst this official definition is somewhat prosaic, in reality 'alien' as a term is redolent with negative connotations. Psychologist Helen Haste argues, 'The "threats" posed by immigrants are more usually expressed in terms of their cultural difference, or in terms of

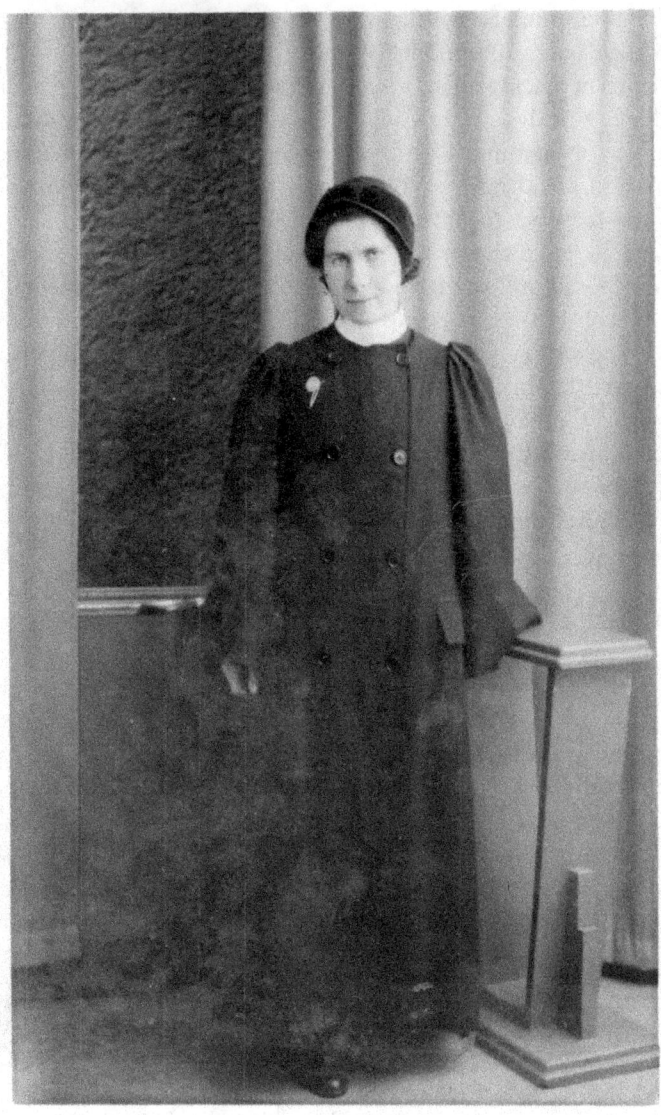

Figure 3.1 Lisbeth Hockey in her London Hospital uniform, *c.*1938–39. Reproduced with kind permission of the Royal College of Nursing Archives [fo. 154]

potential criminality arising in part from "alien" codes and in part from their reduced economic status.'[27]

The term 'enemy alien' found its way into the English lexicon in the First World War. In August 1914, Anna Freud, the youngest daughter of Sigmund Freud, was trying to return to her home in Austria, just as the First World War was starting. For the first time, she was required to have a personal document in which she was designated 'alien enemy'. It did not take too long for the words to be transposed and the term 'enemy alien' logged into officialdom. The person ceased to be just a foreigner; they were now foreign and an adversary. This status became the 'primary distinguishing characteristic' for immigrants.[28] Given the trauma of exile, it is not surprising that young Jewish nurses were hurt by the nomenclature. When France fell to the German army in June 1940, the psychological responses to their change of status would be matched by a very real and profound alteration in their physical condition.

Dismissal

The 1940 Report of the Central Council for Refugees was cautious in its description of the dire situation in which many refugees found themselves after the fall of France: 'The Jewish and Christian Councils did not think it right to oppose the general Government policy.' Instead it acknowledged that reports of treachery by German residents in the Netherlands and France, which had aided the fall of France, had brought about 'A change of feeling and of policy in England ... Under the stress of "intern the lot," the Government felt compelled to disregard the distinction that had been made by it in favour of refugees.'[29] On 1 May 1940 a special meeting of the Executive of the Central Council for Jewish Refugees recorded its concerns over the loss of employment for refugee doctors, dentists, nurses and professional men 'who were not at present allowed to engage in their normal vocations'.[30] The Committee acknowledged that at that time, nothing could be done to alleviate the problem. The inclusion of nurses among this list of professional men is of interest. Nurses were women in an occupation that sat in the interstices between the learned professions and family carers or domestic servants. This is the only document I have found that places refugee nurses alongside male refugee doctors and dentists as equals. As employees in the nation's hospitals, unlike most of their compatriots, refugee health workers were visible to the public and had potential access to members of the armed forces. Their dismissal was part of the strategy to placate Britons who were fearful of spies.[31] Despite the reality that as Jews they were deemed enemies of the German and Austrian states, the belief that no German or Austrian could be trusted pervaded.[32]

A few weeks later, on 25 May 1940, the news section of the *Nursing Times* announced that all hospitals and similar institutions must send details to the Aliens War Service Department of 'all German, Austrian and Czech females employed in any capacity'.[33] A month later, on 15 June 1940, both *Nursing Mirror and Midwives' Journal* (hereafter *Nursing Mirror*) and the *Nursing Times* reported that all German, Austrian and Czech nurses had to be dismissed from their hospital positions.[34] On 22 June, the *Nursing Times* printed a letter offering sympathy for those alien nurses who had been dismissed: 'This has involved 800 to 900 nurses, many of whom are friendly to this country ... While we all recognise that our national safety must be protected, we offer our sympathy to all these nurses who share our ideals; they will understand as well as we do, the essential need for care in the very difficult position now facing us.'[35] Despite the words of sympathy, it is clear that the profession was unable to counter the edict that all refugees from Germany, Austria and Czechoslovakia were to be dismissed.

In July 1940, a letter to the *Nursing Times* reported that the Minister of Health had decided 'All persons of either sex of German, Austrian, or Italian nationality who are engaged in any capacity at any hospital in the Emergency Scheme which is providing treatment for members of the Forces must still be dismissed.'[36] The letter added that in those hospitals where members of the Forces were not being treated, alien personnel could be retained and that those of Czech nationality did not need to be dismissed from any hospital. In reality, the vast majority of alien personnel were dismissed; matrons did not take into account the provenance of their Czech nurses.

Aviva Gold was dismissed from the Princess Margaret Rose Hospital in Edinburgh because of fears of refugees so close to the

Firth of Forth. The Firth provided vital access to the North Sea and therefore towards enemy territory. There were, therefore, particular concerns with refugees who lived or worked near the coast or airports, where they potentially had easier access to the enemy. Gold returned to London, seeking new training opportunities across the capital. Like other refugees, she was turned away by all the hospitals because of her enemy alien status. She was called to a tribunal. Instead of being interned, as she feared, she discovered that because her parents had become citizens of British Mandated Palestine in 1936 when she was still a child, she qualified for British citizenship. No longer an enemy alien, she started training at the Royal Cancer Hospital in Fulham before transferring to University College Hospital in 1941 or 1942.[37] Few of her compatriots were so fortunate.

Susi Loeffler recalled the matron of the cottage hospital where she was working telling her that she needed to leave: 'and the matron said to me, after about, er, two months, ah, I can't remember how long, she said, "we can't have enemy aliens in this hospital"'.[38] Loeffler replied that she was not an enemy alien, that she had a Czech passport, but to no avail. She was on her own again. Josephine Bruegel, also Czechoslovakian, was working at a convalescent home in Bognor Regis when the British Expeditionary Force fled the Continent:

> Then came Dunkirk and I was on the south coast. All the nurses who were not British had to leave ... I was called to the matron. A policeman was waiting there for me to take me to the police station. I asked, 'Why? I am a Czechoslovakian citizen. I belong to the Czech Refugee Trust Fund and they know me. Before you imprison me, you had better contact the Czech Refugee Trust Fund', which they did. The Czech Trust Fund told the police to put me on a train and send me straight to London.[39]

Once in London, Bruegel was given accommodation in Bloomsbury, with a number of other refugees who had been evacuated from the coast. She admitted that Bloomsbury still had the intellectual atmosphere for which it was famous, and despite the bombs she was not unhappy. Bruegel met her husband, also a Czech refugee, in August 1940, and by the following year she was admitted to the Royal Free Hospital to complete her medical studies. The London Hospital where Hockey was training was evacuated to Rochford in Essex soon after the declaration of war.[40] Her time there was short-lived. Reflecting on this and her dismissal from her medical studies in Austria in 1938, she commented: 'it was the second time that my career had been abruptly broken ... without my intervention and totally beyond my control'.[41]

Annie Altschul was dismissed from her training hospital in Ealing. In her oral history interview, she stated that she had never forgotten the day France fell to the Germans: 'One of my most vivid memories of Ealing actually was looking out the window onto lilac and red bushes which were quite magnificent in the grounds and being quite sure that I'd never see them again; that was the end of the world as far as I was concerned.'[42] The defeat of France, a country only 22 miles away from Dover, was a moment of fear for all in the British Isles. For Jewish refugees, the certain knowledge of what would happen to them should Germany invade was terrifying.

Only two of the nurses whose narratives comprise this book were not dismissed from the profession in 1940. Although the matron of the Miller Hospital was not able to keep Fink, she arranged for her transfer to a maternity hospital. In her oral history, Fink was judicious in her recollection of this decision. She was, she stated, 'lucky' not be interned.[43] Hodge was found a position at Killingbeck Fever Hospital by her matron at St James's. Sadly, this was not a success, as she was bullied and ostracised by her co-workers whilst there.[44] This difficult period only came to an end when she was interned on the Isle of Man.[45]

Internment

On the declaration of war, only those in Category A were interned, but fear of spies after the fall of France led to far more draconian measures against refugees. According to historian Glyn Prysor, fear rather than the reality of fifth columnists had been a major influence in the defeat of the British Expeditionary Force in 1940. The Allied Forces were fearful not only of the possibility of an invasion by the German army, quietly parachuting in behind enemy lines, but also the possibility of traitors within their midst.[46] This fear of internal spies in the army transposed itself all too easily onto fears of internal columnists within the refugee community on the home front. As most of the refugees were Jewish, religious prejudice only added to the anti-refugee rhetoric.

Sonya O. Rose maintains that Jews in wartime Britain were accused of 'engaging in selfish actions' simply because they were Jewish and therefore 'un-British' and 'un-English'.[47] Anti-alien sentiment, Rose continues, persisted during the early twentieth century and may even have increased during the Second World War.[48] As Kushner argues, 'antisemitism was common in daily discourse, literature and the press'.[49] Jews 'threatened British national identity' and were therefore to be treated with suspicion.[50] The young refugee nurses were not viewed as highly suspect as their male compatriots, but they were not immune to public fears of the enemy within. One bright moonlit night during her nursery-nurse training, Marianne Parkes left nappies on the washing line. They were seen by RAF pilots, and she was reported to the police for trying to signal to the enemy: '[The policeman] decided I was too stupid to be a spy, so let me go.'[51] The lack of understanding of the plight of Jews under Hitler meant that the British public were able to believe Jewish refugees in Britain were Nazi spies. The right-wing press in particular fed into the populist fears, whilst the Government did nothing to calm the rising panic.[52] The British press and security services called for all enemy aliens to be interned. Under the headlines 'Collar the lot',[53] all those in Category B were located and sent to internment camps.

Only about 4,000 women were interned compared to 23,000 men. The majority were sent to the Isle of Man, and in keeping with gendered ideas of women's general acquiescence to authority, they were treated more leniently than the male internees.[54] Whereas the men were housed in barrack-type accommodation, the women were sent to two holiday resorts in a remote part of the island.[55] For those women who had been domestic servants and some, like Hodge, who had been bullied in their nurse-training hospitals, internment on the Isle of Man was a welcome relief.[56] Nevertheless, the experience of being arrested and shipped off to an unknown island was a distressing episode for these young women. Having been placed in the B category at the beginning of the war, Elisabeth Katz joined the other interned women on the Isle of Man:

> Then just before Dunkirk ... and I was called ... and they just grabbed everybody, everybody and put them into camps. And that's how I ended up on the Isle of Man, being shipped there in the middle of the night ... I was working and I was called to the administration and there were these people who were detectives or something and I had to pack my stuff up and I had to go with them. There was another refugee girl in the same hospital, she was there too ...We were physically taken care of, but we had no idea where we were going or what would become of us.[57]

The matron of Killingbeck Hospital and a police officer arrived at Hodge's bedroom in May 1940. Hodge was told to pack a small bag and was escorted to Leeds Town Hall basement where other refugees were gathered. They were taken on buses to Liverpool. Hodge recalled the journey itself:

> Our trip to the Isle of Man was horrific. The ship, a Belgian coaster, capable of transporting at most 250 people, was full to bursting. She did not look seaworthy and was filthy. There was no order and no discipline. It was 'first come, first served'. I found a bit of floor space in front of a toilet that was in constant use and stank to high heaven ... There were Jewish refugees and hard bitten Nazis all clumped together on one ship.[58]

The cruelty of placing refugees in such close proximity to Nazis continued once on the Isle of Man. As discussed above, to the British Government they were all German. The persecution of Jews by Nazis was either too poorly understood – or perhaps there was little interest in understanding properly – to prevent such a brutal practice. The situation was clearly challenging for Jewish refugees and fights did occur between them and Nazi women internees. Yet despite this, many of the Jewish refugees remembered their time on the island as relatively happy.[59] Katz remembered the ship docking on the Isle of Man, although at the time she did not know where they were. She admitted that they were apprehensive, but the refugees soon found themselves in a town with beautiful beaches and hotels into which they were dispatched. She spent nine months on the island and even celebrated her twenty-first birthday there. Not used to forced idleness, the interned women organised themselves to provide useful skills to fellow internees, including teaching, hairdressing, medical care, language courses and dramatic productions.[60] As student nurses, Katz's and Hodge's skills were sought after and both were able to work as a nurses throughout their internment.[61] Hodge remained critical of the internment procedure but admitted she learnt much in her nursing work: 'we had a woman in the late stages of TB, a small boy with diabetes, a woman who delivered ... a baby and people with sundry and imagined illnesses which kept us busy'.[62]

In her oral history, Katz voiced a greater acceptance of her internment, seeing the policy as a necessary move to prevent espionage. One cannot be certain whether she was as tolerant of her treatment at the time. I would argue that the overlaying of eighty years of composing herself as a British and then US citizen, and thus perhaps the desire to appreciate the perspective of the Allied governments, were central to the creation of this positive trope.[63] Kushner argues that in many accounts of internment, there is a sense that it was a period of 'temporary aberration in an understandable moment of panic'. This, the refugees appreciated, would be followed by a 'return of a British sense of justice'.[64]

Although none of the other nurses whose narratives comprise this book were interned, some did experience the internment of family and friends. Trudie Moos's father and brother were interned on the Isle of Man. Like Katz, Moos did not express outrage about this treatment in her memoir, stating that they were treated 'courteously' and that her brother Werner 'soon found some occupation in the internment camp office'. What is more distressing is her lack of anger over the deportation of her cousin, Hans, who had a 'mental handicap, [and was] soon shipped off to a camp in Australia'. This deportation triggered the stroke suffered by Moos's aunt, Hans's mother. She died whilst Hans was still overseas.[65] Kitty Schafer's uncle, who had done so much to support her escape, was also interned on the Isle of Man. She reports this action in her oral history and then moves the discussion on to general restrictions placed on refugees: 'We had great restrictions. But it's as I said, somehow you get over it.'[66] Fink was equally as accepting of the possibility of internment, as 'the fear of a German invasion was genuine'.[67] As Kushner argues, most oral and written presentations of internment by refugees are a mixture of humour, understanding and frustration that their time in the camps prevented them from supporting the war effort.[68] Hodge summed up the situation: 'Months went by and as far as we were concerned we could have been on the moon, so little were we in touch with the real war that was going on in England and elsewhere.'[69]

Most of the refugee nurses tried to demonstrate gratitude to the British for offering refuge rather than criticising the Government for the blanket decision to dismiss all nurses and doctors. However, there were refugee nurses who openly questioned the decision to dismiss them from their hospital training programmes. In August 1940, one wrote to *Nursing Mirror* describing herself as 'just an alien nurse' and expressed dismay at being dismissed from her nurse training school: 'We are sent away from hospitals because we are aliens, but we were turned out of our native country because we were enemies of the Nazi regime.'[70] In November that same year, *Nursing Mirror* published another letter in which a refugee nurse set out a heartfelt plea to the hospitals of Britain: 'I thought I was very lucky to get to England at last. Then in June this year I received a letter saying that I had to leave the hospital as well as the town in three days. Destroyed were all my hopes and plans, destroyed all my feelings of having a home.'[71] Even amongst these entreaties, the desire to appease the profession and Government is apparent. Another refugee, who also identified herself as 'just an alien nurse', wrote to *Nursing Mirror* on 29 June 1940. She stated that she appreciated the decision to keep aliens out of hospitals that treated military patients, 'but there is a great demand for nurses just now, and we could relieve British nurses for war work, from county, mental, fever, and general hospitals. We would be only too pleased to do any kind of nursing.'[72]

The loss of nursing appointments was keenly felt. At a special meeting of the Central Council for Jewish Refugees on 1 May 1940, it was argued that the dismissal of professional men and women was not only a waste of 'skilled manpower', but it also threw the responsibility for their upkeep onto voluntary organisations.[73] Whilst accommodated by the Czech Refugee Trust Fund in Bloomsbury, Bruegel admitted that she and other female Czech refugees 'cleaned the rooms for the men and did some mending to make a little bit of pocket money, and when the dining room was damaged by bombing, we did the cooking'.[74] Whilst this work enabled her to maintain a level of independence, it was a waste of her medical and nursing training. Susi Loeffler was forced to attend the labour exchange on her dismissal and found work as a domestic servant:

> So I bought a cookbook (I still have it). Went to the local labour exchange and told them I was an experienced general maid. They asked me could I cook? 'Of course' I said. So I got a job with a lady in a big Tudor mansion, she had two children and employed a nanny. I don't know to this day how I did it. But I did. I lasted three weeks and I didn't get the sack[.] I left of my own accord. I only got about four hours sleep. I was so very slow and inept.[75]

Annie Altschul and Lisbeth Hockey both returned to domestic work on their dismissals. Altschul was employed as a nanny for a wealthy English family. The grandparents lived in a large house and had four sets of grandchildren living with them, 'and each set of grandchildren had a nanny and I was engaged as one of those'.[76] Hockey did not dwell on this period at all; only that she found a position to take care of a little girl for a while.[77] The refugees' discussions of the dismissal period are limited. This is possibly because most were invited to return to nursing within a few months and their dismissals were largely forgotten in the extensive wartime effort. It is also possible that the refugees did not wish to remember a time in which they were once again treated as enemies and obliged to work in other people's homes. Kushner and Cesarani maintain that once internment finished, most refugees needed to manage their lives and the war; those who had been dismissed from their employment probably felt the same.[78]

If the British public and the Government were fearful of spies in their midst, hospital matrons and the Nursing and Midwifery Department were anxious about the loss of vital members of nursing staff in a time of war. On 29 August 1940, the General Committee of the Nursing and Midwifery Department at Bloomsbury House passed a unanimous resolution on refugee nurses' employment:

> The Committee of the Nursing and Midwifery Department asks that the earnest consideration of the Home Office may be given to

its request that Refugee Nurses removed from their Hospitals under Circular 2080 may be allowed to return and remain as long as the Matron is satisfied with their conduct, to such Hospitals as can make arrangements for their working in wards to which soldiers, sailors or airmen of H.M. Forces will not be admitted.[79]

'Aliens may nurse again'

As early as July 1940, *Nursing Mirror* reported that aliens could return to nursing work, provided they did not work in hospitals where there were service personnel.[80] In August that year, the Nursing and Midwifery Department acknowledged the support of the General Nursing Council in helping those refugees who were moved to hospitals not recognised by them as training schools: 'The General Nursing Council is willing to make special arrangements to enable [refugees] to complete their training and obtain State Registration after the war, should their work during it be mainly confined to women and children.'[81] I have not found any data to suggest this resolution was ever put into effect, but only two months later, general hospitals started to relax restrictions, probably making such a decision unnecessary. On 18 October 1940, Miss Frey, secretary to the Nursing and Midwifery Department, wrote to Mr E. N. Cooper of the Home Office. Frey informed him that the situation within the London County Council (LCC) Hospitals had altered. LCC hospitals were now willing to accept Czech refugees back into their establishments.[82] An anonymous letter to *Nursing Mirror* on 9 November acknowledged that 'Aliens may nurse again'.[83] According to Frey, the LCC also agreed that German and Austrian nurses could return to hospitals for the chronically sick as assistant nurses, provided those hospitals did not admit military personnel: 'This latter form of employment is of course not training, but in this way our candidates will be able to take a share in the country's need for nurses and it will also enable them to continue their practical experience.'[84] It also enabled the nursing profession and the Government to staff unpopular hospitals cheaply. Eva Flatow found work in a psychiatric hospital:

> Banned from working in a general hospital, [Flatow] was assigned work in a mental asylum. This she found unbearable, carrying a large bunch of keys to enter locked wards, never knowing what disturbed behaviour she would have to deal with. But there she made friends with a fellow refugee, and together they took French leave and found work in London, in a private nursing home.[85]

Whilst living in London, Flatow met a fellow Jewish immigrant and they were married the following year. She did not return to nursing. In September 1940, Lisbeth Hockey had also returned to nursing, having been given a position at a fever hospital in London. Her oral history suggests that she was offered this work during the Blitz 'because it was dangerous'.[86] After nine months interned on the Isle of Man, Elisabeth Katz returned to St Luke's Hospital in Bradford: 'And I was told that St Luke's would have me back and an arrangement was made with the Board of Nursing that we could step back into our training.'[87] Hodge returned to St James's, but they would only credit her with three months' previous training, despite having trained for much longer. In the end, she had to do the full three years:

> I was helpless and very disappointed as this was the third time I had to begin my nursing career. I had fifteen months in Germany, started again in England in 1939, been transferred to a fever hospital in 1940, had been taken to the Isle of Man, had been nursing there and gaining experience and it all counted for very little.[88]

Although Hodge acknowledged the value of her nursing work and the training that was provided, her memoir brings into stark relief the opportunism of the profession. By ensuring that she start at the beginning each time, St James's acquired her skills for additional years at a lower pay scale. Margaret Marflow's memoir recalled her personal feelings about the return of Jewish refugee nurses to the hospitals of Britain: 'A few months later there was an acute shortage of Nurses and someone remembered all these "redundant" Refugee Nurses and the London Country Council Hospitals decided to take many of us on.' Marflow restarted at St Mary's Hospital in Islington: 'By the time I restarted training at St. Mary's Hospital, my father had returned from internment and slowly we became acclimatised, that is to say, British. As also we became acclimatised to the War, the Bombing, the Rationing, and all the hardship, including fire-watching!'[89]

Annie Altschul also decided to return to nursing, despite not enjoying the work. She applied to Epsom Hospital, as they were seeking assistant nurses, but after about a month she was asked to take up her nurse training:

> I said I didn't think I would because I wouldn't be there long enough. But they prevailed, and we were eight I think, who started at the same time. What happened from then on was that people who I think before hadn't gone into nursing, people who would normally have gone to university or who would normally have done other jobs ... Many of them chose nursing because they had to go into one of these things. What happened at Epsom, I think, was that they had never had an intelligent nurse ever before, I'm not sure about ever, but they had a tutor who dictated notes which you wrote out and handed back for correction and who was totally thrown by the arrival of a few people who were capable of thinking.[90]

She did not consider her training at Epsom a full-blown success but only 'wartime training'.[91] According to historian of mental health nursing, Peter Nolan, she thought it was a basic and practical training, which was 'disinclined to encourage reflection, argument or questioning on the part of students'.[92] Altschul was not alone in this analysis of nurse training during the war years. In January 1942, Susi Loeffler also returned to nursing, obtaining a training place at Harefield Hospital in north-west London. This was not a successful return to the profession. She described the lack of support and the very poor staffing levels: 'We were two nurses ... We had to do everything. No help at all. As it was Xmas nobody could get a day off and 12 hour shifts. That was the first and only time in my life I fainted.'[93] In the absence of alternatives, however, she completed the course.

Josephine Bruegel returned to medicine. When refugees were allowed to resume paid employment, she applied for work monitoring German aircraft with the Air Force. However, at her interview, they noted that she had almost finished her medical studies in Czechoslovakia and recommended that she apply to the Government to finish them. She began at the Royal Free Women's Medical School in 1942. Of the refugees whose narratives comprise this book, only Schafer refused to return to nursing work. After a short period at the John Lewis department store, she took a job at the BBC monitoring service, where she worked as a teleprinter, typist and then translator.[94] She remained at the BBC throughout the war, after which she married and, like most women at that time, left paid employment to work in the home.[95]

With the relaxation of regulations, refugees who had been working as domestic servants were able to move into nursing or other war work. Those who had come as Kinder but who were now 18 years old were also eligible to train as nurses. Lee Fischer was working as a maid in Manchester when she decided that she should do something for the war effort and applied for a place to train as a nurse at Booth Hall Children's Hospital in the city.[96] Hortense Gordon left her work as a domestic servant in 1941 and started children's nurse training at Queen Mary's Hospital, Carshalton. She remembered that, since the Blitz continued until June 1941, the nurses were required to go on duty in tin hats and gas masks.[97] The children at Queen Mary's were mostly long-term chronically sick, and according to Gordon, their parents were only permitted to visit once a fortnight.[98] Nevertheless, she clearly thrived in this work and won the silver medal for nursing at the hospital.[99] When she qualified in 1945, she commenced her general nurse training, for which she won the gold medal.[100] Gordon admitted that she felt this was an 'honour and a point of achievement'.[101]

Cilly Haar also left her domestic service position to train as a nurse in 1942, beginning at the City General Hospital in Gloucester. However, ill health and a broken relationship sent her back to London, where she began her training again in 1943 at Lambeth Hospital, part of the LCC hospital group.[102] Haar recalled the matron of Lambeth hospital, who did not have 'any compassion for either patients or staff', and how she and her fellow nurses tried to bring some laughter to the ward of female patients with terminal cancer. On one particular occasion, Haar recalled how she and her friend 'made up' a grapefruit with lipstick and rouge and propped it on the pillows in an empty bed. When the matron came to the ward to do her usual round, she nodded at the 'model patient': 'her face went as red as her hair. All the patients had a supressed grin on their face. The accompanying ward sister felt very uncomfortable and we nurses, although a little scared, were enjoying a bit of fun at her expense.' The matron was not at all amused and removed the late passes from Haar and her friends as punishment. Haar wrote that she never regretted the prank: 'If we did bring a little sunshine and laughter to the patients, then we had achieved our aim and purpose.'[103] However, despite the occasional rebellion, war work for all nurses was hard, with limited time off. Working through the Blitz added bombs to their workload and war work to their limited free time.

War work

Nurses' lives in the Blitz

In her oral history Lisbeth Hockey recalled her work at the fever hospital. In the absence of penicillin, which had been discovered but was not yet available, most of their patients were children.[104] On night duty during the Blitz, they nursed children on the floor under their cots, 'so the bottom of the cot was their shelter'. Hockey continued, 'there was a great big bang one morning ... I remember that to this day and the kids screaming and the bombs dropping and the parents being killed and the kids being left in the hospital because there was nobody to take them home and their home had been bombed'.[105] On qualifying as a registered nurse, Elisabeth Katz moved to London for her midwifery training: 'Half the bloody lot was bombed out. I mean we couldn't use the elevator in the middle of the night unless it was an emergency for a patient.'[106]

The Blitz began on 7 September 1940 and continued for ten months. Histories of the Blitz are by now legendary, 'the Blitz spirit' holding a special place in the narrative of the war on the home front. Historian Angus Calder wrote, 'As heavy bombing of London began in the later summer, the word "Blitz"' became 'almost overnight a British colloquialism for an air raid.' But from the beginning, the words carried resonance as the period was instantaneously and spontaneously 'mythologized' and the 'Blitz spirit' prevailed.[107] However, just exactly how this manifested itself on a collective and individual level is difficult to analyse. As Hockey's recollections above attest, nurses – like much of the civilian population – both struggled with the realities of the situation and accepted the conditions as part of being at war. Yet these oral histories were collected many years later. According to Brad Beaven and John Griffiths, the narratives have been heavily influenced by modern and powerful myths about the war on the home front. Nevertheless, oral histories do give a sense of the demands on the populace and how they coped with ongoing aerial bombardment.[108]

Unlike oral history data, Tom Harrison's study of the Blitz was based on the Mass-Observation project, based on data collected at the time. His findings also identified a genuine sense that the country was determined to maintain itself.[109] As Juliet Gardiner argues in her celebratory but valuable text, there was a very real difference between the public being frightened at times and frustrated with those in power and the desire to 'throw in the towel and bring an end to the bombing on any terms'.[110] The call to the country was to get on with life in as normal a way as possible. Such internalising of the Blitz spirit was vital to the nation's resolve.[111] Government propaganda set Britain's ability to withstand the onslaught of the *Luftwaffe* as the country standing together in recognition of a common enemy.[112] Harnessing the Blitz spirit was useful for the Government, who wanted the country to keep going in the face of the relentless bombing. The need to manage in this time of crisis was critical for the young nurses caring for the nation's sick and in need.

Gertrude Roberts may have argued that the war did not intrude on her nurse training, but she still accepted that there was 'community spirit'.[113] Trudie Moos recalled the challenges of living through the bombing raids and caring for young children when the air-raid sirens sounded. Yet, she maintained, 'I felt that we were all in this together; how different from the years in Germany, when I was one of the despised minority group.'[114] Despite her dislike for nursing work, Altschul admitted that the war was good for collegiality in the hospitals.[115] Healthcare workers across the country pulled together to support a nation under fire. The Blitz had a significant impact on the work of nurses across the country, both on and off duty. Lee Fischer maintained that night duty was better than day duty because at least they were already awake when the bombs fell:

If we were on days and an air raid was on, we had to go on duty and had to put the children under the bed. And of course, Matron was very fussy to make sure we were dressed properly. That was very important. No bobby-pins in the hair and whatever. So we preferred to be on night duty because we were up already. During the day, you know, we needed our sleep. At night, when we had the air raids on it was difficult at the time ... We didn't analyse it, we just took it the way it was.[116]

The Blitz not only gave the nurses extra work, but in some instances altered the way patients were cared for in material ways. Hockey recalled the work during this time at the fever hospital:

The whole fever hospital ... with glass partitions in between and we were supposed to go out of the cubicle and leave all your things, and wash your hands, disinfect your hands, and then go in the next cubicle, out through the door and into the next cubicle, put their gown on and all that. And that was the strictest thing we had to obey, there was no relaxation on that regime ever, ever, ever, always had to do that. And then when the Blitz came the glass partitions were all taken down because of the glass, danger of broken glass and the people popped from one cubicle into the other and nothing happened, no cross infection.[117]

I have not located any data that conceded a direct impact of the Blitz on the decision to allow Jewish refugees to resume nursing. However, once the women were readmitted, hospitals promptly took advantage of their presence. The refugees' return to hospital work was not limited to patient care. Wendy Webster examines the absurdity that male refugees felt when they were released from internment and almost immediately recruited into the British Army. In their narratives of the episode, the men laughed at the 'sudden switch in meaning of their nationality – from enemies to soldiers in British uniform in less than twelve hours'.[118] Female refugees were encouraged to return to work but with far fewer alternatives than their male compatriots. Refugee nurses were now deemed sufficiently trustworthy not only to return to the profession but also to engage in the various forms of unpaid war work expected of the whole population.

Air raid precaution (ARP) work had been established before the war in anticipation of aerial bombardment. Susan Grayzel argues that a vast stream of propaganda was directed towards the women of Britain to take on the mantle of protecting the nation at home, as war workers, air-raid wardens and fire-watchers. Yet their gendered positions were reinforced.[119] Women were expected to fulfil their roles as citizens in war but only within existing notions of femininity.[120] As Grayzel maintains, the Home Office film unit's *Do It Now* heralded the primacy of women's role and their work in civil defence.[121] Nevertheless, men remained in charge.[122] The Air Raid Precautions Bill was enacted in December 1937, presaging the civilian effort in expectation of aerial bombardment. The ARP enrolled 200,000 civilians. This volunteer workforce included doctors, nurses and non-professional workers who would distribute gas masks, train in anti-gas measures and ensure, if and when war was declared, that blackout orders were followed.[123] The Act estimated that almost half of the ARP workers required would be women.[124] In 1938, a year before the commencement of war, the national movement of women to join the ARP was well under way. By the end of the year, 32,000 had enrolled with the Women's Voluntary Services for Air Raid Precautions, or WVS, as they became known.[125]

On 14 September 1942, the 'Fire Prevention (Business Premises) (No. 3) Order, which included women in the fire watching service, came into force'.[126] According to the exemption rules, 'Whole-time nurses and midwives' were exempt, but this does not appear to have applied to nurses in training.[127] Whilst nursing in the fever hospital, Hockey recalled, 'We had the different buildings for the different diseases ... scattered throughout a very large sort of complex and we used to have to go from one to another to do fire watching ... and it was a fascinating experience – quite dangerous.'[128] Hockey's somewhat spirited analysis of the danger and the fascination inherent in it belied the fear that she and the nation felt at the possible incursion of German forces. Trudie Moos admitted that her greatest fear 'was the possibility of German paratroops being dropped on British soil'.[129] For the refugees, the thought of a German invasion must have been terrifying. Many were only too aware of the situation for their families and friends in Nazi territories. Even as the Blitz seemed to come to an end, no one could be sure that it had. Anxieties remained high that its purpose was to 'soften' the country in preparation for invasion: 'A state of alertness was maintained and would be reactivated on occasions both as a defence and to encourage the war effort.'[130]

'Straight to the wards'

The Blitz ended in the spring of 1941 as Hitler turned his attention to Russia. The war continued into its third year. With so many qualified nurses volunteering for military service, great responsibility was placed on probationer nurses. In the absence of modern treatments and drugs, particularly penicillin, a probationer nurse's work was physical, arduous and sometimes technically demanding. The loss of men to the Forces and working-class women to the factories meant that the nursing staff needed to undertake orderly and ward domestic duties as well. Whilst nursing was nominally a profession, the lack of academic study and the requirements to undertake domestic duties added to its unpopularity amongst British young women. Few hospitals even had any sort of preliminary training for probationer nurses; their work on the ward started immediately and this usually meant menial tasks for the first few months. In her oral history, Edith Bown was asked, 'Was there any teaching before you went to the wards?' Her reply was, 'No, of course not. Straight to the wards.' She continued, 'I don't know about the training, I don't know what the sluice is like now but it was pretty grim.'[131]

Mia Ross recalled arriving at the Nurses' Home at the Keighley and Victoria Hospital and being shown to her room. The very next day she was sent to the matron's office for a short interview and from there, straight to the children's ward. She admitted that the work was hard and the hours long: 'I was not used to physical work – being on your feet all day so I got very tired and had no trouble sleeping. But you knew there was a war going on and everybody had to work hard and so you carried on.' By 1942 Ross passed her preliminary examination and moved into her second year. Now with more responsibility, she was expected to take her turn on medical and surgical wards: 'I have a vivid memory of those days when penicillin was discovered but not available for use. Patients who had pneumonia usually suffered a crisis and that happened in the early hours of the morning. Some managed to conquer it and survived and others did not and died.'[132]

The lack of access to antibiotics in this early war period is a recurrent theme in the narratives of the refugee nurses, as it is in testimonies of British nurses working during the war. With the almost total relaxation of restrictions, Lisbeth Hockey was able to return to general nursing, completing her general training at Watford General Hospital in Hertfordshire. Without antibiotics, they just had 'basically good nursing' and the sulphonamides: 'You were given a patient to care for and you cared for that patient. You did everything that patient needed.'[133] Hortense Gordon recalled the chronically ill children and the time-consuming nursing care required: 'It was total care and gradually they improved, and, of course, don't forget, it was the days before antibiotics.'[134] Lee Fischer remembered nursing without antibiotics during the war: 'I call myself a nurse before penicillin because we had no IVs during the war, nothing. And whenever we pulled a patient through, it was our work, what we did for them.'[135] Penny Starns, a historian of Second World War nursing, cites Sister Monica Baly of the Princess Mary's Royal Air Force Nursing Service recalling the importance of good nursing care before antibiotics. Doctors, she maintained, would say, 'I can't do anything, but nursing will do a great deal.'[136] Nurses may have been poorly paid, their conditions of work debilitating, but they were a vital part of the healthcare system, needed by doctors, hospitals and the public.

The need for nurses on the home front continued even as the bombs ceased. Nursing was seen as a valuable contribution for women towards the war effort.[137] As the war progressed into its middle years, more refugees turned to the profession as a means of independence. On 1 January 1942, Trudie Moos started her nurse training at the Royal Free Hospital in London. Unlike Ross, who trained at a small local hospital, entering a major London teaching hospital meant that Moos was able to spend the first eight weeks in the preliminary training school learning fundamental nursing skills.[138] Moos was impressed with the system, describing Miss Sheehan as a 'good tutor [who] gave us a lot of useful instruction during the weeks of the Preliminary Training School. The subjects included Anatomy and Physiology, Hygiene, Practical Nursing and

First Aid ... During the weeks of the Preliminary Training School, we all became good friends.'[139] Once on the wards Moos accepted that the work was hard, though interesting, and the patients were friendly:

> The physical work was hard. Few patients were allowed to do anything for themselves. We had to bathe them in bed, make their beds at least twice a day, lift the patients, feed the helpless ones, clean their mouths and attend to their pressure areas. The bed baths gave us a splendid opportunity to listen to the patients' worries ... As chatting to patients was not generally encouraged unless you were actually doing something for them physically, junior nurses had the best chance to listen.[140]

Like Moos, the other refugee nurses continued with their training, working alongside their British counterparts, helping the population of Britain manage wartime illness and injury. As her quote above identifies, war work for all nurses, refugees and their British colleagues was hard and demanding, with little free time, and in many cases limited educational input. However, despite the assertion of several refugee nurses that they were all in it together, it is clear from both written and oral narratives that they had a much more challenging war than British nurses. The refugee nurses had to manage the great shifts in culture and language from their lives in Continental Europe to the new world of the British hospital. They also needed to cope with anti-Jewish and anti-German hostility and the knowledge that they had nowhere to go if they did not like nursing or if they were not liked. Most importantly, they needed to live with the knowledge of the situation in Nazi territories, the dwindling contact with their families left behind and ultimately the knowledge of their almost certain deaths. Reports of their families' deportations and deaths infiltrated their lives in a devastating manner. Most hospitals did not understand the impact of what had happened and matrons were not always sympathetic.

'I had no one'

Bown was the only refugee and only Jew at her hospital in Northern Ireland, a country ridden with sectarian hatred between the Catholics and Protestants. She thought that she had made one friend, the only Protestant student nurse in the hospital:

> She said, 'I am going to see my grandmother, would you like to come with me?' And when we got to the front door, she said you will have to wait out here, my grandmother wouldn't like a German Jew to come in. So I waited an hour while she visited. And the other thing, she invited me to her wedding ... and three days before the wedding she said 'my parents don't want you to come.' That was my friend. No, I had no-one.[141]

This part of her oral history was not full of the stories of torture, murder and brutality that form many narratives of Holocaust survival, but it was the one I found most difficult to read. Indeed, Anna Sheftel and Stacey Zembrzycki argue that it is often not the 'gory details' that are the hardest to hear but the politicising of the personal.[142] The absence of all that a young woman's life should have – home, family and kindness – are replaced by the harsh realities of antisemitic and anti-foreign actions. Edward H. Powley, an academic from a business and policy background, highlights the importance of close relationships when the 'physical place to call "home"' is missing.[143] This is particularly important when one considers Holocaust survivor expert Henry Greenspan's analysis that 'the present and absent sense of "home" is always part of the survivors' accounts'.[144] With their homes destroyed, these young refugees would have relied on the kindness of their work colleagues and those in positions of authority. Instead, Bown is alienated twice, once by the girl whom she thought her friend and by once by the hospital chaplains, who said she would 'go to hell' for being Jewish.[145]

Even if other refugees did not describe such stark forms of alienation, they experienced the challenges brought about by estrangement from family and home. Lisbeth Hockey admitted, 'I had no home and no money or anything. I was totally dependent on my nursing livelihood for anything.'[146] The matron's report from her early training period at the London Hospital, Whitechapel, acknowledged that when she 'received [a message] to say her father had died, she was greatly distressed about this, and much concerned about her mother[;] in consequence her health suffered'.[147]

Unlike British girls who could leave nursing if they did not like it and return home, the refugee nurses had limited alternatives and no family to return to. Furthermore, Hockey could not go home to care for her bereaved mother. The lack of familial support created financial difficulties as well. Edith Bown recalled, 'and I was told the first three months there would be no pay and I would have to supply the uniform. So I had to go cap in hand to the [refugee] Committee and I think ... they had to fit me out.'[148] Stephanie Homer argued that for the Kinder, 'the separation from family and dislocation from everything familiar was emotionally scarring'.[149] To then continue the struggle as an adult trying to survive and create a place for themselves in Britain must have only increased the 'overwhelming despair' of these young women. Bown's emotional dislocation continued into her training. In the absence of other refugee nurses, no one was concerned about her situation; the matron did not even address her by her correct name. Bown recalled that she 'fell into every difficulty, like saying "OK" and Matron saying "that is not correct English, nurse Jacobs" ... Nobody of course pronounced my name.'[150]

Other refugees were keen to show that they were part of the war effort, as essential to the Allies as their British nursing colleagues. Gertrude Roberts maintained that when she began her nurse training, 'And still the war didn't intrude, being Jewish didn't intrude, I was kind of beginning at the beginning.'[151] But this relative ease changed later:

> I was a junior probationer, I had to scrub bed pans, I had to scrub bed wheels, I had to do all sorts of menial works which wasn't pleasant. I remember lying, practically on my stomach, under beds cleaning bed wheels while the doctors were doing the rounds. It was very demeaning again.[152]

The unwillingness to lay any blame on the British for the situation they were in reverberates across many refugee narratives. Marion Berghahn describes being '"grateful for" [as] a recurrent theme used by the older generation'.[153] Refugees were encouraged to be thankful that Britain had saved their lives. The desire therefore for the refugee nurses to make claims that all nurses were in the same position resonates throughout their stories. Yet if allowed and encouraged to be the subject of their story rather than its object, the narratives highlight the challenges of the wartime hospital world to their young lives.[154] Much of what Roberts described was the experience of every junior probationer. Yet the 'demeaning again' moments of lying on her stomach cleaning under the beds echoes the humiliation of Jews in Nazi ghettos who were forced to clean streets on their hands and knees. As the oral history was conducted by someone else, I was not able to probe this with her, but it is difficult not to make the connection. Judith Tydor Baumel refers to the 'feminine degradation' to which Jewish girls and women had been subjected whilst in Germany.[155] Working on her hands and knees under patients' beds, whilst the male medical staff moved around the ward, must have echoed the treatment that Roberts and other Jews experienced under Nazi rule.

The impact of being estranged in these ways placed the experience of the refugee nurse in war into a very different space than her British colleagues. The horror of their situation multiplied as they began to realise their parents had been murdered. According to Greenspan, when one's family had been killed, it might have been too unbearable to recall or recount the trauma: 'the anguish of being helpless to help others and above all bottomless loss and grief' were too hard to endure.[156] For Ross the ongoing terror of war and the reduction in correspondence from her parents coupled with rumours of atrocities were recalled with increasing emotion. Her description of her parents' death is raw and devastating: 'This is very difficult to put into words. I had a letter from my sister Lisl telling me that my parents had been transported to Minsk and presumed dead ... I was so shocked that I told nobody in the hospital.'[157]

As Ross took her preliminary exams to enter her second year of training, she received one of the last messages from her parents, in which they 'wished me luck in my exams'.[158] Before Cilly Haar commenced her nurse training, she regularly received Red Cross messages from her parents:

> We used to go to the Red Cross Office in Luton every month. I was happy, I wrote a message and often thanked my parents for the handwriting, that was important to me. Until I had the last message and I

was already in Gloucester [as a probationer nurse]. 'We are about to go on a journey where friends of ours were.' That was Poland ... and I knew what they meant.[159]

In her oral history, Haar immediately moved the talk on to her brother's life, unable to dwell on the unbearable sadness of her parents' deportation to a concentration camp. Bown received the final letter written to her by her mother through the Red Cross: '"I must go now, we won't see each other again, have a good life. Go to the hairdresser sometime. Love Mum". Kind of thing.'[160] In contradiction to Greenspan's theory that there are aspects of our lives that are too traumatic to speak about, it was Bown who felt that she was upsetting the interviewer with her narrative and wondered if the interviewer wanted her to continue. As Sheftel and Zembrzycki argue, oral historians are not always able to take the time to understand the fullness of a life. We may move the interview on to safer ground without allowing the participant to reflect on difficult periods.[161] We need, however, to pursue 'the subjective experience of the past more rigorously',[162] to uncover the life that has been led. We need to listen not only to what is said but to the meaning that the participant makes of what they are saying. Haar may not have been able to speak her words of grief, but in her memoir she recalled, 'I knew that I would never hear from my family again, but I always, even now, have hope that my sister is alive somewhere, though extensive searching has proved negative.' In the next lines, Haar returns quickly to happier thoughts, 'Despite this news I tried to get on with my life as best as I could under the circumstances. I was as happy as I could be. I led a very full life and did like nursing very much.'[163]

Foundations for their future careers

For most refugee nurses this period was one of challenges, extreme sadness and a real sense of fracture in their young lives. However, the war years also laid the foundations for their future careers. Towards the end of her general training, Annie Altschul considered what sort of work she wanted to do. In her oral history she mentioned a ward sister with whom she worked who had a sister at Mill Hill emergency psychiatric hospital. The ward sister asked Altschul if she would be interested in applying for her psychiatric training. Altschul commenced at Mill Hill in 1944 and stayed there until moving back to the Maudsley Hospital at the end of the war: 'I certainly knew I would stay the moment I arrived at Mill Hill.' She admitted that she enjoyed everything about the work, 'the patients, the fact that one was expected to think and there was opportunity to think, the patients were fascinating and you were encouraged to talk to them'. At Mill Hill, she marvelled that doctors would ask nurses about the patients: 'I enjoyed the feeling of being expected to contribute something but certainly it was the patients rather than that that caused me to feel I had a future in psychiatric nursing.'[164] But Mill Hill was critical for Altschul in other ways. She did not discuss the hospital as a safe space for Jewish refugees in her oral history. However, Peter Nolan commented on how important the Maudsley's Jewish community was to her, where open discussions were 'like a Jewish prayer meeting'.[165]

Several of the refugees whose narratives form this book found spaces for themselves in other areas of the nursing profession, routes that would be their life's work. Rarely were these places in the rigid world of the general hospital. Edith Bown went to Liverpool Tropical School of Medicine. Alice Fink, also keen to expand her education, took her theatre training between 1943 and 1944 at the North London Fever Hospital and then further instruction at the Brompton Chest Hospital. In 1944 she began her midwifery training. Rosa Sacharin was given the opportunity to attend a symposium on child psychology and initially faltered: 'I felt totally lost. The language was something I simply did not understand. What were they all talking about?' Still, eager to comprehend these new ideas, she was fortunate to find a book on the shelves in the nurses' recreation room. She asked the sister tutor if she could borrow it, 'and it was the first time anybody had ever asked for books ... and that got me very interested in psychology'.[166]

By 1943 the war appeared to be turning in favour of the Allies. But this did not make the lives of nurses easier. In the same year, the Government imposed restrictions on certain senior members of the nursing profession and those in community practice to volunteering for the military. The Control of Engagement Order, which took effect on 10 April in the same year, made the movement of junior nurses to new jobs more difficult.[167] Despite these ongoing challenges, the end of the war in the Middle East, the overthrow of Mussolini and Italy's signing an armistice with the Allies on 3 September 1943 raised the spirits of the nation.[168] The optimism was not to last.

The final year and the V1 and V2 missiles

Between June 1944 and March 1945, Britain was subjected to the bombing campaign of V1 and V2 missiles. Trudie Moos recalled that one ward was kept empty at the Royal Free Hospital in preparation for air-raid victims. The V1 bombs, or doodlebugs, as they were colloquially known, were pilotless missiles. The first one struck Britain just one week after the Allied troops landed at Normandy.[169] Of the V1s that were launched, only 23 per cent exploded with impact in the London region, but that still amounted to 2,420 bombs.[170] Moos recalled, 'The doodlebugs made an uncanny whistling noise which suddenly stopped, and then, after an eerie silence, there would be a loud explosion.'[171] She lamented the results:

> Again we were inundated with terrible casualties. At seven minutes past ten on 7th June 1944 in the evening, the Royal Free received a direct hit. The exact time was remembered as all the electric clocks stopped and the hands remained in that position ... A student nurse on night duty had been killed and so had one of the patients.[172]

Josephine Bruegel had left medicine by 1944 and was a mother with a baby. In her memoirs she admitted that V1 bombardment had become so unbearable that she and her infant were evacuated to Cardiff, where they lived with a mining family who had an outside lavatory and no bath.[173] In September 1944, the defeat of the Allies at the Battle of Arnhem and the failed assassination attempt on Hitler gave rise to growing pessimism in Britain. Bruegel felt that she should return to London, work as a doctor once more to support the war effort and be close to her husband during the bombing campaign: 'One evening I was called urgently to the hospital. A hotel housing some American soldiers had been hit and there were lots of casualties.'[174]

According to Martin Gilbert, the British Government announced the end of the V1 missile campaign on 7 September 1944. No bomb had been sent across the Channel for a week, but the Government's optimism was too hasty; the V2 rockets were unleashed one day later on 8 September. The first ones landed on the outskirts of the capital, killing three people.[175] The V2s were more deadly than the V1s because, although they were less accurate, they travelled at the speed of sound. There was no warning of their impact. There was no defence against them. The campaign lasted six months.

The V2 rockets finally stopped in March 1945. By this time the true horror of the extermination of the Jews of Europe began to be realised. Auschwitz was liberated in January 1945, though knowledge of the atrocities there was only slowly released. Then in April 1945, the British Army liberated Bergen-Belsen. The BBC sent the journalist Richard Dimbleby, who reported on 19 April, only four days after Derrick Sington, a captain with the Intelligence Corps, first entered the camp.[176] Images of the camp were circulated in the press and the British population started to realise just what had been happening in Nazi territories. Refugee nurses, like all refugees in Britain and across the globe, started to try to find out what had happened to their families and friends who had not managed to escape. Fink recalled, 'And then the waiting started. We didn't know where to turn. We wanted to find out what happened to our people, to our families. But it was a long, long wait.'[177] In 1946, Rosa Sacharin learned that her mother had survived and she arrived in Glasgow to live with her daughters in February 1947. According to Sacharin, one of the first things she said when she arrived in Britain was that she would never set foot in Germany again:

> And I can understand that ... when she told me that my aunt and her children were gassed, I said to her 'but how do you know that?' And she then told me that a German soldier came home on leave and she went to him and said to him that her sister and her nephews and nieces were on the transport to Riga: I have never heard from them ... he laughed cynically and he said, 'Riga? They never reached Riga; they were gassed in the trains.'[178]

Given the sheer horror of the unfolding tragedy, it is probably not surprising that the personal testimonies of the refugee nurses are relatively silent regarding their families' murders. Of all the narratives used for this book, only Trudie Moos wrote about the developing knowledge of the camps:

> Soon news reached us of the horrors discovered by the allied forces in the concentration camps. Ruth learned that her mother and father had not survived but could never discover the details of their deaths. Similarly Carla's parents, my uncle and aunt, had both perished. My father's brother and aunt had survived the concentration camp, but both their sons and families had been killed. Gradually we heard about the deaths in camps of so many of our friends and relatives. It was difficult to imagine what they all must have suffered.[179]

Conclusion

The declaration of war on 3 September 1939 changed the lives of many women in Britain, but not in the watershed way that historians have often suggested. Women might have been encouraged and then conscripted into spaces usually reserved for men, but mostly their lives persisted within the accepted gendered system.[180] Nursing was considered a critical profession for women's support of the war effort. For the refugee nurses, the six years of war were a time of stark contrasts. In 1938, they were wooed by the nursing leadership, who saw their presence as a valuable way to bolster the profession's numbers. With the fall of France, all refugee nurses lost their nursing positions, though some did manage to continue in fever, maternity and psychiatric institutions, places which did not treat men and women from the Services. Less than six months later, the Government and profession once again called on refugees to support the health of the nation and war effort and return to nursing. Most willingly returned. For some, this was a real choice because they liked nursing; for others; it was pure pragmatism. They needed to do something for the war effort and nursing was better than some of the alternatives.

The 'courting' of refugees for the profession was clear opportunism on the part of the Government and nursing leadership. Nevertheless, many refugees saw it as an opportunity and were pleased to be given the chance to support the Allied effort and train for a profession at the same time. By the end of the war, several of the refugees were qualified and looking forward to a professional future. The growing knowledge of the extermination of European Jewry and the realisation that their parents, families and friends had been murdered in the most brutal fashion precluded any real joy for the end of the war. However, as will be demonstrated in the next chapter, refugee nurses accepted their place within the nursing profession and worked to support the post-war world and the birth of the National Health Service.

Notes

1 Kitty Schafer, oral history interview by Jane Brooks on 30 August 2017. Personal archive.
2 Brian Bond, 'The calm before the storm: Britain and the "Phoney War" 1939–40', *RUSI Journal* 135, 1 (1990): 61.
3 Arthur Marwick, *War and Social Change in the Twentieth Century: A Comparative Study of Britain, France, Germany, Russia and the United States* (London: Macmillan, 1974), 152.
4 Penny Starns, *Nurses at War: Women on the Frontline, 1939–45* (Stroud: Sutton Publishing, 2000), 8.
5 Starns, *Nurses at War*, 8. See also Susan McGann, Anne Crowther and Rona Dougall, *A History of the Royal College of Nursing, 1916–90: A Voice for Nurses* (Manchester: Manchester University Press, 2009), 104.
6 Susan R. Grayzel, *At Home and Under Fire: Air Raids and Culture in Britain from the Great War to the Blitz* (Cambridge: Cambridge University Press, 2012), 277.
7 Joel Morley, 'The memory of the Great War and morale during Britain's phoney war', *Historical Journal* 63, 2 (2020): 437–67.
8 Margaret Marflow (Weiss), 'For my Grandchildren' (2001), 52. A biographical database of European Medical Refugees in Great Britain, 1930s–1950s.: Oxford Brookes University, Oxford.
9 Marflow, 'For my Grandchildren', 52.
10 Sheer Ganor, 'Forbidden words, banished voices: Jewish refugees at the service of the BBC propaganda to wartime Germany', *Journal of Contemporary History* 55, 1 (2020): 102.
11 Colin Holmes, 'Enemy aliens?', *History Today* (September 1990): 26.

12 Central Council for Jewish Refugees, 'Report for 1940' (24 June 1941), 6. ACC/2793/5/A/85, London Metropolitan Archives (LMA).
13 Margot Hodge (Pogorzelski), 'My Life, 1920–1943', 2004.633. Library and Archives, Rubenstein Institute, USHMM, Washington, DC.
14 Jennifer Craig-Norton, '"We had the most marvellous time": Jewish refugee domestics' narratives of internment in Britain during the Second World War', *Jewish Historical Studies: Transactions of the Jewish Historical Society of England* 52, 1 (2021): 41; Rachel Pistol, '"Heavy is the responsibility for all the lives that might have been saved in the pre-war years": British perceptions of refugees, 1933–1940', *European Judaism* 40, 2 (2017): 38.
15 Tony Kushner, *The Holocaust and the Liberal Imagination: A Social and Cultural History* (Oxford: Blackwell, 1994), 155.
16 Central Council for Jewish Refugees, 'Report for 1939', 13. ACC/2793/5/A/84, LMA.
17 Kushner, *Holocaust and the Liberal Imagination*, 155.
18 Kushner, *Holocaust and the Liberal Imagination*, 157.
19 Juliette Pattinson, *Behind Enemy Lines: Gender, Passing and the Special Operations Executive in the Second World War* (Manchester: Manchester University Press, 2007), 137.
20 These prohibitions were recalled in a number of refugees' testimonies. Trudie Moos, 'I Remember: My Life Story' (printed 1995). A biographical database of European Medical Refugees in Great Britain, 1930s–1950s, Oxford Brookes University, Oxford, 41; Hodge, 'My Life 1920–1943', 62; Lotte Heyman, oral history interview with Barbara Mortimer at her home in Buckinghamshire on 15 September 2009. Interview T235, Oral History Collection, RCN, Edinburgh; Elisabeth Katz (Rosenthal), oral history video interview by Sandra Bendayan on 4 August 1994. Gift of Jewish and Children's Services of San Francisco, the Peninsula, Marin and Sonoma Counties, USHMM, Washington, DC.
21 Marion Berghahn, *Continental Britons: German-Jewish Refugees from Nazi Germany* (Oxford: Berg, 1988), 139.
22 Moos, 'I Remember', 41.
23 Alice Fink (Redlich), oral history interview by Lyn E. Smith in November 1997. Interview 1775, Sound Archive, Imperial War Museum, London.
24 Moos, 'I Remember', 41; Marflow, 'For my Grandchildren', 52.
25 1951 United Nations Convention on the Refugee, as discussed in Andrew E. Shacknove, 'Who is a Refugee?', *Ethics* 95, 2 (1985): 275. It is acknowledged that this declaration was made twelve years after

the commencement of the Second World War. It is highlighted here because of the language used and the post-war developing understanding of alien status.
26 James C. Hathaway and Michelle Foster, 'Alienage', in James C. Hathaway and Michelle Foster (eds), *The Law of Refugee Status* (Cambridge: Cambridge Core 2014), https://www.cambridge.org/core/books/law-of-refugee-status/alienage/D1BEC5D910910E9AF870DBA82641D9ADb [accessed 29 September 2023].
27 Helen Haste, 'Asset, alien or asylum seeker? Immigration and the United Kingdom', *Prospects* 36, 3 (2006): 328.
28 Michael Molnar, 'Portrait of an alien enemy', *Psychoanalysis and History* 10, 2 (2008): 171.
29 Central Council for Jewish Refugees, 'Report for 1940', 7.
30 Executive of the Central Council for Jewish Refugees, 'Minutes of special committee meeting' (1 May 1940), 7. ACC/2793/01/01/07, LMA.
31 Tony Kushner, *The Persistence of Prejudice: Antisemitism in British Society during the Second World War* (Manchester: Manchester University Press, 1989), 144.
32 Louise Burletson, 'The state, internment and public criticism in the Second World War', in David Cesarani and Tony Kushner, *The Internment of Aliens in Twentieth Century Britain* (London: Frank Cass, 1993), 102.
33 Anonymous, 'News in brief: Employment of aliens', *Nursing Times* (25 May 1940): 554.
34 Anonymous, 'Alien nurses dismissed', *Nursing Mirror and Midwives' Journal* (15 June 1940): 258; Anonymous, 'To leave at once', *Nursing Times* (15 June 1940): 629.
35 Anonymous, 'Alien nurses', *Nursing Times* (22 June 1940): 653.
36 Anonymous, 'Employment of aliens', *Nursing Times* (13 July 1940): 725.
37 Dina Gold, *Stolen Legacy: Nazi Theft and the Quest for Justice at Krausenstrasse 17/18, Berlin* (Chicago: American Bar Association Pubishing, 2016), 76.
38 Susi Loeffler, oral history interview by Jane Brooks from Australia on 18 January 2018, via Zoom. Personal archive.
39 Josephine Bruegel, 'Reminiscences': oral history interview by Sylva Simsova between 1998 and 2001. 'The War Years', 1. OSP 2122, Wiener Holocaust Library, London.
40 Lisbeth Hockey, oral history interview at her home (interviewer not specified) in Edinburgh on 27 December 1987. Interview T26, Oral History Collection, RCN, Edinburgh.

41 Hockey, oral history interview, 1987. Hockey's first dismissal was from the University of Graz, Austria. She was expelled along with all other Jews and non-Aryans in 1938, following the Anschluss.
42 Altschul, oral history interview.
43 Fink, oral history interview.
44 Hodge, 'My Life, 1920–1943', 64.
45 Hodge, 'My Life, 1920–1943', 67.
46 Glyn Prysor, 'The "fifth column" and the British experience of retreat, 1940', *War in History* 12, 4 (2005): 418–47.
47 Sonya O. Rose, *Which People's War? National Identity and Citizenship in Wartime Britain 1939–1945* (Oxford: Oxford University Press, 2003), 92.
48 Rose, *Which People's War?*, 93.
49 Kushner, *Persistence of Prejudice*, 12.
50 Rose, *Which People's War?* 103.
51 Marianne Parkes, 'The Past and other Pastimes' (no date), 8. A biographical database of European Medical Refugees in Great Britain, 1930s–1950s, Oxford Brookes University, Oxford.
52 Tony Kushner, 'Clubland, cricket tests and alien internment, 1939–40', in David Cesarani and Tony Kushner (eds), *The Internment of Aliens in Twentieth Century Britain* (London: Frank Cass, 1993), 90.
53 Holmes, 'Enemy aliens', 25.
54 Miriam Kochan, 'Women's experience of internment', in David Cesarani and Tony Kushner (eds), *The Internment of Aliens in Twentieth Century Britain* (London: Frank Cass, 1993).
55 Craig-Norton, '"We had the most marvellous time"', 38.
56 Craig-Norton, '"We had the most marvellous time"', 50.
57 Katz, oral history video interview.
58 Hodge, 'My Life, 1920–1943', 67.
59 Craig-Norton, '"We had the most marvellous time"', 55.
60 Kochan, 'Women's experience of internment'.
61 Katz, oral history video interview.
62 Hodge, 'My Life, 1920–1943', 69.
63 Pistol, '"Heavy is the responsibility for all the lives that might have been saved"', 39.
64 Tony Kushner, 'Finding refugee voices', in Anthony Grenville and Andrea Reiter (eds), *Political Exile and Exile Politics in Britain after 1933* (Amsterdam: Rodopi, 2011), 127.
65 Moos, 'I Remember', 43.
66 Schafer, oral history interview.
67 Fink, oral history interview.

68 Tony Kushner, *Journeys from the Abyss: The Holocaust and Forced Migration from the 1880s to the Present* (Liverpool: Liverpool University Press, 2017), 93.
69 Hodge, 'My Life, 1920–1943', 69.
70 Just an alien nurse, 'Aliens wish to serve', *Nursing Mirror and Midwives Journal* (3 August 1940): 415.
71 U. Herz, 'Refugee nurse's plea', *Nursing Mirror and Midwives' Journal* (9 November 1940): 142.
72 Just an alien nurse, 'Alien nurse wishes to serve', *Nursing Mirror and Midwives Journal* (29 June 1940): 317.
73 Executive of the Central Council for Jewish Refugees, 'Minutes of special committee meeting', 7.
74 Bruegel, 'Reminiscences', 36.
75 Susi Loeffler, 'The Family Löffler: Part V – 1939: Escape of Susi' (unpublished ms, 2017), 10–11. The interview was undertaken by Susi Loeffler's nephew.
76 Annie Altschul, oral history interview at her home in Edinburgh. No date. Interview T8, Oral History Collection, RCN, Edinburgh.
77 Hockey, oral history interview, 1987.
78 Tony Kushner and David Cesarani, 'Alien internment in Britain during the twentieth century: An introduction', in David Cesarani and Tony Kushner (eds), *The Internment of Aliens in Twentieth Century Britain* (London: Frank Cass, 1993), 5.
79 General Committee of the Nursing and Midwifery Department, 'The following resolution was unanimously passed' (29 August 1940). Aliens Home Office Department, HO 213/521, National Archives, Kew, London.
80 Anonymous, 'Alien nurses in hospitals', *Nursing Mirror and Midwives' Journal* (13 July 1940): 342.
81 General Committee of the Nursing and Midwifery Department, 'The following Resolution was unanimously passed'.
82 A. M. Frey to E. N. Cooper, 'Dear Mr Cooper' (18 October 1940), 1–2. Aliens Home Office Department, HO 213/521, National Archives, Kew, London.
83 Anonymous, 'Aliens may nurse again', *Nursing Mirror and Midwives' Journal* (9 November 1940): 121. It is worth noting, that in the same issue of the journal, a letter was published by a refugee, U. Herz, who wrote of her dismay at being dismissed. It is not clear why there is one letter saying that aliens could return to nursing employment and a letter saying the opposite. It is possible that the letter from Herz was written earlier, before the regulations

were relaxed. It is also possible that some hospitals were quicker to reinstate their refugee nurses.
84 Frey to Cooper, 'Dear Mr Cooper' (18 October 1940), 1–2.
85 Yarm School Assembly, A talk on the theme of 'Great Lives', 2 June 2014. A talk given by Eva Flatow's son, Dr David Gordon, 2. 'French leave' refers to a departure without ceremony, permission or notice.
86 Hockey, oral history interview, 1987.
87 Katz, oral history video interview. According to Katz's interview, it was normal at that time to go back to the beginning of your training if you interrupted it for any reason.
88 Hodge, 'My Life, 1920–1943', 71.
89 Marflow, 'For my Grandchildren', 54.
90 Altschul, oral history interview. No date. Trudie Moos noted that whilst most of the probationers in her 'set' at the Royal Free Hospital were between 19 and 24 years of age, there were two women of about thirty years old, one who was a teacher and the other a vet. Moos, 'I Remember', 47.
91 Peter Nolan, 'Annie Altschul's legacy to 20th century British mental health nursing', *Journal of Psychiatric and Mental Health Nursing* 6 (1999): 268.
92 Nolan, 'Annie Altschul's legacy', 268.
93 Susi Loeffler, 'Extract from draft: Appendix 4', unpublished ms, July 2017, 3.
94 The BBC employed a number of Jewish refugees as translators and some also for the German service, which broadcast propaganda into Nazi Germany to instil defeatism in the populace. See for example, Ganor, 'Forbidden words, banished voices'.
95 Schafer, oral history interview.
96 Lee Fischer (Liesl Einstein), oral history interview by Jane Brooks on 12 October 2017. Personal archive.
97 Hortense Gordon, oral history interview by Sharon Rapaport in London on 3 July 2004. Interview 65, Refugee Voices: Association of Jewish Refugees (AJR) Audio-Visual Testimony Archive, British Library, London.
98 Parental visits to children in hospital remained limited until the work of John Bowlby, Mary Ainsworth and James Robertson paved the way for unlimited parental visiting from the 1950s. Graham Mooney and Jonathan Reinarz, 'Hospital and asylum visiting in historical perspective: Themes and issues', in Graham Mooney and Jonathan Reinarz (eds), *Permeable Walls: Historical Perspectives on Hospital and Asylum Visiting* (Amsterdam: Rodopi, 2009), 10. See also, Inge

Bretherton, 'The origins of attachment theory: John Bowlby and Mary Ainsworth', *Developmental Psychology*, 28, 5 (1992): 759–75.
99 Hortense Gordon, oral history interview by Jane Brooks at her home in London on 27 October 2017. Personal archive.
100 Medals were issued by many nursing schools up until the 1980s and were awarded to the best nursing student of the year.
101 Gordon, oral history interview, 2017.
102 Cilly Haar (Brauer) oral history interview by Jane Brooks at her home in London on 4 September 2017. Personal archive.
103 Cilly Haar, *Then and Now: The Memoirs of Cilly Haar, nee Brauer*, 2. There is no further information about this publication.
104 Penicillin was first trialled and used for military patients only in the desert war from 1943. According to medical historian Peter Neushul, it was probably the 'most significant achievement of the Second World War science and technology'. Peter Neushul, 'Fighting research: Army participation in the clinical testing and mass production of penicillin during the Second World War', in Roger Cooter, Mark Harrison and Steve Sturdy (eds), *War, Medicine and Modernity* (Stroud: Sutton Publishing, 1998), 204. It was not until 1946 that there was sufficient penicillin in Britain to make it available to the civilian population. Robert Bud, *Penicillin: Triumph and Tragedy* (Oxford: Oxford University Press, 2007), 75.
105 Hockey, oral history interview, 1987.
106 Katz, oral history video interview.
107 Angus Calder, *The Myth of the Blitz* (London: Random House, 1991), 171.
108 Brad Beaven and John Griffiths, 'The blitz, civilian morale and the city: Mass-Observation and working-class culture in Britain, 1940–41', *Urban History* 26, 1 (1999): 71–88.
109 Tom Harrisson, *Living Through the Blitz* (London: Penguin, 1990).
110 Juliet Gardiner, *The Blitz: The British Under Attack* (London: Harper Press, 2010), 170.
111 Jane Brooks, 'The bombing Blitz of London and Manchester, England, 1940 to 1944', in Arlene W. Keeling and Barbra Mann Wall (eds), *Nurses and Disasters: Global, Historical Case Studies* (New York: Springer, 2015), 122.
112 Rose, *Which People's War?*, 11.
113 Gertrude Roberts, oral history interview by Alan Dein on 23 January 1982.Audio 184. Oral History Collection, Jewish Museum, London.
114 Moos, 'I Remember', 43.
115 Altschul, oral history interview.

116 Fischer, oral history interview.
117 Hockey, oral history interview, 1987.
118 Wendy Webster, 'Enemies, allies and transnational histories: Germans, Irish, and Italians in Second World War Britain', *Twentieth Century British History* 25, 1 (2014): 64.
119 Lucy Noakes, *Women in the British Army: War and the Gentle Sex, 1907–1948* (London: Routledge, Kindle edition, 2006), 14.
120 Noakes, *Women in the British Army*, 52.
121 Grayzel, *At Home and Under Fire*, 278.
122 Harrisson, *Living Through the Blitz*, 35.
123 Grayzel, *At Home and Under Fire*, 218.
124 Lucy Noakes, '"Serve to save": Gender, citizenship and Civil Defence in Britain, 1937–41', *Journal of Contemporary History* 47, 4 (2012): 743.
125 Gail Braybon and Penny Summerfield, *Out of the Cage: Women's Experiences in Two World Wars* (London: Pandora, 1987), 152.
126 Labour Research Department, 'Fire watching for men and women: Worker's pocket book series' (London: Labour Research Department, 1942): 2, CP/ ORG/MISC/11/01: Labour History Archive Study Centre: People's History Museum, Manchester. Although this booklet postdates the Blitz, it was the updated version of previous booklets on fire-watching, the first which was published in May 1941. Labour Research Department, 'Fire watching for men and women', 2.
127 Labour Research Department, 'Fire watching for men and women', 12.
128 Lisbeth Hockey, oral history interview by Helen Sweet at her home in Edinburgh on 13 August 1996. Interview T221, Oral History Collection, RCN, Edinburgh.
129 Moos, 'I Remember', 43.
130 Gardiner, *Blitz*, 43.
131 Edith Bown (Jacobowitz), oral history interview by Barbara Mortimer in Maidstone on 24 May 2008. Interview T379, Oral History Collection, RCN, Edinburgh.
132 Mia Ross (Maria Fuchs), 'War memories', 13–14. Personal archive.
133 Hockey, oral history interview, 1987.
134 Gordon, oral history interview, 2017.
135 Fischer, oral history interview. IVs are intravenous infusions.
136 Starns, *Nurses at War*, 72. The advent of penicillin raised concerns with the nation's nursing staff that their work would no longer be important. Barbara Mortimer cites Winifred Hector, a ward sister at St Bartholomew's Hospital in London. It was as if 'nursing had gone

out of the window'. Barbara Mortimer, *Sisters: Extraordinary True-Life Stories from Nurses in World War Two* (London: Hutchinson, 2012), 196.
137 Penny Summerfield, *Reconstructing Women's Wartime Lives: Discourse and Subjectivity in Oral Histories of the Second World War* (Manchester: Manchester University Press, 1998), 57.
138 The first preliminary training school was founded by Rebecca Strong at the Glasgow Royal Infirmary in the last decade of the nineteenth century. Strong, a key protagonist of the need for educated nurses, felt that all probationers required theoretical knowledge before they entered the ward environment. St Thomas's Hospital in London did not begin theirs until 1910 after the death of Florence Nightingale, who was against learning that did not happen in the ward environment. By 1913, St Thomas's had appointed its first sister tutor to lead the probationers' learning in these preliminary weeks of training. Miss Coode, 'The Nightingale Home, 1903–1910.' H1/ST/NTS.Y13/4/14, LMA. For a broader discussion of the training of nurses in the late nineteenth and early twentieth centuries, see for example, Anne Marie Rafferty, *The Politics of Nursing Knowledge* (London: Routledge, 1996); Jane Brooks, '"Visiting Rights Only": The Early Experience of Nurses in Higher Education', PhD thesis, London School of Hygiene and Tropical Medicine, 2005.
139 Moos, 'I Remember', 47.
140 Moos, 'I Remember', 48.
141 Bown, oral history interview.
142 Anna Sheftel and Stacey Zembrzycki, 'Only human: A reflection on the ethical and methodological challenges of working with "difficult" stories', *Oral History Review* 37, 2 (2010): 203.
143 Edward H. Powley, 'Reclaiming resilience and safety: Resilience activation in the critical period of crisis', *Human Relations* 62, 9 (2009): 1299.
144 Henry Greenspan, 'The unsaid, the incommunicable, the unbearable, and the irretrievable', *Oral History Review* 41, 2 (2014): 241.
145 Bown, oral history interview.
146 Hockey, oral history interview, 1987.
147 Matron's remarks, 'Register of probationers entering training in 1938–39', cited in Laurence Dopson, 'Obituary: Lisbeth Hockey – Pioneer of nursing research', *Independent* (25 June 2004). C300/1/9/3, RCN, Edinburgh.
148 Bown, oral history interview; Jennifer Craig-Norton highlights the fiscal concerns of the Refugee Committee which shouldered much of

the burden of the Kinder. Jennifer Craig-Norton, *The Kindertransport: Contesting Memory* (Bloomington: Indiana University Press, 2019), 45.

149 Stephanie Homer, 'The resilience of the refugee: How Kindertransport memoirs complicate understandings of "resilience"', *Transactions of the Jewish Historical Society of England* 51 (2019): 107.
150 Bown, oral history interview.
151 Roberts, oral history interview.
152 Roberts, oral history interview.
153 Berghahn, *Continental Britons*, 174.
154 Judith Tydor Baumel, '"You said the words you wanted me to hear but I heard the words you couldn't bring yourself to say": Women's first-person accounts of the Holocaust', *Oral History Review* 27, 1 (2000): 17.
155 Baumel, '"You said the words you wanted me to hear"', 38.
156 Greenspan, 'The unsaid, the incommunicable, the unbearable', 239.
157 Ross, 'War memories', 15. On the next page of her memoirs, Ross wrote that she had only recently had it confirmed that they were shot in the woods just outside Minsk: 'There were no survivors.'
158 Ross, 'War memories', 14.
159 Haar, oral history interview.
160 Bown, oral history interview.
161 Anna Sheftel and Stacey Zembrzycki, 'Who's afraid of oral history? Fifty years of debates and anxiety about ethics', *Oral History Review* 43, 2 (2016): 348.
162 Kathryn Anderson, Susan Armitage, Dana Jack and Judith Wittner, 'Beginning where we are: Feminist methodology in oral history', *Oral History Review* 15, 1 (1987): 108.
163 Haar, *Then and Now*, 25.
164 Altschul, oral history interview. No date.
165 Peter Nolan, personal conversation on 22 September 2022 regarding Annie Altschul, via Zoom.
166 Rosa Sacharin, oral history interview by Barbara Mortimer on 28 April 2010. Interview T407, Oral History Collection, RCN, Edinburgh.
167 Anonymous, 'Ministry of Labour and National Service: The Nurses and Midwives (Registration for Employment) Order, 1943', *British Journal of Nursing* (April 1943): 44.
168 Joanna Bourke, *The Second World War: A People's History* (Oxford: Oxford University Press, 2001), 118.
169 Gabriel Moshenska, 'Moaning Minnie and the doodlebugs: Soundscapes of air warfare in Second World War Britain', 3. https://

discovery.ucl.ac.uk/id/eprint/1549850/1/Moshenska_Moaning%20Minnie%20and%20the%20Doodlebugs.pdf [accessed 28 September 2023].

170 Stephen G. Evans and Keith B. Delaney, 'The V1 (Flying Bomb) attack on London (1944–1945): The applied geography of early cruise missile accuracy', *Applied Geography* 99 (2018): 44.
171 Moos, 'I Remember', 57.
172 Moos, 'I Remember', 57. Moos wrote that this student had been in her set; she was under 24 years of age.
173 Josephine Bruegel, 'Memoirs', Wiener Holocaust Library, London, 45. https://wiener.soutron.net/Portal/Default/en-GB/RecordView/Index/23314 [accessed 29 September 2023].
174 Bruegel, 'Memoirs', 46.
175 Martin Gilbert, *The Second World War: A Complete History* (London: Phoenix, 2009), 589.
176 Christine Lattek, 'Bergen-Belsen: From "privileged" camp to death camp', in Jo Reilly, David Cesarani, Tony Kushner and Colin Richmond (eds), *Belsen in History and Memory* (London: Frank Cass, 1997), 39.
177 Fink, oral history interview.
178 Sacharin, oral history interview.
179 Moos, 'I Remember', 60. Ruth Pfifferling was a fellow refugee and trained with Moss at the Royal Free Hospital. Miss Cockayne, the matron, arranged for them to start their training together to be a support for each other. In her memoir, Moos wrote, 'She must have anticipated that we would become friends, a friendship which lasted until Ruth's untimely death' (p. 45).
180 Noakes, *Women in the British Army*.

4

From the post-war world to a nursing legacy

Refusing to surrender under any circumstances, Adolf Hitler committed suicide on 30 April 1945.[1] Eight days later, General Jodl signed for an unconditional surrender with General Eisenhower. The following day, on 9 May, Field Marshal Keitel signed an unconditional surrender to the Russians.[2] The war in Europe ended on 8 May 1945. With the cessation of hostilities, the demobilisation of Allied and Axis troops began. British troops experienced delays and challenges, but their discharge was more orderly than in 1918.[3] As men returned from the war, the women who had taken on home-front work returned to home and hearth. For many of them, wartime work had been a welcome opportunity, but with the 'regendering' of the post-war world, the labour of women in the public world of work was no longer wanted.[4] As Beate Fieseler and colleagues note, women's participation in war duties, such as anti-aircraft batteries – work which had been so vital to the war effort – needed to be forgotten quickly. Their actual removal from such work began even before the end of hostilities.[5] Official propaganda, such as *Rebuilding Family Life in the Post-War World*, encouraged or perhaps coerced women to return to the home and make way for demobilised soldiers to find work.[6]

Nursing was and remains a predominantly female occupation. There was, therefore, no requirement for nurses to leave their jobs for returning soldiers. Nor did the end of hostilities mean the end of nurses' war work. Many were not demobilised until as late as 1947; the need to care for sick and injured soldiers and civilians at home and overseas continued. The requirement for nurses to support work with prisoners of war, the inmates of liberated concentration camps and the starving children across Europe did not cease for several years.[7] For the Jewish refugee nurses, this work persisted as the realities of the fate of European Jewry unfolded.

The National Health Service, which was inaugurated on 5 July 1948, offered refugee nurses new possibilities for nursing the sick. The opening of borders enabled emigration, and many simply chose to marry. These seemingly positive elements to their professional and personal lives were blighted with a growing understanding of the extermination of European Jewry at Auschwitz, Bergen-Belsen and many more places of death. In his account of the work of the Friends Committee for Refugees and Aliens, Lawrence Darton argued, 'Reports of the brutal treatment of prisoners in concentration camps had begun to reach England and other countries very soon after Hitler came to power.'[8] Nevertheless, Bernard Wasserstein maintained, 'It was only with the liberation of the concentration camps in Western Germany by the British and American troops in the final weeks of war that there was a dawning realisation in Britain of the magnitude of the catastrophe that had befallen European Jewry.'[9]

This chapter explores how refugee nurses searched for meaning and peace after the horror of Nazism, as they forged a life for themselves in Britain and beyond. I examine the work and lives of the Jewish refugee nurses from the early post-war period and consider the significance of nursing to their lives and their influence on nursing within the gendered expectations of the time. Nursing was encouraged as a legitimate means for British women to support the war effort, but at the cessation of hostilities many decided to leave. In the decades following the Second World War, there were profound changes in the position of women and their access to higher education and professional work. Nursing, with its petty discipline, poor pay and long hours, lost out to more attractive work. Once again, the profession struggled to recruit and retain nursing staff. Yet, as I argue, nursing did witness slow but inexorable change, brought about as the Government, profession and higher education were forced to accede to the alterations in women's social and economic space. This chapter considers the impact and influence of refugee nurses on new ways of nursing within the gendered relationship of the nurse/doctor dyad and the place of women in the academy.

From the post-war world to a nursing legacy

I begin with a discussion of the extermination of European jewry and consider the inability of the British public to conceive murder on such an industrial level.[10] The failure to comprehend the scale of the lethal Nazi regime exacerbated the loneliness of the refugees as they came to terms with the loss of their families and friends and the knowledge of the murder of over six million Jews. The chapter explores the responses of the young nurses to this developing knowledge and the reactions of those around them to their suffering. It then examines the 'use' the refugee nurses made of their professional lives in order to find some sense of peace in the post-war world. The chapter considers the distinct 'spaces' in which the refugee nurses influenced the profession and those in their care. First, I assess their work as clinical nurses by exploring the work of Eva Minden and Alice Fink as part of the rehabilitation of the survivors of Bergen-Belsen concentration camp. Next I examine the work of others in Britain as part of the newly instituted National Health Service, both as hospital staff and in the community. I then consider the changing social, professional and educational sphere of women and the ramifications these changes had on the nursing profession. Using the experiences of Hortense Gordon and Lisbeth Hockey, this chapter explores the altering of relationships between the medical and nursing staff in community settings, to highlight the shifting expectations of women and the sometimes intransigent attitude of their medical colleagues. Finally, the chapter examines changes to nurse education, first through the progressive attitudes of Rosa Sacharin and Trudie Moos, and concludes with a discussion of the embryonic university departments of nursing and the development of nursing research. As I argue, these early manoeuvres into higher education enabled the profession to begin its shift towards an academic and evidence-based discipline, but this was not without its detractors.

The destruction of European jewry

The British Government was acutely aware of the mass murder of the Jews of Europe as early as 1942. According to Tony Kushner, the press frequently reported on the atrocities. On 27 October 1942, the

Manchester Guardian informed its readers of the ghettos and labour camps appearing across the Continent.[11] Two months later, C. J. Wright wrote in the same newspaper, 'The magnitude of the tragedy being perpetrated on the Jewish population of Nazi occupied Europe defies imagination. Two million European Jews according to reliable sources have already perished; 5,000,000 more are being hunted to their doom. What more can be done?'[12] The Government might not have wished to consider the reports of the left-wing press, but even the *Daily Telegraph* noted the atrocities. On 25 June 1942, it reported that 'More than 700,000 Polish Jews have been slaughtered by the Germans in the greatest massacre in the world's history.'[13] The Government received reports, which were sent directly to them, highlighting the extermination of Jews. No reply or acknowledgement was forthcoming.[14] Whilst some of the refusal to act on the knowledge was linked to the war itself, there was also a certain amount of incredulity. People simply could not believe the sheer enormity of the scale of murder that was being perpetrated.[15]

The extent of the rehabilitation required for those still alive, refugees and camp survivors alike, was beyond the comprehension of the Allies until images of the liberation of Bergen-Belsen were published. Kushner and colleagues maintain that at war's end, 'even those in the comfort of the cinemas, front rooms and libraries of the Home Front exposed to the newsreels, press and radio reports were left in a state of emotional shock by the attempts to communicate the horror of Belsen'.[16] According to David Cesarani, although the Allies may have been aware of the potential refugee problem, they were barely 'prepared or equipped' for the relief and rehabilitative organisation that was required.[17]

'I was still suffering from the trauma of losing my parents'

For the refugee nurses, many of whom were still very young women, the images and growing knowledge carried unimaginable terror. In her oral history, Edith Bown described receiving what she instinctively knew was the final letter her parents would ever send. Asked how she knew it was their last correspondence, Bown admitted to being very aware of the political situation, even in the early years of the war, 'because when we were on the farm, and I still visited the farm on days off, we had these sort of letters coming, we always knew and then the person whoever it was went to say the prayer for the dead'. Thus, when the final letter came, Bown broke down, devastated by the news. The response from the matron of her hospital demonstrated a complete lack of empathy: '"No English girl would have behaved like that." They gave me a dose of morphine and put me to bed.'[18] If Bown as a young woman was aware of the situation, it is inconceivable that the matron of a hospital was unaware and insensitive to the obvious consequences of learning that one's parents had been murdered. Perhaps it was her desire to not know. The knowledge that other European countries could have committed such atrocities on their own people was overwhelming for the majority of the population. Why not the matron of a small Irish hospital? Susi Linton's analysis of the situation frames the world of many of the refugees:

> I wanted to read the newspapers to see what's going on, the main interest what was going on in Germany, never mind what I did here. What was going on? What am I going to hear next? Well, slowly and slowly it came to light – concentration camps, no survivors. I didn't hear anything; I had no communication, so I had to come to the conclusion. Well that was unbelievable, we all went through – That's why we had to be together with other people with the same fate.[19]

Linton suggested that she was able to find others with whom she could share the burden of knowledge and therefore manage the grief. Not all refugees were so fortunate. Gertrude Roberts's narrative demonstrated the determination to keep going, the silence involved in such determination and the reality of the pain generated by this resolve:

> Hmmm, and then all we were told was [that my parents were] transported to an unknown destination. And here the whole problem, is one had to put it out of one's mind in order to survive, I went through years and years and years of kind of stunning myself into not knowing, not being able to know, not wanting to find out, because if I had found out I couldn't have gone on. So, I just threw myself in my job, I took a training in midwifery.[20]

If work was able to help her in the early years after the war, this was not to last. She admitted later: 'Ten years into my marriage I started gradually having nervous breakdowns ... I just went down, down, down, down the more I came towards facing the truth. Until, you know, in 1980 I nearly killed myself and that was the beginning of the way up.'[21] Susi Loeffler described similar trauma in the face of her parents' murder: 'I worked with a lot of Jewish refugee nurses and none of us ever talked about our past, we couldn't, I couldn't [inaudible], I never talked about it until I was about 40 or 50. I just couldn't do it. I couldn't read my parents' letters, I just couldn't, I was really [? bereft] you know. Anyway, um, you have to live with it.'[22] This silencing of traumatic experiences resonates through many of the narratives, particularly the oral histories. As psychologist and Holocaust interviewer Henry Greenspan argues, survivors have many reasons for their silences. The 'unsaid' maybe because they cannot speak of the trauma, but often it is simply because they choose not to.[23] Even the relief of the end of hostilities did not help. As Roberts asserted, 'I remember very little about VE Day, it didn't seem to matter to me very much. I was still suffering from the trauma of losing my parents.'[24]

Despite the developing knowledge of the extermination of European jewry, the impulse of most of the refugee nurses was to settle into the relative security of post-war Britain and their professional future. For two of the refugees whose narratives comprise this book, the end of the war created a critical moment in their lives and one which, far from removing them from this security, placed them directly in the face of the horror of the genocide. In 1946 the Government began to permit non-British nationals to support the displaced persons' programmes on the Continent. Alice Fink and Eva Minden both applied and were posted to Bergen-Belsen to help with the rehabilitation of the former inmates of concentration camps. Both saw this work as an opportunity to use their nursing skills to help other Jews, those who had not escaped but had miraculously managed to survive.

The relief and rehabilitation work of Fink and Minden

Bergen-Belsen originated as a transfer camp for influential Jews who could be used to barter with German prisoners of war in British and

American camps.²⁵ According to Hannah Craven, a historian of the liberation of Belsen, the camp retained this privileged status until 1943.²⁶ By 1944, the number of inmates had increased from 2,000 to 7,000. In December of that year, Josef Kramer, the ex-commandant of Auschwitz, was appointed to govern Belsen and immediately established it as a 'proper' camp.²⁷ With the disintegration of the Third Reich in early 1945 and the progression of the Russian Army, Nazi forces started the Death Marches. The Marches forced inmates from concentration and extermination camps across eastern Nazi territories to camps such as Belsen. The vast majority did not survive, but some did, and they arrived at Belsen as the numbers grew exponentially.²⁸

By the time the British Army arrived on 15 April 1945, Belsen was divided into two camps. Camp 1, which became known colloquially as the 'Horror camp', housed approximately 22,000 women and 18,000 men, 90 per cent of whom were of Jewish origin. Camp 2 held approximately 27,000 inmates. About 50,000 had died in the previous two months and 12,000 to 14,000 more were to die following liberation.²⁹ Yet, despite the camp's inmates being predominantly Jewish, apart from the Jewish chaplain, Lesley Hardman, none of the early relief teams included Jewish nurses, doctors or welfare workers.³⁰

Ben Shephard argues that Jewish organisations failed to influence the relief efforts abroad.³¹ This may have been, he suggests, because of the military's suspicion of sectarian organisations.³² Jane Leverson, one of the earliest Jewish welfare workers to arrive, had originally volunteered with the Jewish Committee for Relief Abroad (JCRA). She became increasingly frustrated by the reluctance of the authorities and she joined the Quaker relief team instead.³³ In her oral history, Alice Fink, who eventually arrived with the Jewish Relief Unit (JRU) in 1946, maintained that before that time, only the British could go into the Occupied Zone and that was why she was delayed; not only was she in a reserved occupation, she was also an enemy alien.³⁴

The opportunity to use her nursing background to help the survivors also impelled Eva Minden to apply to the JRU on 17 June 1946. In her application she stated that she had qualified as a State Registered Nurse in 1945 and had been working as a district nurse. Both her parents were alive and living in London. Minden had dual nationality at birth, both German and British, but had been educated at the Jewish secondary school in Hamburg. She stated that she wished to be considered for relief work for a six-month period.[35] By September that year, the JRU had posted her to Belsen to work in the Glyn Hughes Hospital. Her memoir recalled that before welfare and other volunteers were sent to Belsen, they needed to undergo a preparatory course to prepare them for the horror: 'as I was a trained nurse, they thought I did not need a course'.[36] The mid-twentieth-century nursing world placed its community in a highly ambiguous physical and psychological 'space'. Nurses were simultaneously treated like children, with petty rules and regulations, and expected to shoulder huge burdens and responsibilities. The decision, therefore, that nurses did not require the preparation given to other workers, whilst unfortunate, is not surprising. It is clear from testimonies from many nurses who volunteered for Belsen that they were traumatised by the experience and that this trauma continued throughout their lives.[37] Minden anticipated that she would be one of several Jewish staff to go and support the rehabilitation effort.[38] In a letter to Miss Glover of the JCRA written on 14 October, she stated:

> I for one have been sent out under false pretences. When XXX [name unclear] wrote to me first, she gave me to understand that the hospital will be staffed by entirely Jewish staff, with trained nurses as sisters over DP [displaced persons] staff. That is not the case and will not be so either now or ever.[39]

The presence of Minden, Leverson and Fink might have provided some succour for the ex-inmates, but three Jewish women alongside eighty German nurses was a poor ratio, given the psychological trauma of Jewish survivors. In a report written in 1948 when back in England, Minden gave a full account of her time at Belsen:

> I was taken to the ward with these words of introduction: 'this is your staff nurse, sister is on leave. Don't criticise, but supervise and control. For three terrible days I gazed at the wall in my office. Gradually I recognised the ward work ... The third day I spent in the labour ward. Sterility poor, the women crawling about the floor screaming. (A sepsis soon developed from all this). A premature baby was born.

On her third day she collapsed. The young nurse almost knocking the life out of her, trying to make her breathe! She was almost black with cyanosis when I came in, with this my work began. I knew now that without criticism I would not be able to do the work. I had come to help the babies – not the nurses, and a certain amount of correction had to be done. I took charge of the baby, called the doctor, gave oxygen. The child soon recovered and several days of extreme care and gentleness saved her life.[40]

Although supporting the nurses working on the wards tested the skills of trained nurses like Minden, the work was certainly valued by her. Holocaust historian Jo Reilly argues that Minden was glad to work on the maternity ward, for at least here the young mothers started to learn to care again. Minden used her nursing expertise to support these young women to invest their long-abandoned aspirations for the future in their babies, creating a place of hope.[41] Initially Minden's work kept her in the maternity ward, but after a short while she decided to organise nursing courses for female inmates and was asked to support the children's ward as well. It was here that she met Alice Fink (then Redlich) who was in charge of the mothers and childcare in the camp.[42]

When the war ended in 1945, Fink had been working in a maternity hospital in Britain. Her experiences in this area of nursing made her an ideal choice to work with the children and women at Belsen. She arrived at Belsen in 1946, over a year after liberation. In her oral history, she recalled how the surviving inmates had started to organise themselves into groups, and the JRC worked with and supported them in their rehabilitative ventures. Fink set to work with children:

> By this time some of the younger people who have survived had gotten married, but had grown up without mothers, without families and needed to be taught how to live a normal life, especially if they had babies. In the simple matters of hygiene in their rooms, they needed to be taught ... many of them who had [lived] in the woods, if they hadn't been in the camps. Another friend who had come just a little before me, who was working in the hospital. We did many things together ... many people were working with the children and we tried to teach them general basics of clean living, hygiene and helping bringing up the children. Baby care was something that many of them were not really knowledgeable about.[43]

Like Minden, Fink found great value in helping these new mothers learn to care for their babies. Thus, when Minden returned to Britain in the spring of 1948, Fink took over the supervision of the maternity ward and nursing courses that Minden had established. Minden recalled her departure from Belsen in her memoir. One of the young nurses whom she had trained came to her in tears and told her of witnessing the murder of her mother and sisters at Auschwitz and her being saved by a woman who had dragged her away and brought her to Belsen, where she eventually enrolled in the nursing course organised by Minden. This course, she believed, gave her back a measure of self-esteem.[44]

When the British liberated Belsen, the original plan was to use those inmates who had been doctors and nurses to support the hospital work. Whilst there were some who had been able to manage this, most were unable to engage with even the most basic work. Many were not trained nurses, having volunteered for the work in the camps, possibly for additional rations, better sleeping arrangements and access to water and cleaning products.[45] But most were too weak, too debilitated and too sick themselves to cope with the work. Tragically, the years of Nazi rule and camp life left many unable to act for anyone but themselves and they could not give their patients even the most fundamental care.[46] The ability of Minden and Fink to start a nursing school a year later with survivors is therefore even more remarkable. Nursing work and the nursing profession were arguably not only able to rescue refugees like Minden and Fink and provide them with an escape route and worthwhile work; nursing work also provided rehabilitation for those who had survived the extermination and concentration camps.

Fink returned to Britain in 1947 to organise her citizenship, after which she returned to Belsen and married Hans (later John) Fink, who had been an inmate at Belsen before offering his services to the United Nations Relief and Rehabilitation Administration (UNRRA). Alice became pregnant – initially an obstacle to travel – but after gaining permission, she made her way to Chicago on 1 September 1949. Her daughter was born a few weeks later, after which she rescinded her British nationality and became a US citizen.[47]

Minden and Fink stand out in the story of post-war refugee nurses. There are no other records of refugee nurses returning to Germany to support surviving Jews. Nor are there any sources that provide insight into why they did not help. Probably, as suggested above, many simply wanted to return to a normal life. Some refused to return to what had been Nazi Europe. Annaliese Pearl admitted in her oral history that she refused to teach her children German and would never return to Austria.[48] Some married and could not leave their families. Others were employed by hospitals that might not have been able to relinquish valuable staff to work on the Continent. One critical factor that prevented nurses from moving into other work was the continuation of the Control of Engagement Order.[49] As Fink argued, nurses were part of a reserved occupation; they could not simply leave their jobs. Importantly, the new National Health Service (NHS), which was instituted on 5 July 1948, would need more nurses – a tall order given the haemorrhaging of professional staff.

A 1947 memorandum on the shortage of nurses by the Socialist Medical Association agreed with these reasons for poor recruitment and retention but felt they were not the only ones. Other criticisms included the deprivation of home life, living arrangements in a building usually within the hospital grounds, so that the nurse can never 'get away' from the hospital, poor and inadequate food, virtually no redress for understandable grievances and complaints and the unapproachability of the matron. Whilst these criticisms appear to be laid at the feet of the nursing profession, the SMA was not blind to the complicity of the medical profession: 'Those most intimately concerned, i.e., nurses and doctors show a continued lack of initiative in analysing the causes of this unsatisfactory state and in removing them.' The SMA then made several suggestions to improve the situation, including higher pay, building hostels away from the hospital and introducing a six-hour day to allow student nurses time to study, but none were put into practice.[50]

Nurses across the country volunteered to support the liberation of Europe and sought work across the Commonwealth.[51] Others left to marry or decided to leave a profession they entered solely to support the war effort.[52] The 1944 Education Act had expanded secondary education. More girls were staying on at school and hoping for places at universities or in teacher-training colleges.[53] Nursing also competed with the additional demands for teachers to educate extra female pupils. Teaching was better paid and had fewer petty restrictions than nursing.[54] Nurses were therefore not only leaving the profession, but recruitment from the educated middle-class population that the leadership sought did not materialise. The number of nurses across the country fell in the years between the end of the Second World War and the founding of the NHS. In March 1945, there were approximately 11,000 nursing vacancies across the country.[55] In 1948, that number had risen to between 40,000 and 50,000.[56] Refugee nurses might have been keen to support the NHS, but like their native British colleagues, they did not wish to remain in the confines of the civilian hospital ward.

Returning to normal: the National Health Service

Prior to the founding of the NHS in 1948, district nursing had been independent from the hospital service and funded through local nursing associations.[57] Families would pay a subscription fee to be a member of an association and have access to the service, or they would be required to pay for individual visits.[58] In this, as in many aspects of life, the disparities between the urban and rural populations were brought into stark relief. Patients in rural areas in Britain were less able to pay their subscriptions and were likely to be more reliant on the nurse's good will.[59] In her oral history, Lisbeth Hockey reflected on the changes to the nation's access to healthcare and therefore their own work:

> Didn't enjoy the pre-National Health Service days so much because you had to ask the patient for money. You know we had a receipt book and it was half a crown a visit and so you might have to give an old lady an enema and charge her half a crown when you've caused her a lot of misery and embarrassment. So that worried me, and some patients really couldn't afford it because [of] the little insurance scheme that they could have, but many of them didn't have it. And I remember that several of us ... used to put our own money in the bag and not charge the patient, which we could ill afford ourselves ... Horrible times. I remember with great delight the 5th of July 1948,

which was the day the National Health Service came into operation and that day, all our receipt books were done away with and there was no more money to be collected, and that was a very jubilant day.[60]

Nursing historian Rosemary White argued that the foundation of the NHS was one of the most important pieces of legislation in bringing profound change to nurses.[61] Clearly it had a substantial impact on Hockey, working as a domiciliary nurse. Nevertheless, Martin Gorsky and colleagues have pointed to the privileging of hospital medicine over community care in the newly established service.[62] This was and undoubtedly remains a problem for those keen to encourage preventative rather than curative health provision. However, Hockey's words suggest that community nurses were more immediately impacted by the advent of the NHS than their hospital-based colleagues.

According to Stephanie Snow and Angela Whitecross, opinion polls conducted when the Beveridge Report was first published in 1942 were enthusiastic for health reforms.[63] Voting in a Labour Government in 1945 suggests that the nation was ready for a more egalitarian country. Trudie Moos was as enthusiastic as Hockey for the NHS, calling it a 'shining example for and the envy of many countries, including the United States'.[64] Yet, despite the initial enthusiasm for the reforms and the momentous change to the healthcare of the nation, refugee nurses were less than effusive about its impact on them. The biographical questionnaire sent to refugee medics and nurses by Paul Weindling asked the respondent to describe the 'Impact of National Health Service (1948–) on career'. Of the approximately fifteen forms completed by those who worked or trained as nurses, only two filled in this section. Ilse Lewen wrote an emphatic 'none'.[65] Only Bettina Cohn made any comment about the value of the NHS: 'Improved conditions for patients and primitive outlook for preventative medicine.'[66] The latter criticism is particularly salient when considered against the analysis of Gorsky and colleagues. It appears that despite their claims that the new NHS was detrimental to preventative medicine, there were those who thought it helpful. Both Hockey and Cohn seem to suggest that community and primary care were very much beneficiaries.

The new NHS was to be paid for out of citizens' taxes. The whole population of Britain had equal access to it, whether they were young or old, or needed surgery or long-term care.[67] The nursing profession included those with a broad range of abilities, to those with barely any educational qualifications, to those with university-level entrance credentials. The breadth of nursing activities was considerable, and nurses worked in multiple and diverse locations. It is therefore to be expected that the new service was perceived in a number of different ways by the nation's nurses. It is only to be speculated on, but it appears the value the nurses saw in the new NHS depended on whether they worked in hospitals or the community, long-term care or the more prestigious acute care, which had always been better funded. What is perhaps surprising is that the profession's leaders did not embrace all the changes, soon realising that they would continue to be marginalised in policy debates. In his 1990 essay on the NHS, Charles Webster declared that 'the medical profession is regarded as the prime mover in health service reform. Whether acting in a technical capacity or as a professional pressure group, the medical profession is granted a predominant voice.'[68] Webster's article only refers to nursing twice, thus emulating the marginalisation of key nursing protagonists.

The establishment of the NHS was led by predominantly male doctors, politicians, intellectuals and pressure groups. Women's voices, specifically those of nurses, are largely silent, despite making up the largest single body of workers.[69] For Hockey and others in community practice, the changes the NHS brought to their daily working lives might have been substantial, but for many nurses, especially those in the hospital sector, the personal impact was not as obvious. Writing of her memories of the advent of the NHS, former Queen Alexandra's Imperial Military Nursing Service nursing sister Kitty Hutchinson recalled, 'Possibly the majority of nurses, including myself, were enthusiastic about universality and no payments.' But, she continued, 'I cannot recall any ceremonies or celebrations when the NHS became fact in July 1948 ... Things seemed to go on in exactly the same way for us nurses.'[70]

In 1947, Annie Altschul listened to the debates about the new health service. She was concerned that the system would be organised around medical schools, making training hospitals the places to train and be treated.⁷¹ The patients and staff in those hospitals without medical schools would be second-class citizens in much the same way as the municipal hospitals had been in the 1930s. As a member of the Socialist Medical Association (SMA), Altschul was excited about a healthcare system that would be free for all at the point of delivery.⁷² The contribution of left-wing medical practitioners and politicians cannot be ignored in the development of the NHS.⁷³ SMA members were themselves highly influential in the move to national health service provision, believing that health was a right.⁷⁴ The SMA was also an important friend to nursing, judging nurses to be professional colleagues to doctors rather than docile handmaidens.⁷⁵ According to Stephanie Snow, the historian at the centre of 'NHS at 70', 'The core purpose of the NHS is grounded in humanitarianism; it alleviates suffering through giving care and treatment to those in need.'⁷⁶ It is not surprising, therefore, that refugees like Hockey, Moos and Altschul were excited by its promise. The NHS represented all that was the negation of their younger lives. Prior to its institution, kindness to patients was not assured.⁷⁷ However, despite the enthusiasm of NHS proponents, it is not clear that the ethos actually altered much after 1948. In his analysis of chronic-care beds in the early post-war period, Webster describes wards as places where patients were 'exposed to humiliating conditions arguably little better than the concentration camps'.⁷⁸ Hockey's recollections offer a clear picture of the treatment of patients in the nation's public hospitals. Hospital nursing, she argued, was not sympathetic to patients: 'In the London hospital in those days … beds were numbered, we didn't even know the names of patients … they knew the patient by the disease they had.' She continued, 'That's why I got out of hospital as soon as ever I could to go into the community.'⁷⁹ In the years following the end of the Second World War, public health work was increasingly popular with nurses disillusioned by the warehousing of hospital patients and keen for greater professional autonomy.⁸⁰

'It wasn't so much ambition. I think it was much more'

Hortense Gordon qualified as a State Registered Nurse in 1947, having previously qualified as a State Registered Children's Nurse.

She had won both silver and gold medals during her nurse training days and was considered by her matrons as one worthy of promotion. However, after six years of hospital-based training, she admitted that she did not really like hospital nursing. Like Hockey, her goal was to work in the community, so she applied for her health visitor training: 'The first health visitor's course that the London County Council did [was at] London University, and I got a place. There were, I think, about 20 places and about 250 applicants, but I did get a place and, of course, I had a good record because of the London County Council, I had awards. So, I got this.'[81]

Hockey started her midwifery training at the North Middlesex Hospital in Edmonton, North London. If she had thought midwifery would take her away from the misery that she had experienced in hospitals that cared for the sick, she was mistaken. Her midwifery training, undertaken in the pre-antibiotic era, coincided with a gastroenteritis epidemic and eleven otherwise healthy babies died in three weeks. Hockey's desperation to get out of hospital care only increased and she moved to Essex to do her Part II, which was on the district; 'I was never a very good midwife, but I loved just being a friend to a woman in labour.'[82]

On qualifying as a midwife, Hockey returned to nursing and was working in the community as the NHS was established. Hockey maintained, 'in those days you know you weren't really a nurse unless you were a Midwife as well. It was very much, you know, every Sister had a Midwifery qualification.'[83] Stephanie Kirby maintained that the matrons of London County Council (LCC) hospitals would select certain nurses on qualifying for midwifery training. Such a practice suggests that midwifery was seen as a route for those who had shown unusual abilities or talents.[84] Because many senior positions in nursing required candidates to be certified midwives as well as registered nurses well into the second half of the century, this cherry-picking would ensure that the best nurses were groomed for senior positions.

The requirement to be both a nurse and midwife was not just custom and practice but written into the prerequisites for some nursing work. Historian Janet Greenlees argues that in order to be accepted on to a Queen's Nursing (i.e., district nursing) training, a candidate had to be a registered nurse 'with a Central Midwives'

Board (CMB) certificate'.[85] In the early to mid-twentieth century, it was not unknown for community practitioners to take on what was called 'triple-duty' employment. These jobs required the nurse to be district-nursing, midwifery and health-visitor trained – highly valuable assets in more rural areas.[86] As rural district nurses sometimes shared patients with the general practitioner in the area, such postings offered an unusual level of autonomy and demanded highly skilled and knowledgeable nurses.[87] Given the number of refugee nurses who had either been medical students or wished to train as doctors, it is not surprising that several felt positively about the opportunity for greater autonomy and the value placed on a broader range of healthcare skills. The need for practitioners with these abilities increased with the proliferation of scientific discovery and changing expectations in the post-war years.

Later twentieth-century lives

The latter decades of the twentieth century witnessed significant shifts in British nurses' professional and personal lives as the economic and social position of women altered. A new Nurses' Act became law in 1949, just one year after the founding of the NHS. The Act led to a number of changes, the most important of which were the separation of finance for training from the needs of the hospital and the establishment of experimental courses for nursing.[88] From this point, at least in theory, student nurses' educational needs would not be constantly subsumed into the service requirements of the hospital.[89] Yet as McGann and colleagues argue, despite the loss of reciprocity of registration with British Columbia and ongoing anxieties that British nurses were losing out on the international stage to those from the United States and Canada, the opportunities from these changes, at least in the short term, were limited.[90] The Act nevertheless eventually paved the way for the early university programmes. It was in these courses that many of the refugees solidified their positions as leaders of the profession. Before they could achieve their ambitions and create a hoped-for academic space for nursing, they had to overcome numerous obstacles, including conflict over married nurses' work, the opposition of universities to nursing as a discipline and the desire of the medical profession to keep nurses as subordinates rather than colleagues of equal standing.

Penny Summerfield argues that married women's participation in the labour market grew throughout the 1950s.[91] However, unofficial bans on married and particularly, pregnant women continued to be enforced, especially in the professions.[92] By the late 1960s attitudes started to change and the number of working married women doubled between 1951 and 1971.[93] Still, the preference for single women endured in nursing, even though this reduced the pool of experienced nurses. Hortense Gordon did not leave the profession upon marriage, unlike many others. In a short piece she wrote entitled 'Marriage versus carreer' [sic], she remembered, 'When I got married two years after completing my Health Visitor's course, many people I knew in the profession shook their heads in surprise. Nobody thought that I would give up my work for the sake of domestic life. However, I was happy to be able to continue in my job inspite [sic] of marriage.'[94] Later in the essay, she shared that she even returned to work after the birth of her first child: 'My decision of returning to work and leaving my baby was frowned upon by many.'[95]

Like Gordon, Cilly Haar continued to work after her marriage, admitting that she did not know any other married nurses at the time. The response of the ward sister to her marital situation highlights the friction this decision caused: 'And she said to me, now listen to me Staff I don't want to hear about your honeymoon or your marriage, you're just here to nurse. I said, "Yes, Sister I realise that."'[96] Such hostility to married nurses both from within the profession and from their medical colleagues did little to support recruitment and retention.[97] Women and girls could increasingly choose from a wider occupational base, although the feminine professions dominated the discourse.[98] Universities maintained quotas and created obstacles to women studying medicine until the 1970s. It was only after the Sex Discrimination Act of 1975 that women's numbers in medicine and the law increased. By 1990, the number of women in medicine finally reached 50 per cent; in law it remained only a quarter of all students.[99] Nevertheless, other 'feminised' professions started to develop more progressive attitudes. Teacher-training colleges even ran courses specifically for married women.[100] Nursing continued to lose out to professions like teaching and social work, which had far more family-friendly policies.[101]

Gordon spent her working life as a health visitor and retired in 1997. When asked if she thought that being a refugee had any bearing on her ambitions, Gordon responded, 'No, I don't honestly think so, it was just me. It wasn't so much ambition. I think it was much more. I needed to work. I worked all my married life. I enjoyed the work.'[102] Despite her denials of ambition, Gordon published an article in *Nursing Mirror* in 1983 about her work as a liaison health visitor for the elderly in Barnet, North London, a role which was at the time unusual and pioneering. Her abilities were once again noted by those with whom she worked when she started to participate in 'geriatric outpatient clinics. I am introduced to patients and relatives by their doctors and am often able to advise on management and problems.'[103]

Relationships with medical staff, particularly in community care, started to change in the latter half of the twentieth century, as Gordon's comments above indicate. However, whether they became as egalitarian as some nurses wished to believe is a moot point. The doctor–nurse dyad retained both professional and gendered relations, in which the female nurse was subservient to the male doctor. In the early years of the NHS, the Queen's Institute for District Nurses agreed with the British Medical Association that community nurses would work under the direction of the general practitioner (GP).[104] Whilst community nurses might have articulated that their motivation for working on the district was to 'be my own boss', in practice they were aware of the power of the GP and would concede to their medical judgement.[105] Hockey admitted feeling particularly annoyed when GPs treated nurses 'like a bit of dirt'.[106] This was especially galling to her because she would have become a doctor herself had Hitler not come to power.

The reorganisation of district nurses, which attached them to GP surgeries, began in the late 1960s. Community nursing officers argued that GP attachments should place community nurses alongside the GP as colleagues and not subordinates. By 1974, NHS reforms theoretically supported the idea that nurses managed nurses, but in practice many GPs continued to view community nurses as subservient.[107] Gordon's medical colleagues might have been keen to work collaboratively with her, but not all were. Nursing's movement out of the shadows of the medical profession could only be achieved with better education and a research base. Several of the refugee nurses were at the forefront of both. Nevertheless, nursing's foray into the academy was not popular with medicine or the universities themselves. Even within nursing, the endeavour to place its professional preparation on a solid educational foundation rather than in-service training had its detractors. Such was the insularity of nursing education that even those who tried novel teaching methods within the hospital training system were subject to derision from their colleagues.

Education work

Despite her initial dislike for nursing and her near-resignation, Rosa Sacharin stuck with it and qualified in 1946, settling into professional life in Glasgow. She trained as a midwife and spent six years working in the city at Redlands Hospital. In 1952 she took a posting as a children's nurse in Israel, at this point a young country keen to establish itself and its people. When family illness brought Sacharin back to Scotland, she returned to York Hill and was promoted to ward sister, after which she pursued a career in teaching. Her somewhat maverick ideas and professional past made teaching in a general hospital untenable.

As nurse historian Rosemary Weir argues, training hospitals across Scotland varied in size and the type of nurse training offered. There was also a huge gulf between those schools in cities and urban areas and those in remote rural locations like the Hebrides. But two things they all had in common were their integration with the hospital and their isolation from higher education.[108] After Sacharin was urged by the senior tutor to 'not teach to such a high level', she understood the impossibility of her situation.[109] She successfully applied for a sister tutor post in Ayrshire. She described this move as one that enabled her to develop her ideas and teaching skills: 'I introduced my own ideas, I felt the way a Sick Children's nursing course should really be taught and supported.'[110] She published two books on children's nursing before she retired in 1988. Sacharin was ultimately appointed an examiner to the General Nursing Council and the Northern Ireland National Board.[111]

Trudie Moos also trained as a midwife following her nurse training. On qualifying, she applied to King's College Hospital in London for a staff midwife post. After about a year, she made the decision to move into teaching, like Sacharin. Knowing she would need experience as a ward sister before she could embark on a career as a sister tutor, she returned to general nursing.[112] Moos was promoted quickly, being appointed night sister by the matron Miss Opie soon after her naturalisation in 1947. Opie's request for Moos to assume the sister tutor position was a critically important moment in changing British attitudes towards Continental Jews. Moos had her original application to train as a nurse refused by the earlier matron at King's 'on the grounds of being foreign'.[113] This profound change of attitude after only ten years is not something that Moos even mentions in her memoir. It is possible that this is because she wanted to put her 'foreignness' behind her. Only a few lines before, she had reflected that for a while she became '"150% British" and nobody was allowed to run down my newly acquired homeland'.[114]

Moos's descriptions of her work as a ward sister suggest that she was innovative and enthusiastic about training students. Perhaps her most important improvement was to insist that the nursing students join the medical students on teaching rounds. Moos dealt with this in a perfunctory manner in her memoir. It was, however, a crucial shift in the thinking of the position of student nurse and one which some in the hospital likely did not approve. Historian Celia Davies argues that nurses were generally happy to be subordinate to their medical colleagues.[115] But Moos's ideas identify alteration in the thinking of some nurse educators, ideas under discussion amongst the profession's revolutionary thinkers. According to Susan McGann and colleagues, Gladys Carter, research fellow at the University of Edinburgh and author of the radical 1939 text *A New Deal for Nurses*, argued that nursing students should be treated like medical students.[116] This was not a widely held view or one that was popular with hospital matrons and administrators, even into the latter half of the twentieth century. Moos admitted that she received criticism from the assistant matrons for the more relaxed manner of her ward. She maintained that she 'bore the gibes [sic]' because she knew her priorities were unassailable.[117] Whether Moos's ability to ignore the criticisms of the senior nurses was associated with her professional abilities, her personality and upbringing, or her resilience as a refugee is not important. Whatever gave her the confidence, there is little doubt that it was useful for the development of King's College Hospital student nurses when she entered teaching. Despite her professional accomplishments, however, and the wholesale adoption of her new country, the shadow of the Holocaust never fully left her.

Moos maintained contact with her friend, compatriot and fellow refugee Ruth Pfillering. Tragically, despite her own professional success, Pfillering could not ignore the pain wrought by the murder of her parents. Nazi commander Adolf Eichmann's trial in 1962 brought back all the sadness and according to Moos, Pfillering admitted then that if she could not cope, she would end her life. She managed another eight years. Pfillering took a sister tutor's post on the Wirral, near Liverpool, in 1969. Then, in 1970, Moos recalled, 'She had sealed off the bungalow door and windows and had turned on the gas. She was not found until two days later when she had not turned up for work.'[118] Moos reflected on the guilt she felt at not being able to help Pfillering but also expressed anger: 'We had been friends for so many years and I felt very shut out and quite angry. She had confided in no-one in those last years and must have gone through hell.'[119]

Suicide by Holocaust survivors was not unknown, even after several decades of security and safety. Most famously, Primo Levi committed suicide in 1987. In *The Lost and the Saved*, originally published in 1986, Levi posits, 'I might be alive in the place of another; I might have usurped, that is, in fact killed ... Preferably the worst survived, the selfish, the violent, the insensitive, the collaborators of the "grey zones", the spies.'[120] In the introduction to the text, Paul Bailey maintains that these words were not written in anticipation of suicide, but it is difficult not to read them and experience the horror of survivor guilt.[121] Pfillering's knowledge that she survived when so many did not was one struggle too many for her. Even the most resilient refugee nurses were not able to suppress their memories of Nazi persecution. Altschul was never able to rid herself of the spectre of Hitler.[122] However, most refugees tried to regain some normality and peace after the horror. Craig-Norton provides a focus on the Kinder of both sexes who achieved educational and professional goals, many of whom did so through correspondence courses, night classes and part-time courses.[123] Both Moos and Sacharin studied for degrees on retirement, an opportunity they saw as a validation of their life's work. Moos admitted that studying philosophy also enabled her to 'make sense of life situations', a rare nod to reflections about her past.[124] However, neither degree would have any impact on the nursing students they had taught, or the profession more widely.

Nurses had been given the opportunity to study in the academy in Britain from 1918. The sister-tutor and health-visiting courses were both taught within the higher education system. Leeds and London Universities both had Diplomas in Nursing from 1921 and 1925, respectively, and Bedford College, London, ran international courses with the Red Cross. Nevertheless, all these programmes were post-registration and none were at graduate level. Many of the nurses on the Diplomas and sister-tutor courses struggled with the transition to more liberal educational principles.[125] Moreover, as with access for women to universities in general, the numbers were low. Well into the 1960s and 1970s, the number of women attending university on all courses was small compared to that of men.

In her 1957 study of graduate nurses, Gladys Carter reported that there were only about fifty working in the profession throughout the country.[126] According to education historian Roy Fisher, in the 1960s and 1970s, women constituted about 15 per cent of the total undergraduate population, although Carol Dyhouse quotes the Robbins Report's figure of 25 per cent.[127] It is therefore striking that during this period, four of the refugee nurses made the transition to degree study. It was these four women who were at the forefront of nursing research and education for at least the next three decades. Altschul studied for her degree in evening classes at Birkbeck College, London.[128] Hockey studied for a degree in economics as an evening student at the London School of Economics and did so whilst carrying on with her full-time job.[129] Charlotte Kratz returned to Britain in 1963 after developing the district nursing service in Dar es Salaam, Tanzania. She quickly registered for the nurse-tutor course at the RCN. By the mid-1960s she realised that she needed a degree, at which point she gained a place as an external student at Goldsmiths, London (then Goldsmiths' College), to read Sociology. Like Hockey, she studied at night during the week whilst working full time as a tutor.[130] Marion Ferguson was awarded an MA some time before the mid-1970s, working first as a lecturer in nursing at the Welsh School of Medicine in Cardiff and then as Director of Nursing Studies at Bedford College, London.[131] Despite the pioneering work of some, nurses with degrees remained an anomaly until the last decade of the twentieth century. As nurse historian Nicola Ring maintains, there was an ongoing debate, 'whether academic learning was a necessary requirement for "good" nurses'.[132]

'A small but influential group'

The first degree associated with nursing – the degree was a BA Social Sciences (Nursing) – was established at the University of Edinburgh in 1960.[133] The University of Manchester followed in the late 1960s, with the first course in which nursing was an academic discipline in its own right.[134] In 1963, in the midst of these developments in the higher education of nurses, the Robbins Committee on Higher Education published its report. The remit of the Committee was to review the nature and manner of higher education in the UK and consider if any changes were required for its long-term development. Its reference to nursing was perfunctory: 'We received evidence about training for nursing and some of the occupations associated with medicine. Since this does not form part of higher education as we have defined it, we have not specifically considered this wide area of opportunity for girls.'[135] At the same time, the report acknowledged 'certain points of contact with universities and colleges' which had been established.[136]

The 1960s and 1970s witnessed phenomenal change in the social make-up of Britain and the Western world.[137] The role of women in the public world of work and their increasing visibility in universities and professional careers had a slow but significant impact on nursing.[138] In 1987, Altschul published an article on the higher education of nurses since the 1950s. She observed that up to that decade, when few people and even fewer women were admitted to institutions of higher education, the chances of the profession being able to recruit from the elite group were slim. However, once the school-leaving age was raised to 16, as it was in the early 1960s, most children had the opportunity to gain O levels. As more children stayed on at school, the ambition of a place at university became 'a hallmark of youth culture'.[139] The Robbins Report acknowledged that whilst almost as many girls as boys took their O levels, fewer stayed on for A levels, the entry requirement for higher education. Nevertheless, of those who did, the proportion of girls to boys accessing university was equal.[140] In 1999, Altschul returned to the same theme, this time with a more robust analysis:

> What is important is that for better or for worse, more than 50 per cent of school leavers go into tertiary education. If you leave nursing out of this sector, you're telling schools that you want idiots for nursing – don't send us any of those who are capable of undertaking tertiary education, send us the ones who are incapable.[141]

By this point, all nurse education had moved out of the hospital training school and into the higher-education sector, though most nurse education remained at sub-degree level. It was not until 2013 that nursing became an all-graduate profession. This decision was followed by complaints in the press about nurses being 'Too posh to wash', comments completely at odds with the research.[142] Clearly the desire to keep nurses – as women – in their 'place' was a powerful trope, even after over fifty years since undergraduate education for nurses was first established.

Refugee nurses from the 1950s onwards seized on the growing argument for a better-educated workforce in nursing, as degrees in nursing became available.[143] The opportunities that higher education presented enabled those who had originally wanted medical careers to find stimulation within the nursing profession. Kratz proclaimed, 'The fact that I, having become educated ... for the first time, I saw nursing as challenging and exciting. Never again did I want to be a doctor, I was quite happy to be a nurse.'[144] Nevertheless, whilst the new university departments considered themselves 'avant-garde', they were not necessarily popular at a time when most nursing students were still trained within the confines of the hospital training school.[145] The medical profession was not generally supportive of degree nursing courses but neither were many nurses, and nursing had not yet established a research base.[146]

In 1959, the RCN's annual general meeting considered the challenges nurses faced in their attempts to conduct research.[147] According to McGann and colleagues, the outcome of this discussion was an informal research group for college members headed by Gertrude Ramsden, with Marjorie Simpson appointed as the RCN's first research officer.[148] The meetings took place in members' homes; ten people attended the first.[149] Doreen Norton's research on the care of older people was inspired by one of the early meetings. Despite the importance of this research, Norton was not able to conduct it without a consultant physician as both the instigator of the funding call and as part of the research team.[150] In her oral history, Hockey recalled joining this group early in its incarnation and the influence of three of its members, Elsie Ensing, Marjorie Simpson and importantly for her later career, Margaret Scott Wright.[151] Hockey was cautious about the value of these meetings, suggesting that the group did little more than 'belly ache and regret we couldn't do more'. She was more upbeat later in the interview, adding that members 'switched each other on, you know we gave courage to each other ... We still had to go back to our own institutions where we were very solitary in a large group of people who just thought of us as being ... well troublemakers, too academic and heavenly minded to be of earthly use.'[152] Despite her ambivalent recollections of the value of the group, it gave Hockey the confidence to continue to ask difficult questions about nursing. This confidence enabled her to undertake her first research project as Queen's Nursing Institute (QNI) research officer. She admitted that she was unsure of whether the project itself was of any benefit, but she acknowledged that it convinced the 'paymasters' that research was valuable.[153] It also put her back in contact with Margaret Scott Wright, who was involved in the QNI. In 1968, Scott Wright was appointed as head of the Department of Nursing Studies at the University of Edinburgh.[154]

The Department of Nursing Studies at the University of Edinburgh was the brainchild of three people: Professor Francis

A. E. Crew, Chair of Public Health and Social Medicine at the University; Gladys Carter, a Boots Scholar under the supervision of Crew; and Margaret Lamb, Education Officer at the RCN, Scotland, and a Rockefeller Travelling Scholar.[155] This triumvirate of reformers wanted to develop the academic nature of nursing and place it alongside other disciplines in the academy. The Faculty of Medicine were hostile, refusing to countenance nursing as a discipline appropriate for university.[156] An eventual home was found in the Faculty of Arts, with students being taught through the University's Department of Education.[157] The *Nursing Times* advertised the position of Director on 2 December 1955.[158] When the Nurse Teaching Unit was established the following year, Elsie Stephenson was appointed to the post.[159] When she died at the age of 51 in 1967, she was succeeded by Scott Wright, who was keen to promote nursing as a research discipline. Scott Wright approached Hockey about becoming the research director, and Hockey was appointed in 1971, becoming the first director of nursing research in Europe and joining fellow refugee, Annie Altschul, in the department.

Altschul completed her tutor's course in 1950 and returned to the Maudsley as its senior and then principal tutor. In 1951 she graduated from Birkbeck with a degree in psychology.[160] The following year Hildegard Peplau published her groundbreaking study, *Interpersonal Relations*. Altschul was immediately aware of the force of this work on the field of psychiatric nursing.[161] In 1960 she was awarded a scholarship to study in the United States and took leave from the Maudsley for a year.[162] The 1960s started to see a shift in psychiatric practice and Altschul's scholarship enabled her to witness these changes first-hand.[163] Within three years of her return to the UK, Altschul moved from her post as principal tutor in a traditional hospital training school to a university department. She joined the staff of the Nursing Studies Unit at Edinburgh University in 1964 and was promoted to senior lecturer in 1974. In 1976, on the departure of Scott Wright, Altschul took over as Director of the Department,[164] and two years later, she was awarded one of the first fellowships of the Royal College of Nursing (see Figure 4.1).

With Altschul in charge and Hockey as research director, the Department of Nursing Studies and its research unit gained

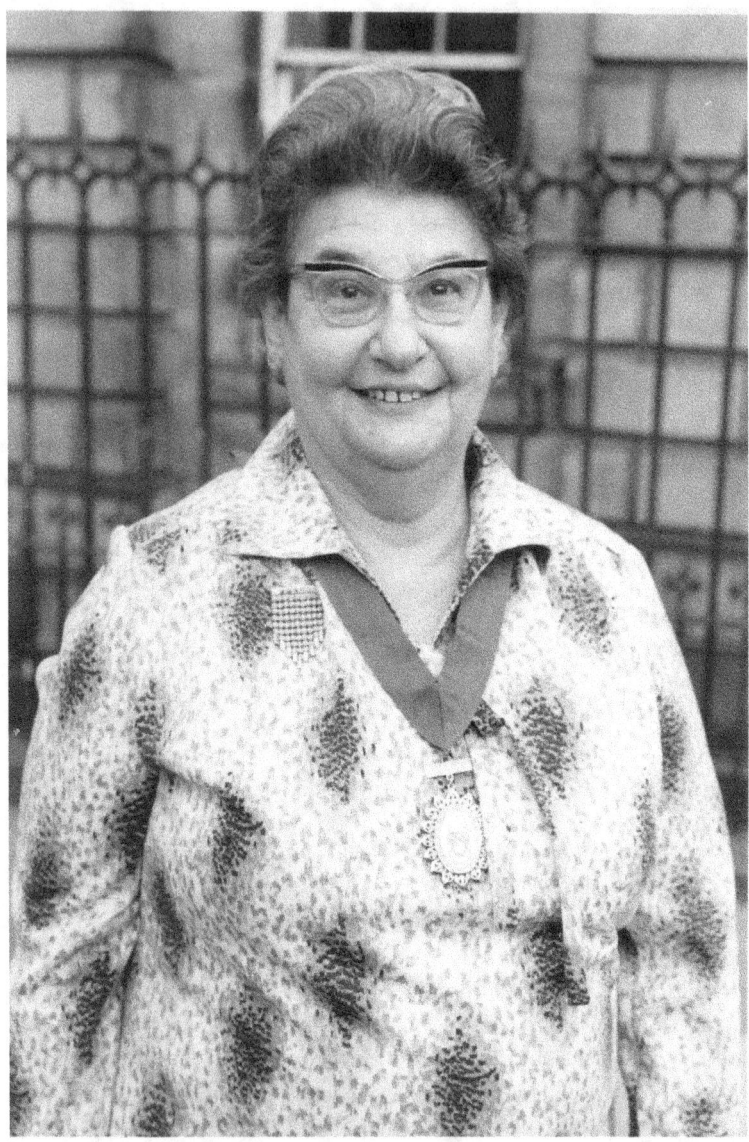

Figure 4.1 Annie Altschul with her Fellow of the Royal College of Nursing (FRCN) medal, 1978. Reproduced by courtesy of The Scotsman Publications Ltd [fo. 235]

credibility across the University of Edinburgh and the wider country. After the first three years, there were twelve research students.[165] Hockey was convinced that the unit was beginning to show its value to senior nurses in the UK and Europe. In 1976 the General Nursing Council for Scotland considered that approximately 5 per cent of nurses should have a university degree. There was, the Council felt, a growing appreciation of graduate nurses, and that this was therefore a possibility.[166] Despite Hockey and others' enthusiasm for the unit, a note of caution was raised: 'Nursing research, though a growth area, has limited resources, a factor which, in a vicious circle, has resulted in limited implementation of findings, thereby attracting criticism of the purpose and value of the research.'[167] This phenomenon was not limited to Edinburgh. As Director of Nursing Studies at Bedford College, London, Marion Ferguson was determined to see nursing as an accepted subject for university education. Described as being part of 'a small but influential group', alongside Altschul, Hockey and Kratz, she was vocal about the place of nursing in the university sector.[168] In 1986, she wrote to Altschul, offering her the draft of a paper on the college and its connections to nursing.[169] Ferguson's goal was for nursing to create 'a new way of organising academic work in Institutions of Higher Education', ways that would be mindful of wider social issues and interdisciplinarity.[170] Her untimely death that same year stymied any attempts to bring her ideas to fruition.[171]

A year before Hockey arrived at Edinburgh, 48-year-old Charlotte Kratz applied to the University of Manchester. Her position and that of her co-worker Dorothy Baker were paid for through a fellowship instituted by Marjorie Simpson. Simpson's influence on both Kratz and Hockey is important. By 1968 Simpson had moved from the RCN to the Department of Health as its principal nursing officer in charge of research.[172] Given that the RCN headquarters were in London, as was the Department of Health, it might have been expected that the nascent developments in university education for nurses and nursing research would have been made in the capital. Kratz recalled attempts to develop a degree in nursing in the 1960s at the University of London and that institution's lack of interest in the discipline.[173] Manchester and Edinburgh already had small nursing departments; early nursing research thus began in those two locations. Kratz's time at Manchester was, however, short-lived.

The research fellowship did not have a remit, so Kratz's first task was to write the proposal and estimate the costs of the project. She had no support for this, and with only a first degree, had very little experience. Kratz tried to resign after two months, but Simpson persuaded her to stay. Like the Edinburgh department, the Manchester Nursing Department had also been instigated originally by professor of social medicine, Fraser Brockington. He was a longstanding supporter of health visiting who believed that the discipline should have a place in the university.[174] But as with Edinburgh, the development of the department was challenging. There were continued debates as to the academic nature of nursing as a discipline and the 'fit' of its curriculum in the university system. There were also those fearful of the influx of a critical mass of women into the hallowed walls of higher education. Ferguson might have hoped that the academy would move into line with the interdisciplinarity of nursing, but nursing departments needed to be sensitive to their hosts.[175] By the time Kratz joined the department, Brockington had retired and was superseded by Alwyn Smith. Smith was supposed to support the new fellows, but according to Kratz, Smith's demanding work schedule meant that 'we were literally on our own and it was a very hard time'.[176]

The enforced independence meant that Kratz had to develop her own research study. She decided to concentrate on district nursing, 'as there wasn't much work done on it apart from Lisbeth's work'.[177] Despite the difficulties, Kratz stayed and completed her PhD in 1974, becoming the first nurse to be awarded a PhD at the University of Manchester.[178] Kratz might have found academic success, but the fellowship on which she was employed was never converted into a tenured position. According to Cree and colleagues, even in the twenty-first century, women academics are less likely to have permanent contracts than their male colleagues.[179] Other feminised professions such as social work, which were established university subjects, struggled to be valued in higher education.[180] It is also possible that because the nursing department at Manchester was located within the medical faculty, its staff were considered somewhat infra dig. Kratz left Manchester in 1976 and took up a post at the *Nursing Times*. Whilst this position was not academic, it potentially placed her in a position to influence the profession more widely. She acknowledged that at this point she still thought she would return to academia but soon realised:

> I have never been an establishment figure and that just came out again and again and again ... I think it had something to do with the fact, probably that I was never seen as being completely anglicised and that I was just too honest and I think I was in a way too stupid to see the sort of deviant ways one had to use to get on ... I became more politically aware when I got to the *Nursing Times*.[181]

The lack of finances to retain Kratz's research fellowship in what was to become one of the foremost nursing research departments in the world might have stymied both her personal advancement and her research programme, but the department continued to develop. In 1987, the University of Manchester, in collaboration with the Queen's Nursing Institute, created the Chair in Community Nursing. Despite the difficult end to her employment at Manchester, Kratz was generous in her analysis. It was, she stated, 'fortuitous' that the Chair had been inaugurated at Manchester.[182] In the same year, long after she had retired from her position at the University of Edinburgh, Lisbeth Hockey visited a former student in Galena, Illinois. The *Galena Gazette* published a piece on her visit, quoting Hockey's beliefs about the importance of research:

> [Research] is the attempt to create new knowledge ... For many years, nursing was a passive kind of profession. Certainly, in the United Kingdom, nurses were less inclined to explore scientifically their own profession ... The importance of nursing research is to see where we are going. Professional people, whatever their field, should question their own activity, otherwise, we become static and not dynamic.[183]

Hockey's analysis that nursing is a 'passive kind of profession' might be a valid criticism.[184] But it appears that this passivity might not have been solely a nursing problem. Lynda Grier, Principal of Lady Margaret Hall, Oxford, was concerned about the 'docility' of women students.[185] What Hockey failed to identify were the huge obstacles that individual nurses and the profession as a whole faced in their pursuit of a credible knowledge base to their discipline.

Conclusion

This final chapter charts the creation of lives in British nursing by the refugees who entered the nursing profession in the 1930s and during the Second World War. It follows their early post-war choices and their determination to develop nursing skills in the face of the horror and tragedies of the Holocaust. Some, like Ruth Pfillering, were unable to shoulder the burden of survivor guilt and committed suicide. Most others struggled for years to cope with the knowledge that their families had perished in the Holocaust. Yet, as I demonstrate, they found some solace and purpose in their professional lives.

The shift from being viewed as suspicious 'foreigners' in the late 1930s, to their almost vilified status following the fall of France, to posts at the very pinnacle of the profession is testament to their resilience, bravery and fortitude to make a life for themselves. Most had no family to support them and once they were no longer able to perform domestic service, they had few career options. As legitimate war work, nursing was a better occupational choice than most. By the middle war years, employment opportunities for refugees had multiplied, yet many remained in nursing. The Nurses' Act of 1949 did not lead to the rapid changes that some wanted and many of the innovations remained constrained by the conservatism of the General Nursing Council.[186] However, the Act enabled courses for nurses to be created outside the confines of the hospital system for the first time. Once again, refugee nurses seized the opportunities that were offered, seeking entrance into the early degree programmes, despite higher education's antipathy to the discipline of nursing.

Universities in the second half of the twentieth century were keen to maintain their status and thus placed significant obstacles to the entrance of women, obstructions that were seen particularly in medical schools.[187] The incursion of nursing into the hallowed academic environment would, they believed, damage their prestige. However, as I argue, despite this antipathy, changes in the position of women were unalterable. By the 1970s, graduate refugee nurses had established themselves not only as students but also as academic staff in the new departments of nursing. Once there, they exercised their considerable influence on the profession, in practice, education and research. The impact of the refugee nurses on the profession far outweighed their numbers within it. Their enquiring minds supported the development of a new way to think about nursing. Yet, the movement to develop nursing from 'an intuitive act that expresses women's caring or moral nature' to a science-based one remains moot, even in the current century.[188]

Notes

1 Martin Gilbert, *The Second World War: A Complete History* (London: Phoenix, 2009), 681.
2 Joanna Bourke, *The Second World War: A People's History* (Oxford: Oxford University Press, 2001), 172.
3 Rex Pope, 'British demobilization after the Second World War', *Journal of Contemporary History* 30 (1995): 65–81.
4 Penny Summerfield, '"They didn't want women back in that job": The Second World War and the construction of gendered work histories', *Labour History Review* 63, 1 (1998): 92.
5 Beate Fieseler, M. Michaela Hampf and Jutta Schwarzkopf, 'Gendering combat: Military women's status in Britain, the United States and the Soviet Union during the Second World War', *Women's Studies International Forum* 47 (2014): 115–26.
6 Arthur Salusbury MacNalty, 'Influence of war on family life', in Sir James Marchant (ed.), *Rebuilding Family Life in the Post-War World: An Enquiry with Recommendations* (London: Odhams Press, 1945), 133.
7 Jane Brooks, *Negotiating Nursing: British Army Sisters and Soldiers in the Second World War* (Manchester: Manchester University Press, 2018), 170.
8 Lawrence Darton, 'An account of the work of the Friends Committee for refugees and aliens, first known as the Germany Emergency Committee of the Society of Friends, 1933–1950', 9. Issued by the Friends Committee for Refugees and Aliens, 1954. Friends Meeting House Library, Euston Road, London.
9 Bernard Wasserstein, *Britain and the Jews of Europe, 1939–1945* (London: Clarendon Press, 1979), 343.
10 Despite the British public's reluctance to face what has become known as the Holocaust, there was a realisation in some arenas

that those Jews who had been given sanctuary in Britain could not possibly return home. Most had no home to go to. In May 1945, Winston Churchill himself spoke against repatriation. In the final chapter in his account of the Friends Committee, 'Naturalization', Darton states, 'in a reply to the House of Commons, the Prime Minister made it clear that it was not the Government's intention to compel refugees from political oppression to return to their country of origin'. Darton, 'An account of the work of the Friends Committee for refugees and aliens', 133.
11 Anonymous, 'Extermination', *Manchester Guardian* (27 October 1942): 4.
12 C. J. Wright, 'Jews' extermination', *Manchester Guardian* (14 December 1942): 4.
13 *Daily Telegraph* Reporter, 'Germans murder 700,000 Jews in Poland: Travelling gas chambers', *Daily Telegraph* (25 June 1942).
14 Tony Kushner, *The Holocaust and the Liberal Imagination: A Social and Cultural History*. Oxford: Blackwell, 1994), 169.
15 For a detailed discussion of the response both of and to the British press's publication of the extermination of the Jews, see Andrew Sharf, *The British Press and Jews under Nazi Rule* (London: Oxford University Press, 1964).
16 Tony Kushner, David Cesarani, Jo Reilly and Colin Richmond, 'Approaching Belsen: An introduction', in Jo Reilly, David Cesarani, Tony Kushner and Colin Richmond (eds), *Belsen in History and Memory* (London: Frank Cass, 1997), 3. Personal testimonies from those who had supported the liberation suggest that those who were there could not talk about their experiences. Even those who had been on active service during the war could not talk about the horror of the camps. See for example, the testimony related to Ethel Bardsley: 'On the 18th May 1945, when the war in Europe ceased, Ethel was posted, with other personnel, to Belsen Concentration Camp. The scenes that faced the team were so horrific that everyone was lost for words. The work of caring for and moving the living skeletons horrified them but they all worked with dignity and respect. Ethel refused to discuss what she had witnessed at Belsen – not even with her family.' 'Ethel Bardsley, a Queen Alexandra nurse at Belsen. WW2 People's War: An archive of World War Two memories', written by the public, gathered by the BBC. www.bbc.co.uk/history/ww2peopleswar/stories/98/a2758098.shtml [accessed 6 October 2023].
17 David Cesarani, *Final Solution: The Fate of the Jews, 1933–1949* (London: Pan Macmillan, Kindle edition, 2017), 895.

18 Edith Bown (Jacobowitz), oral history interview by Barbara Mortimer in Maidstone on 24 May 2008. Interview T379, Oral History Collection, Royal College of Nursing (RCN), Edinburgh.
19 Susi Linton, oral history interview by Rosalyn Livshin on 19 October 2004. Interview 78, Refugee Voices: Association of Jewish Refugees (AJR) Audio-Visual Testimony Archive, British Library, London.
20 Gertrude Roberts, oral history interview by Alan Dein on 23 January 1982. Audio 184. Oral History Collection, Jewish Museum, London.
21 Roberts, oral history interview by Alan Dein.
22 Susi Loeffler, oral history interview by Jane Brooks from Australia on 18 January 2018, via Zoom. Personal Archive.
23 Henry Greenspan, 'The unsaid, the incommunicable, the unbearable, and the irretrievable', *Oral History Review* 41, 2 (2014): 229–43.
24 Roberts, oral history interview by Alan Dein.
25 Ben Shephard, *After Daybreak: The Liberation of Belsen, 1945* (London: Pimlico, 2005), 30.
26 Hannah Craven, 'Horror in our time: Images of the concentration camps in the British media, 1945', *Historical Journal of Film, Radio and Television* 21, 3 (2001): 208.
27 Craven, 'Horror in our time', 2009.
28 Ellen Ben-Sefer, 'Surviving survival: Nursing care at Bergen-Belsen 1945', *Australian Journal of Advanced Nursing* 26, 3 (2009): 101–10.
29 Jane Brooks, '"The nurse stoops down…for me": Nursing the liberated persons at Bergen-Belsen', in Jane Brooks and Christine E. Hallett (eds), *One Hundred Years of Wartime Nursing Practices* (Manchester: Manchester University Press, 2015), 213.
30 Lesley Hardman entered Belsen two days after its liberation. For a full and detailed account, see Lesley H. Hardman and Cecily Goodman, *The Survivors: The Story of the Belsen Remnant* (London: Vallentine Mitchell, 1958).
31 Ben Shephard, 'The medical relief effort at Belsen', in Suzanne Bardgett and David Cesarani (eds), *Belsen 1945: New Historical Perspectives* (London: Vallentine Mitchell, 2006), 34. Despite Shephard's long-ago critique of the lack of research into this issue, it is not clear that any further insights have come to light.
32 Shephard, *After Daybreak*, 160.
33 Levy, 'Appendix: Belsen testimonies', 239; appendix to Johannes-Dieter Steinert, 'British relief teams in Belsen concentration camp: Emergency relief and the perception of survivors', *Holocaust Studies: A Journal of Culture and History* 12, 1–2 (2006): 62–78.

34 Alice (Redlich) Fink, oral history interview by Lyn E. Smith in November 1997. Interview 1775, Sound Archive, Imperial War Museum, London.
35 Eva Minden, 'Application for the Jewish Committee for Relief Abroad' (17 June 1946), 1407/17/4/1, Wiener Library, London.
36 Eva Minden, *How it all Started with the Shoes: Memoirs of a Career in Nursing from 1934–1951* (Baltimore, MD: Novice Publishers, 2021), 133. F. M. Lipscomb, Lieutenant-Colonel with the Royal Army Medical Corps, acknowledged in a medical report on 13 June 1945 that doctors had not been trained to provide the mass treatments required for the patients in Belsen. Given this, it would perhaps have been useful to have offered training to all personnel, whatever their professional background. F. M. Lipscomb, 'Medical aspects' (13 June 1945). McFarlane Documents. 9550–2, 9. Imperial War Museum. For a discussion on the expected training of relief workers, see for example, Steinert, 'British relief teams in Belsen concentration camp'.
37 For a description of how postings to Belsen affected nurses, see, Mary Morris (ed. Carol Acton), *A Very Private Diary: A Nurse in Wartime* (London: Weidenfeld & Nicolson, 2014), 221–2.
38 Minden, *How it all Started with the Shoes*, 134.
39 Eva Minden, 'Correspondence: "Dear Miss Glover"' (14 October 1946), 1407/17/4/4, Wiener Library, London. Minden recalled gathering a list of two hundred Jewish nurses from all over Britain to form an unofficial association. She was hoping that eighty would be able to join her in Belsen to replace the eighty German nurses currently working there. Ultimately only two others arrived. Minden, *How it all Started with the Shoes*, 134.
40 Eva Minden, 'Untitled account of some of the details and course of nursing work in Glyn Hughes Hospital, Belsen' (1948), 1407/17/4/22, Wiener Library, London.
41 Jo Reilly, 'Cleaner, carer and occasional dance partner?: Writing women back into the liberation of Bergen-Belsen', in Jo Reilly, David Cesarani, Tony Kushner and Colin Richmond (eds), *Belsen in History and Memory* (London, Frank Cass, 1997), 155.
42 Minden, *How it all Started with the Shoes*, 163. Alice Redlich would become Alice Fink whilst at Belsen. For the purposes of the book, I will continue to refer to Alice Redlich as Fink, as this is the name under which all her archives are located.
43 Fink, oral history interview.
44 Minden, *How it all Started with the Shoes*, 196.

45 For an excellent detailed account of nursing in the camps see for example, Anna Hajkova, 'Medicine in Theresienstadt', *Social History of Medicine* 33, 1 (2018): 79–105; Margalit Shlain, 'Nursing in the Theresienstadt Ghetto', *Nashim: A Journal of Jewish Women's Studies & Gender Issues* 36, 5780 (2020): 60–85.

46 Brooks, '"The nurse stoops down … for me"', 216.

47 Fink, oral history interview. A testimonial written by Captain (equivalent) J. C. Baldry, Chief Supply Officer for UNRRA, on 1 March 1947, described Fink's work: 'he has shown such genuine ability, perseverance and loyal devotion to his duties that he was enrolled in UNRRA and through his good work and attention to duty in often difficult situations was promoted to Magazine Officer with the rank of Lieutenant (British Army Equivalent status)'. J. C. Baldry, 'To whom it may concern: A brief appreciation of the services of H Fink' (1 March 1947), Alice and John Fink papers, John Fink, 1947–1949. Document I Accession Number: 1990.247.13, United States Holocaust Memorial Museum (USHMM). collections.ushmm.org/search/catalog/irn710964#?rsc=210435&cv=1&c=0&m=0&s=0&xywh=-343%2C85%2C5914%2C3875.

48 Annaliese Pearl (Stift), oral history interview by Patrick Gyasi in Queens, New York, on 29 May 2012. Interview 2087, AHC Oral History Archive, Leo Baeck Institute, Berlin and New York.

49 Richard Paul Hatchett, 'The History of Workforce Policy and Planning in British Nursing, 1939–1960', PhD thesis, London School of Hygiene and Tropical Medicine, University of London (2005), 90.

50 Socialist Medical Association, 'Memorandum on the Nursing Problem' (16 September 1947). www.sochealth.co.uk/1947/09/16/memorandum-nursing-problem [accessed 14 September 2023].

51 Susan McGann, Anne Crowther and Rona Dougall, *A History of the Royal College of Nursing, 1916–90: A Voice for Nurses* (Manchester: Manchester University Press, 2009). McGann and colleagues suggest that British nurses were keen to support the relief and rehabilitation of camp survivors.

52 McGann et al., *History of the Royal College of Nursing*.

53 Roy Fisher, 'Gender, class, and school teacher education from the mid-nineteenth century to 1970: Scenes from a town in the North of England', *History of Education* 48, 6 (2019): 806–18.

54 The expectation that even qualified nurses would live in continued. In a pamphlet on staffing in the new NHS, Aneurin Bevin, Minister of Health; Joseph Westwood, Secretary of State for Scotland; and George Isaacs, Minister of Labour and National Service, argued

that married nurses should be able to continue in their profession and that married student nurses be allowed to live out, if they were able to 'meet the reasonable requirements of the hospital'. This caveat enabled most hospitals to prevent student nurses from getting married. Aneurin Bevin, Joseph Westwood and George Isaacs, 'Staffing the hospitals: An urgent need' (London: HMSO, 1945). Reprinted pamphlet, *International History of Nursing Journal* 3, 3 (1998): 11.

55 McGann et al., *History of the Royal College of Nursing*, 129.
56 Charles Webster, 'Nursing as the early crisis of the NHS', *International History of Nursing Journal* 3, 3 (1998): 38.
57 Julie Bliss and Alison While, 'Team work and collaboration: The position of district nursing, 1948–1974', *International History of Nursing Journal* 5, 3 (2000): 22–9.
58 Helen M. Sweet with Rona Dougall, *Community Nursing and Primary Healthcare in Twentieth-Century Britain* (London: Routledge, 2008), 42.
59 Carrie Howse, '"The ultimate destination of all nursing": The development of district nursing in England, 1880–1925', *Nursing History Review* 15 (2007): 81. The disparities in rural and urban healthcare were not specifically British. Historian Jennifer L. Gunn highlights the difficulties in the US with a shortage of physicians, nurses and other healthcare professionals as well as hospitals. Jennifer L. Gunn, 'Meeting rural health needs: Interprofessional practice or public health', *Nursing History Review* 24 (2016): 90.
60 Lisbeth Hockey, oral history interview at her home (interviewer not specified) in Edinburgh on 27 December 1987. Interview T26, Oral History Collection RCN, Edinburgh.
61 Rosemary White, *Social Change and the Development of the Nursing Profession: A Study of the Poor Law Nursing Service, 1848–1948* (London: Henry Kimpton, 1978), 1.
62 Martin Gorsky, John Mohan and Tim Willis, 'Hospital contributory schemes and the NHS debates, 1937–46: The rejection of social insurance in the British welfare system', *Twentieth-Century British History* 16, 2 (2005): 170–92.
63 Stephanie Snow and Angela F. Whitecross, 'Making history together: The UK's National Health Service and the story of our lives since 1948', *Contemporary British History* (2022).
64 Gertrud (Trudie) Moos, 'I Remember: My Life Story' (printed 1995), 71. A biographical database of European Medical Refugees in Great Britain, 1930s–1950s, Oxford Brookes University, Oxford.

65 Ilse Lewen, A biographical database of European Medical Refugees in Great Britain, 1930s–1950s, Oxford: Oxford Brookes University.
66 Gertrud Miriam Bettina Caroline Sylvia Camille Cohen, A biographical database of European Medical Refugees in Great Britain, 1930s–1950s, Oxford: Oxford Brookes University.
67 Charles Webster, *The National Health Service: A Political History* (Oxford: Oxford University Press, 2002). It should be noted that, although in theory the whole population had access to the same care, in reality there were significant differences between the treatment, accommodation and equipment provided for different sectors. Those patients who had historically been cared for in Poor Law establishments remained in old and poorly appointed buildings and wards. According to Charles Webster, the elderly and infirm were cared for in hospitals, some of which had been condemned during the Second World War. Charles Webster, 'The elderly and the early National Health Service', in Margaret Pelling and Richard M. Smith (eds), *Life, Death, and the Elderly: Historical Perspectives* (London: Routledge, 1991), 178.
68 Charles Webster, 'Conflict and consensus: Explaining the British health service', *Twentieth-Century British History* 1, 2 (1990): 117.
69 Martin Gorsky, 'The British National Health Service, 1948–2008: A review of the historiography', *Social History of Medicine* 21, 3 (2008): 437–60.
70 Kitty Hutchinson, 'Memories of the founding of the NHS in 1948', *International History of Nursing Journal* 3, 4 (1998): 34.
71 Peter Nolan, 'Annie Altschul's legacy to 20th century British mental health nursing', *Journal of Psychiatric and Mental Health Nursing* 6 (1999): 269.
72 Annie Altschul, oral history interview at her home in Edinburgh. No date. Interview T8, Oral History Collection RCN, Edinburgh.
73 Gorsky, 'British National Health Service, 1948–2008', 442.
74 Gorsky et al., 'Hospital contributory schemes and the NHS debates, 1937–46', 180.
75 McGann et al., *History of the Royal College of Nursing*, 134.
76 Stephanie Snow, 'The NHS at 70: The story of our lives', *Lancet* 392 (2018): 22.
77 Nick Hayes, '"Our hospitals?" Voluntary provision, community and civic consciousness in Nottingham before the NHS', *Midland History* 37, 1 (2012): 84–105.
78 Webster, *National Health Service*, 6.
79 Hockey, oral history interview, 1987.

80 Jane Brooks, 'Managing the burden: Nursing older people in England, 1955–1980', *Nursing Inquiry* 18 (2011): 226–34.
81 Hortense Gordon, oral history interview by Jane Brooks at her home in London on 27 October 2017. Personal archive.
82 Hockey, oral history interview, 1987. According to historian Tania McIntosh, the Central Midwives Board demanded that all trainee midwives did their Part II or district element to test their 'confidence, clinical judgement, and skills'. The reality was that to gain these skills, student midwives were often left to deal with deliveries on their own. Tania McIntosh, '"I'm not a tradesman": A case study of district midwifery in Nottingham and Derby, 1954–1974', *Social History of Medicine* 27, 2 (2014): 227.
83 Lisbeth Hockey, oral history interview by Helen Sweet at her home in Edinburgh on 13 August 1996. Interview T221, Oral History Collection, RCN, Edinburgh.
84 Stephanie Kirby, 'A splendid scope for professional practice: Leading the London County Council Nursing Service, 1929–1948', *Nursing History Review* 14 (2006): 41.
85 Janet Greenlees, 'To care and educate: The continuity within Queen's Nursing in Scotland', *Nursing History Review* 26 (2018): 99. The Queen's Nursing Institute was founded as the Queen Victoria Jubilee Institute for Nursing and received its Royal Charter in 1889. Its purpose was to train nurses for community work, and by the end of the nineteenth century there were over nine hundred trained Queen's Nurses. Sweet with Dougall, *Community Nursing and Primary Healthcare*, 25. The Queen's Nursing Institute continued to train nurses until 1968. Queen's Nursing Institute, 'History of The Queen's Nursing Institute' (2020) https://qni.org.uk/explore-qni/history-of-the-qni [accessed 15 June 2022].
86 Sweet with Dougall, *Community Nursing and Primary Healthcare*, 40.
87 Greenlees, 'To care and educate', 104. The amount of autonomy that district nurses were afforded depended greatly on the willingness of GPs to share their work in a collegial manner. Frank Honigsbaum argued, 'GPs in their community work were to be at the head of wide-ranging teams, embracing district nurses, midwives, health visitors, and social workers – all of whom would be ready to relieve them of the more menial tasks required.' Frank Honigsbaum, *The Division in British Medicine: A History of the Separation of General Practice from Hospital Care, 1911–1968* (London: Kogan Page, 1979), 311.
88 Anonymous, 'The Nurses' Act 1949: Its educational scope and potentialities', *Nursing Times* (8 July 1950): 13–15. For a discussion of the

Act, see for example, Rosemary White, 'The Nurses' Act, 1949: 2 – Service priorities', *Nursing Times* 78, 5 (1982): 48–50.
89 For a useful discussion on the contradictory position of the student nurse, see Jane Salvage, *The Politics of Nursing* (Oxford: Butterworth-Heinemann, 1985), esp. 68–73.
90 McGann et al., *History of the Royal College of Nursing*.
91 Penny Summerfield, *Reconstructing Women's Wartime Lives: Discourse and Subjectivity in Oral Histories of the Second World War* (Manchester: Manchester University Press, 1998), 205.
92 Laura Jefferson, Karen Bloor and Alan Maynard, 'Women in medicine: Historical perspectives and recent trends', *British Medical Bulletin* 114 (2015): 5–15.
93 Helen McCarthy, 'Women, marriage and paid work in post-war Britain', *Women's History Review* 26, 1 (2017): 46–61; Sarah Stoller, 'Forging a politics of care: Theorizing household work in the British Women's Liberation Movement', *History Workshop Journal* 85 (2018): 95–119.
94 Hortense Gordon, 'Marriage versus carreer' [sic]. Unpublished document given to me at our interview.
95 Gordon, 'Marriage versus carreer'.
96 Cilly Haar (Brauer), oral history interview by Jane Brooks at her home in London on 4 September 2017. Personal archive.
97 McGann et al., *History of the Royal College of Nursing*, 127.
98 Stephanie Spencer, 'Women's dilemmas in postwar Britain: Career stories for adolescent girls in the 1950's', *History of Education* 29, 4 (2000): 329–42.
99 Carol Dyhouse, 'Troubled identities: Gender and status in the history of the mixed colleges in English universities since 1945', *Women's History Review* 12, 2 (2003): 169–94; Pat Thane, 'Afterword: Challenging women in the British professions', *Women's History Review* 29, 4 (2020): 748–58.
100 Fisher, 'Gender, class and school teacher education'.
101 Vivienne Cree, Fiona Morrison, Mary Mitchell and Jackie Gulland, 'Navigating the gendered academy: Women in social work academia', *Social Work Education* 39, 5 (2020): 650–64.
102 Gordon, oral history interview, 2004.
103 Hortense Gordon, 'Supplement. Community forum 7 – Liaison: The vital link', *Nursing Mirror* (3 August 1983): iii.
104 Bliss and While, 'Team work and collaboration', 23.
105 Rona Ferguson, 'Autonomy, tension and trade-off: Attitudes to doctors in the history of district nursing', *International History of Nursing Journal* 6, 1 (2001): 10–17.

106 Hockey, oral history interview, 1987.
107 Bliss and While, 'Team work and collaboration', 28; Sweet with Dougall, *Community Nursing and Primary Healthcare*, 97.
108 Rosemary I. Weir, *Educating Nurses in Scotland: A History of Innovation and Change, 1950–2000* (Penzance: Hypatia Trust, 2004), 12.
109 Rosa Sacharin (Goldschal), oral history interview by Barbara Mortimer on 28 April 2010. Interview T407, Oral History Collection, RCN, Edinburgh.
110 Sacharin, oral history interview.
111 Rosa Sacharin, 'CV.' A biographical database of European Medical Refugees in Great Britain, 1930s–1950s, Oxford: Oxford Brookes University.
112 McGann et al., *History of the Royal College of Nursing*, 183. Sister Tutor was the title of the nurse who taught probationer or student nurses in the nurse training school.
113 Moos, 'I Remember', 45. It is clear from the timeline that Miss Opie had not been the matron in 1941 when Moos's application for nurse training had been refused. It was not possible to locate any literature on the matrons of King's Hospital. However, correspondence with the archivist suggests 'The King's Annual Report 1941 lists Miss Blyde ARRC as the Sister Matron. As far as I can see, this is the only Matron listed in the report.' Personal email correspondence with Senior Archives Assistant, Archives and Research Collections, King's College London (5 May 2022). It is not known why King's used the term 'Sister Matron'; I have not come across this title before.
114 Moos, 'I Remember', 68.
115 Celia Davies, 'Continuities in the development of hospital nursing in Britain', *Journal of Advanced Nursing* 2 (1976): 479–93.
116 McGann et al., *History of the Royal College of Nursing*, 169.
117 Moos, 'I Remember', 73.
118 Moos, 'I Remember', 103.
119 Moos, 'I Remember', 103.
120 Primo Levi, *The Drowned and the Saved* (London: Abacus, 2013), 87.
121 Paul Bailey, 'Introduction', in Primo Levi, *The Drowned and the Saved* (London: Abacus, 2013), xv.
122 Peter Nolan, personal conversation on 22 September 2022 about Annie Altschul, via Zoom.
123 Jennifer Craig-Norton, *The Kindertransport: Contesting Memory* (Bloomington: Indiana University Press, 2019), 204.
124 Moos, 'I Remember', 113.

125 For a full analysis of nurses' access to these courses, see Jane Brooks, '"Visiting Rights Only": The Early Experience of Nurses in Higher Education', PhD thesis, London School of Hygiene and Tropical Medicine, University of London, 2005.
126 Gladys B. Carter, 'British nurses with university degrees or diplomas', *Nursing Mirror* (1957): 1117–18.
127 Fisher, 'Gender, class and school teacher education', 812; Dyhouse, 'Troubled identities', 173. See the Robbins Report, 'Higher Education: Report of the Committee appointed by the Prime Minister under the Chairmanship of Lord Robbins' (London: HMSO, 1963), 43.
128 Altschul, oral history interview, no date.
129 Hockey, oral history interview, 1987; Revd Jeremy R. H. Middleton, 'Thanksgiving service for Lisbeth Hockey', Davidson's Mains Parish Church Edinburgh (21 June 2004): 8. C300/1/9/1 Misc. papers and correspondence. RCN Archives, Edinburgh.
130 Charlotte Kratz, oral history interview at her home in Eastbourne on 16 September 1988. Interview T37, Oral History Collection, RCN, Edinburgh.
131 There are fewer details of Ferguson's life than for the other three pioneers discussed in this section. In an article she published in 1976, she is listed as Ferguson MA and a lecturer at the Welsh School of Medicine. Marion C. Ferguson, 'Nursing at the crossroads. Which way to turn? A look at the model of a nurse practitioner', *Journal of Advanced Nursing* 1 (1976): 237–42.
132 Nicola Ring, 'A personal and historical investigation of the career trends of UK graduate nurses qualifying between 1970 and 1989', *Journal of Advanced Nursing* 40, 2 (2002): 200.
133 Margaret Scott Wright, 'The nurse/graduate in nursing: Preliminary findings of a follow-up study of former students of the University of Edinburgh degree/nursing programme', *International Journal of Nursing Studies* 16 (1979): 205–14; Rosemary Weir, *A Leap in the Dark: The Origins and Development of the Department of Nursing Studies, The University of Edinburgh* (Penzance: Jamieson Library, 1996), 24.
134 Christine E. Hallett, 'The "Manchester scheme": A study of the Diploma in Community Nursing, the first pre-registration nursing programme in a British university', *Nursing Inquiry* 12, 4 (2005): 287–94.
135 Robbins Report, 'Higher Education', 2.
136 Robbins Report, 'Higher Education', 2.
137 It is not the intention of this book to discuss the movement known as 'Second Wave Feminism'. For discussion of the changes to the role

of women in the 1960s and 1970s, see for example, Ina Zweiniger-Bargielowska, *Women in Twentieth-Century Britain* (Harlow: Pearson Education, 2001); Sheila Rowbotham, *A Century of Women: The History of Women in Britain and the United States* (London: Penguin, 1999). Sarah Crook, 'In conversation with the women's liberation movement: Intergenerational histories of second wave feminism', British Library, 12 October 2013, *History Workshop Journal* 77, 1 (2014): 339–42. For a useful analysis of the impact of education on Second Wave Feminism, see Phillida Bunkle, 'The 1944 Education Act and Second Wave Feminism', *Women's History Review* 25, 5 (2016): 791–811.
138 For an excellent analysis of women's access to higher education, see Carol Dyhouse, *Students: A Gendered History* (London: Routledge, 2006).
139 Annie T. Altschul, 'Why higher education for nurses?: Issues and developments', *Nurse Education Today* 7 (1987): 11. For additional discussion on nursing in higher education, see Grace M. Owen, 'For better, for worse: Nursing in higher education', *Journal of Advanced Nursing* 13 (1988): 3–13. The O level was the public examination taken at the age of 16 in the UK. It was disbanded in the 1980s and replaced with GCSEs.
140 Robbins Report, 'Higher Education', 17.
141 Alex Mathieson, 'Chief nurse', *Mental Health Nursing* 19, 2 (1999): 29.
142 See for example the *Daily Mail*: 'Nurses told, "you're not too posh to wash a patient": Minister orders student nurses back to basics to improve compassion in NHS' (25 March 2013), www.dailymail.co.uk/news/article-2299085/Youre-posh-wash-patient-Minister-orders-student-nurses-basics-improve-compassion-NHS.html [accessed 6 October 2023). For a detailed analysis of the value of highly educated nurses, see for example, Linda H. Aiken, Douglas Sloane, Peter Griffiths, Anne Marie Rafferty, Luk Bruyneel, Matthew McHugh, Claudia B. Maier, Teresa Moreno-Casbas, Jane E. Ball, Dietmar Ausserhofer and Walter Sermeus: For the RN4CAST Consortium, 'Nursing skill mix in European hospitals: cross-sectional study of the association with mortality, patient ratings, and quality of care', *BMJ Quality & Safety* 26 (2017): 559–68.
143 Helen C. Sinclair, 'Graduate nurses in the United Kingdom: Myth and reality', *Nurse Education Today* 7 (1987): 24–9.
144 Kratz, oral history interview.
145 Christine E. Hallett, 'Colin Fraser Brockington (1903–2004) and the revolution in nurse-education', *Journal of Medical Biography* 16 (2008): 89.

146 In an article in the *Nursing Times* in 1958, E. M. Weir maintained, 'to be a graduate is quite a handicap for a student nurse'. E. M. Weir, 'Nurses with degrees', *Nursing Times* (30 May 1958): 629. Thirty years later, Winfred Logan was still addressing questions related to the value of the university-educated nurse – a reflection of the views of the detractors of degree nurses. Winifred Logan, 'Is education for a nursing elite?: Some highlights in nursing education in Europe and North America', *Nurse Education Today* 7 (1987): 5–9.
147 Margaret Scott Wright, 'Nursing and the universities', *Nursing Times* (15 February 1973): 222–7.
148 This informal group eventually became the RCN Research Forum.
149 McGann et al., *History of the Royal College of Nursing*, 175. In November 2022, there were 5,415 members in the RCN Research Forum.
150 According to Michael Denham, Professor Arthur Exton-Smith 'obtained a £5,000 grant from the National Corporation for the Care of Old People (NCCOP) for [Norton] and her colleague, Sister Rhoda McLaren, to carry out a two-year study of nursing elderly patients based at the Whittington Hospital, London'. This was, he argues, the first time research funds had been awarded to a nurse, but they were only awarded through Exton-Smith's participation. Michael J. Denham, 'Doreen Norton OBE, MSc, SRN, FRCN (1922–2007): Pioneer who revolutionised pressure sore management and geriatric nursing to international acclaim', *Journal of Medical Biography* 24, 2 (2016): 201–6.
151 Hockey, oral history interview, 1987.
152 Hockey, oral history interview, 1987.
153 Hockey, oral history interview, 1996.
154 Weir, *Leap in the Dark*, 29; Margaret Scott Wright, oral history interview by Rosalie Starzomski in Calgary, Canada on 10 February 1984. Audiovisual Recording Collection of the Learning Resource Centre, Faculty of Nursing, University of Calgary.
155 Anonymous, 'University of Edinburgh – Nurse Teaching Unit', *Nursing Times* (29 July 1955): 825; Weir, *Leap in the Dark*.
156 Weir, *Educating Nurses in Scotland*, 70. Not all medical schools were anti-nursing. In 1972 the Medical Faculty of the Welsh National School of Medicine appointed a Director of Nursing to undertake a degree course for nurses there. It is possible, though, that in the nearly twenty years since the Edinburgh Department was established, medical schools were used to the inroads nursing was making in the academy. Scott Wright, 'Nursing and the universities', 222–7.

157 McGann et al., *History of the Royal College of Nursing*.
158 Anonymous, 'Nursing Teaching Unit, Edinburgh University', *Nursing Times* (2 December 1955): 1353.
159 Anonymous, 'Director, Nursing Teaching Unit, University of Edinburgh', *Nursing Times* (20 April 1956): 299.
160 Nolan, 'Annie Altschul's legacy', 269.
161 Nolan, 'Annie Altschul's legacy', 270.
162 Altschul, oral history interview, no date.
163 Annie Altschul, 'Report on a tour of the United States of America, Canada, and Australia to study psychiatric nursing, May 1960–April 1961', in Stephen Tilley (ed.), *Re-Reading Altschul: A Festchrift in Honour of Professor Emerita Annie Altschul, CBE, BA, MSc, RGN, RMN, RNT* (Penzance: Hypatia Trust, 2004).
164 Weir, *Leap in the Dark*, 40.
165 Lisbeth Hockey, 'The nursing research unit after three years.' Manuscript for an article for *Nursing Times* (1974), C300/3/3/1, RCN Archives, Edinburgh.
166 Scott Wright, 'The nurse/graduate in nursing', 206.
167 Lisbeth Hockey, 'The Edinburgh University's Nursing Research Unit: The first four years', *Journal of Advanced Nursing* 1 (1976): 441.
168 Anonymous, 'Marion Ferguson: An appreciation' (1986), C342/1/8, RCN Archives, Edinburgh. By 1981 there were sixteen full-time undergraduate degrees for nursing in the UK. Joan Kemp, 'Graduates in nursing: A report of a longitudinal study at the University of Hull', *Journal of Advanced Nursing* 13 (1988): 281–7; see also Joanne M. Howard and Julia I. Brooking, 'The career paths of nursing graduates from Chelsea College, University of London', *International Journal of Nursing Studies* 24, 3 (1987): 181–9.
169 Marion Ferguson to Annie Altschul, 'Dear Annie', C305/2/3/11, RCN Archives, Edinburgh.
170 Anonymous, 'Marion Ferguson: An appreciation', 2.
171 Anonymous, 'Marion Ferguson: An appreciation'.
172 McGann et al., *History of the Royal College of Nursing*, 268.
173 Kratz, oral history interview. The ambivalence of the University of London to founding a nursing degree in the 1960s is corroborated in an oral history interview by Winifred Hector, who later founded a nursing degree at City University in the capital: 'And, the first place I thought of, of course, was London University, and I went to see the academic registrar, anyway, he listened to me and said, "Well Miss Hector, I can see very clearly what we could do for you, I can't quite see what you would do for us".' Winifred Hector, oral history

interview by Jane Brooks at her home in London on 5 April 2000. Personal archive.
174 Hallett, 'The "Manchester scheme"', 4.
175 Ina J. Bramadat and Karen I. Chalmers, 'Nursing education in Canada: Historical "progress" – contemporary issues', *Journal of Advanced Nursing* 14 (1989): 724.
176 Kratz, oral history interview.
177 Kratz, oral history interview.
178 Anonymous, 'PhD degree for nurses at Manchester University', *Nursing Times* (11 July 1974): 1055.
179 Cree et al., 'Navigating the gendered academy'.
180 Cree et al., 'Navigating the gendered academy'.
181 Kratz, oral history interview.
182 Charlotte R. Kratz, 'Matters for concern – Groves of academe', *Community Outlook* (March 1987), C305/1/1 RCN Archives, Edinburgh.
183 Anonymous, 'Professor visits former student in Galena', *Galena Gazette* (30 September 1987), C300/1/8/4 RCN Archives, Edinburgh.
184 Carolyn Hicks, 'Barriers to evidence-based care in nursing: Historical legacies and conflicting cultures', *Health Services Management Research* 11, 3 (1998): 137–47.
185 Dyhouse, *Students*, 174.
186 Dingwall et al., *Introduction to the Social History of Nursing*, 119.
187 Dyhouse, 'Troubled identities'.
188 Michael Traynor, 'A historical description of the tensions in the development of modern nursing in nineteenth-century Britain and their influence on contemporary debates about evidence and practice', *Nursing Inquiry* 14, 4 (2007): 303. For a detailed discussion of the historical antecedents of and debates around evidence-based practice, see for example, Gary Rolfe and Lyn Gardner, 'Towards a geology of evidence-based practice—A discussion paper', *International Journal of Nursing Studies* 43 (2006): 903–13.

Conclusion

Of all the refugees whose narratives form this book, only three had been nurses before they fled Nazi oppression. Two others admitted that nursing was their ambition. Yet they all chose nursing either as their escape route or for financial independence once in Britain. Although wartime expediencies increased the range of employment options in the service of the Allied cause, most of these nurses remained in the profession. After the war, like many British women, most married.[1] The majority of those who continued to work outside the home retained nursing as their professional identity. *Jewish Refugees and the British Nursing Profession: A Gendered Opportunity* seeks to examine their influence on the profession and the profession's impact on them. My aim in this study has been to make sense of their reasons for choosing and staying in nursing, despite the sometimes insuperable opposition and obstacles they faced.

Using a range of oral and written testimonies, letters and articles in the nursing press and documentary evidence, the book traces the personal and professional lives of Jewish refugees who came to Britain and entered the highly feminised profession of nursing from the late 1930s and into the war years. When the refugees arrived in Britain, nursing was experiencing a substantial crisis in recruitment that appeared to be unassailable. As I argue, whilst the British Government, hospital administrators and nursing and medical professions all agreed that the country required more nurses as the world approached war, there was little agreement on how this should be achieved or what alterations in their working conditions could and would be afforded. In following the uneven chronology of their lives, *Jewish Refugees and the British Nursing Profession* contributes to our understanding of the shifts in attitude of a female profession which, in the mid- twentieth century, was both conservative and insular.

Most refugees who arrived in Britain were required to transmigrate. However, as I argue in Chapter 1, because nurse training lasted three or four years, those who came on nursing visas or became nurses before the declaration of war believed that they would have at least three years of relative security. After the horrors of living under Nazi rule, this offered them some sense of safety. Nevertheless, the recruitment of refugees and the offer of nurse training was not entirely altruistic. Hospital matrons knew they would have willing and cheap labour for the training period. Once qualified and therefore more expensive, these nurses were expected to leave the hospital and the country. Notwithstanding the advantages of recruiting refugees into the profession as the nation faced the imminent threat of war, many of them struggled to gain access to nurse training programmes.

The nursing leadership had long wanted to recruit from the educated middle classes and had largely failed. Most of the refugees whose narratives comprise this book came from markedly more cultured and educated families than most nursing recruits. Jennifer Craig-Norton argues that those refugees who escaped on domestic service visas were 'painfully aware' of their intellectual and cultural superiority to their British employers.[2] For those who worked as nurses, whilst the class division might not have been as great, it certainly existed. However, their refugee status and Jewish heritage marked them as somewhat infra dig. Hospitals across the nation, especially the prestigious voluntary hospitals, refused to take 'foreign' and 'Jewish' probationer nurses into their training schools. However, the municipal hospitals, especially those under the auspices of the LCC (London County Council), realised the benefits they could gain from this cohort of cultured refugees. The requirement for young women across the nation to undertake work to support the war effort meant that hospital training programmes recruited those who would normally have gone to university or into more prestigious professional careers.[3] For those hospitals that accepted them, educated and cultured European Jews were a valuable addition to this cohort of intelligent probationers.

Chapter 2 considers the hospital world in which the refugees attempted to find training and work as nurses. Hospitals were generally not keen to recruit Jewish refugees onto either its medical or nursing staff. If the medical profession were largely successful in their endeavour to prevent Continental doctors from joining them, the nursing profession needed to be less antagonistic. Nurses were needed in greater numbers than doctors and the staffing crisis in the nursing profession was much greater. Several of the refugees were either medical students when they were forced to flee Nazi Europe or had ambitions to be doctors. If medicine was an option for women in Weimar Germany, it was not in Britain, where far more conservative and gendered ideas about medicine existed. The young female refugees educated in a more liberal atmosphere and, forced into nursing as a means of escape and financial independence, brought this cultural milieu into the profession. Thus, whilst German nursing might have been even more conservative than British nursing, most refugees did not come from a nursing background.[4]

Any optimism the refugee nurses may have felt in their new professional lives was shattered after the fall of France in the spring of 1940. As I argue in Chapter 3, all German, Austrian and Czechoslovakian hospital staff were dismissed from their positions following the evacuation of the British Expeditionary Force, fracturing any sense of security these young women felt in their new home. The draconian measures instituted by the Government – which for some included internment on the Isle of Man – played into the hands of the antisemitic and anti-foreign populace. Jews and especially Continental Jews were not to be trusted. Tragically for the refugee nurses, their engagement with this most vital and challenging profession was no antidote to their suspicious backgrounds. Their reinstatement into nurse training programmes after only a few months highlighted the ambiguities over who counted as British. Sonya O. Rose argues that 'all definitions of who "we" are – national identity and concepts of nationhood – are fragile'.[5] The wartime treatment of refugees typifies the arbitrariness of 'togetherness' and the concept of 'The People's War'.[6] Wartime propaganda encouraged a belief that all of Britain was united in the war effort. However, racism did not abate and prejudice towards

Jews, including Anglo-Jews, amid accusations of cowardice and self-serving behaviour, continued.[7] Whilst none of the refugees whose narratives comprise this book dwelt on antisemitism directed towards them, most recalled at least one incident. Tolerating the presence of Jewish refugees was always contingent upon the value they offered to the country. Colin Holmes argues that antisemitism, or perhaps the fear of antisemitism made assimilation difficult.[8] Nevertheless, as the war progressed the need for nurses outweighed the suspicion by which Continental Jews were viewed. The war years and shortage of workers meant that although there was still anti-refugee hostility, their labour was necessary.[9] By 1942, refugee nurses were on wards caring for members of the Armed Forces and in the latter months of the war, were even expected to act as interpreters for German prisoners of war.[10] This latter decision, like the internment of Jews alongside Nazi sympathisers, further exemplifies the lack of vision and understanding of the Government, professional leaders and wider population of Britain to the position of those who had sought refuge in this country. Nevertheless, the refugee nurses persevered, creating themselves as valued and essential members of the nursing community. The developing sense of their place in the British nursing profession and the country more widely paved the way for early naturalisation in the immediate post-war years.

Despite the – at best neglectful and at worse, harsh – treatment experienced by these young women in Britain, they were all keen to become British. Many were naturalised by the late 1940s, though some then rescinded their citizenship as they emigrated to Australia and the United States. The reasons why they were so keen to make Britain their home were varied and a matter of speculation. In his monograph on Jewish refugees in Britain, historian Anthony Grenville argues they stayed because they liked the easy-going attitude of the British.[11] However, the overlaying of nearly eighty years of nostalgia for the country that saved them from almost certain death has probably prevented them from judging accurately why they stayed. As Louise London contends, many had no home to go back to in Continental Europe, so they had no choice but to stay.[12] More pragmatic, some had married and were raising 'British' children and many were simply glad of a quiet and settled life after the devastation of the Holocaust. Others were professionally established and looking forward to the new National Health Service and its benefits for the health of the nation.

In Chapter 4, I consider how the refugee nurses supported the new National Health Service and those who were instrumental in later twentieth-century advances in nursing. The 1949 Nurses Act allowed for experimental nursing schools to be established, but modernising the education of nurses had its detractors.[13] Removing nurse training from auspices of the hospital would lessen the authority of the matron, create challenges to ward staffing levels and reduce the power-base of doctors. In most hospitals the honorary medical staff gave lectures to probationer nurses, so they were thus able to dictate the clinical information nurses learnt and ensure they were taught deference, a position they were reluctant to surrender. Despite the potential of the Act, late twentieth-century educational opportunities in nursing were slow to gestate, stymied by those outside the profession and also many within. In order to come to fruition, they needed determined and critical proponents. It is therefore not surprising that many Jewish refugee nurses were at the forefront of these changes. Within three decades, there were sixteen university departments in nursing across the UK, a quarter of which had refugee nurses on their staff.

The women's movement in the 1960s and 1970s altered the expectations of young women. Changes in educational standards and rapid scientific advances ushered in new ways of thinking and working. These changes impacted other feminised professions such as teaching, which developed more progressive attitudes in its education and working conditions. As more girls stayed on at school, the possibility for the brightest to attend university or teacher training colleges became a genuine option. Nursing was slow in its evolution towards a more liberal education and in the meantime lost out in the bid for educated, intelligent recruits. As the book demonstrates, by the 1970s and 1980s, university departments of nursing, a nascent nursing research movement and pioneering attitudes about the education of the profession's neophytes gained ground. Still, many both within and without the profession continued to contest the need for such developments. Nevertheless, there was an inexorable shift towards change that the detractors could not prevent. Several of the refugee nurses were at the forefront of this transition. Although the number of refugees who entered nursing was not extensive, those who did provided the beleaguered profession with educated, cultured and intelligent young women who would have a significant impact on the profession in the latter decades of the twentieth century.

As the source material exposes, nursing was not an ideal profession and for many not an original ambition, but in a time of limited employment choices for female refugees, it had a number of advantages. I argue that although the refugees were aware of the limitations of nursing as work and a career, they were willing to embrace it as part of the fight against Nazism and as redemptive action: if they could not care for their families who had been murdered in the Holocaust, they could at least care for the sick and ill of Great Britain. Most of the refugees whose narratives comprise this book remained critical of the profession. Yet, instead of leaving it to pursue other ambitions, they worked from within to influence change and advance nursing practice and education through research and innovation. Even those who had originally favoured more academic occupations were satisfied to develop as nurses. As Annie Altschul put it, 'We are different people from doctors and satisfied to be so.'[14]

Through an examination of the refugees' nursing lives, this study thus moves the narrative of women in the Holocaust from that of victims to agency. Much of the current literature, which specifically focuses on the lives of Jewish women under Nazi rule, exposes their experiences as women without power, unable to convince their husbands of the need to emigrate.[15] They are the women who walked with their children into the gas chambers.[16] Even Tony Kushner's and Jennifer Craig-Norton's extensive work on the survival of 20,000 Jewish women through the domestic service visa scheme typify these women as the victims of opportunistic and negligent housewives of Britain, keen to exploit the desperation of German and Austrian Jews.[17] Whilst I am not arguing that the Government and nursing profession were entirely altruistic in their pursuit of Jewish refugees for the nursing profession, at least nursing was able to offer something tangible to their lives.

Craig-Norton's work on the Kindertransport identifies the opportunity for girls to enter 'medical nursing' as the equivalent to boys' chances for a university education and professional future.[18] Most Kinder girls were expected to work as domestic servants and the boys were expected to learn a trade. There were few prospects for any of the Kinder to create a successful and independent future. For many there was little chance for an education on which to scaffold a future career. Nursing, whilst an unpopular profession amongst British girls and women and one that was not supported by a university education like the male professions, did at least provide a training and the chance of interesting work. Nevertheless, as the book demonstrates, the path to a career in nursing was often frustrated by the constellation of anti-German, anti-refugee and antisemitic ideologies of both nursing professionals and hospital authorities. It was also highly gendered. Whilst some talented male Kinder were offered the chance of remaining at school and then attending university, this was not offered to girls. Of those refugees whose narratives comprise this book and were university students before they fled, only Josephine Bruegel returned to her former studies. More common were the expectations exemplified by Otto Hutter and his sister, Doryt (Rita). Otto was awarded a boarding scholarship to Bishop's Stortford College and from there a place at University College London. In 1971 he was appointed the Regius Professor of Physiology at the University of Glasgow, where he remained until 1990.[19] His sister Rita arrived in England as a domestic servant, an experience which left her 'quite traumatised' and was persuaded to enter nurse training.[20] She remained in the profession until ill health rendered her immobile. The maxim was clear: clever male refugees could go to university; their intelligent female compatriots became nurses.

This is the first monograph to examine the engagement of female Jewish refugees in a professional career. It is also the first book to examine nursing as a means of escape and independence for women migrants. I acknowledge that it is not the first monograph to explore the value of nursing as a means of migration. Karen Flynn's excellent work on Caribbean migrant women who came to the UK to nurse as part of the Windrush generation deserves notable commendation.[21] However, Caribbean women came to the UK specifically to nurse, having been courted by the Government as a panacea to the nurse staffing crisis in the post-war period.[22]

Conclusion

For the Jewish refugees, nursing was a means of escape or a suitable alternative to domestic service once in the relative safety of Britain. *Jewish Refugees and the British Nursing Profession* thus breaks new ground in viewing nursing not only as a relative success story for refugees but, importantly, a pragmatic choice. The book also seeks to dispel the notions of the migrants' detractors, who viewed them as inhabiting the 'subversive' camp, or of their supporters, who see them only as victims of corrupt regimes and uncaring immigration policies.[23] According to the late cultural theorist Stuart Hall, refugees are those 'which are constantly producing and reproducing themselves anew, through transformation and difference'.[24] Thus, whilst nursing was not necessarily the profession they would have chosen were it not for the need to escape Nazism, it enabled young women to transition from subjugated refugee to independent womanhood.

The book therefore expands our understanding of how women migrants, particularly forced migrants, negotiate a space for themselves in their new country. Much of the history of Jewish refugees – and indeed current refugee crises – focus on male refugees or gender-neutral displaced persons.[25] I use the lens of nursing to view the movement of women, first escaping the horror of Nazism and then working to create a professional future. The book uniquely sits at the intersections of nursing history and women's history, refugee studies and the histories of the Second World War and the Holocaust. Setting the history of exiled Jewish women who became nurses in the interstices of these disciplines enables a greater understanding of their personal and professional encounters in a new country. By offering a critical eye on the exile of Jewish women and the kaleidoscope of identities they acquired as they reconsidered, re-evaluated and tested their positions as refugee, foreigner and citizen, the book seeks to illuminate the fears and pressures that resound in current refugee crises.[26]

Whilst *Jewish Refugees and the British Nursing Profession* is about the refugees' opportunities as nurses, it also examines the profession's attitude to them as Jewish and 'foreign'. The effects of anti-German and antisemitic feeling created significant obstacles to the refugees' attempts to gain access to nurse training. I hope the exposure of this racially based animosity raises the spectre of the current anti-immigration lobby who seek to damage the reputation of migrant, 'foreign' and non-white nurses in the British health service. The escalation of populist politics has created an environment in which the histories of immigration, escape and asylum-seeking are ever more critical. The migrant workforce in Britain is integral to healthcare provision, despite the reduction in numbers since the Brexit vote in 2016.[27] It is vital that this contribution is acknowledged and valued.

There are, of course, a number of limitations in this research. The first is the nature of the source material. *Jewish Refugees and the British Nursing Profession* uses a range of narrative modalities. I conducted eight oral histories specifically for the study and several families of deceased refugee nurses donated documents. I also engaged with a range of oral and written histories already in the public domain. It is eighty-five years since many of the refugees arrived in Britain: eighty-five years of the knowledge that their lives were saved and of Holocaust education overlaid with the expectation of gratitude. In many of the oral histories, the participants identified the opportunity that nursing presented. Gertrude Roberts spoke of being able to help others when she could not help her family who perished in the Holocaust.[28] Heidi Cowen admitted that the reason she entered nursing was to support her father financially. Yet later in the interview she admitted, 'I enjoyed my training very much ... We were glad it was something which really had potential.'[29] Lee Fischer, who eventually became a health visitor, stated that she loved the work because 'these were people who really needed nursing'.[30] Hortense Gordon wrote, 'When I began my nurse's training at the age of 21 years I did so because I felt that this was the work I really wanted to do for the rest of my life.'[31] The narratives that form the base of the book come from about twenty nurses, though there were probably about 2,000 refugee nurses by the end of the war. How those who did not record their stories felt about the profession is not known.

The second limitation is that I do not read or speak German. This meant that I was unable to review early correspondence by the future refugee nurses, which were written whilst still living on the continent of Europe. It is possible that these may point to a more circumspect view of their choices for escape and financial independence. The final limitation is that I have not reviewed any of the institutional documents from hospitals which employed refugees. Had I done so, I might have uncovered different narratives about the refugees' experiences as nurses. Nevertheless, having made the decision to focus on the words and thoughts of the refugees themselves, this book brings a novel perspective to the lives considered. John Stewart and Paul Weindling have both offered a more political and professional focus to the story of refugee nurses. *Jewish Refugees and the British Nursing Profession* ensures that the personal experiences are more clearly delineated.

The book argues that despite the challenges they faced in their early professional careers, the refugees' intelligence and determination enabled them to seize every opportunity offered to both develop themselves and the profession. University authorities were suspicious of nursing. As a highly gendered profession, it was considered an interloper into the hallowed walls of the male dominated higher education sector. Yet, there is little doubt that the refugees' resolve to engage with nursing and not abandon it for more lucrative or esteemed employment enabled the profession to raise the bar of its educational foundation and establish its nascent research base. As a nation, Britain certainly did more for Jews than other countries of comparable size of population, but it was still meagre. Britain was not indifferent to their plight, but there were 'limits' on what it was prepared to offer.[32] In the final analysis, as refugees to this country they were told to be grateful to the nation for saving their lives. Perhaps the gratitude should be ours, as twenty-first-century nursing and therefore the nation's sick and in need reap the benefits of their work, in practice, education and research.

Notes

1 See for example, Stephanie Spencer, 'Women's dilemmas in postwar Britain: career stories for adolescent girls in the 1950s', *History of Education* 29, 4 (2000): 329–42; Helen McCarthy, 'Women, marriage and paid work in post-war Britain', *Women's History Review* 26, 1 (2017): 46–61.

2 Jennifer Craig-Norton, 'Refugees at the margins: Jewish domestics in Britain, 1938–45', *Shofar: An Interdisciplinary Journal of Jewish Studies* 37, 3 (2019): 302.
3 Annie Altschul, oral history interview at her home in Edinburgh by Jane Brooks on 7 August 2001. Personal archive.
4 Hilde Steppe, 'Nursing in Nazi Germany', *Western Journal of Nursing Research* 14, 6 (1992): 697–800.
5 Sonya O. Rose, *Which People's War?: National Identity and Citizenship in Wartime Britain 1939–1945* (Oxford: Oxford University Press, 2003), 285.
6 Rose, *Which People's War?*
7 Joanna Bourke, *The Second World War: A People's History* (Oxford: Oxford University Press, 2001), 2002.
8 Colin Holmes, *A Tolerant Country?: Immigrants, Refugees and Minorities in Britain* (London: Faber & Faber, 1991), 32.
9 Tony Kushner, *The Persistence of Prejudice: Antisemitism in British Society during the Second World War* (Manchester: Manchester University Press, 1989), 90.
10 Lee Fischer admitted that whilst she would have both cared and interpreted for wounded German soldiers as they were patients like anyone else, it would be a challenge for her. She was glad when none were admitted. Lee Fischer (Liesl Einstein), oral history interview by Jane Brooks on 12 October 2017. Personal archive.
11 Anthony Grenville, *Jewish Refugees from Germany and Austria in Britain, 1933–1970* (London: Vallentine Mitchell, 2010), 60.
12 Louise London, *Whitehall and the Jews, 1933–1948: British Immigration Policy, Jewish Refugees and the Holocaust* (Cambridge: Cambridge University Press, 2000), 258.
13 Anonymous, 'The Nurses' Act 1949: Its educational scope and potentialities', *Nursing Times* (8 July 1950): 13–15.
14 Annie T. Altschul, 'Commitment to nursing', *Journal of Advanced Nursing* 4 (1979): 127.
15 Marion Kaplan, 'Jewish women in Nazi Germany before emigration', in Sibylle Quack (ed.), *Between Sorrow and Strength: Women Refugees of the Nazi Period* (Cambridge: Cambridge University Press, 1995).
16 Jillian Davidson, 'German-Jewish women in England', in Werner E. Mosse, Julius Carlebach, Gerhard Hirschfield, Aubrey Newman, Arnold Pauker and Peter Pulzer (eds), *Second Chance: Two Centuries of German-Speaking Jews in the United Kingdom* (Tübingen: J. C. B. Mohr, 1991).
17 Tony Kushner, 'Asylum or servitude? Refugee domestics in Britain, 1933–1945', *Bulletin of the Society for the Study of Labour History*

53, 3 (1988): 19–27; Tony Kushner, *The Holocaust and the Liberal Imagination: A Social and Cultural History* (Oxford: Blackwell, 1994); Jennifer Craig-Norton, 'Refugees at the margins'; Jennifer Craig-Norton, 'Servitude, displacement and trauma: Jewish refugee domestics in Britain, 1938–45', in Michaels, Paula A. and Twomey, Christina (eds), *Gender and Trauma since 1900* (London: Bloomsbury, 2021).

18 Jennifer Craig-Norton, *The Kindertransport: Contesting Memory* (Bloomington: Indiana University Press, 2019).

19 David Miller and Denis Noble, 'Obituary: Otto Hutter (1924–2020)', *Physiology News Magazine* 121 (2021), https://www.physoc.org/magazine-articles/obituary-otto-f-hutter-1924-2020/ [accessed 29 June 2023].

20 Personal correspondence from Otto Hutter, 1 August 2017.

21 Karen Flynn and Cindy-Lou Henwood, 'Nothing to write home about Caribbean Canadian daughters, mothers and migration', *Journal of the Association for Research on Mothering* 2, 2 (2000): 118–29.

22 Jo Stephenson, 'How nurses of the Windrush generation confounded bias', *Nursing Standard* 36, 7 (2021): 39–41.

23 Tony Kushner, 'Finding refugee voices', in Anthony Grenville and Andrea Reiter (eds), *Political Exile and Exile Politics in Britain after 1933* (Amsterdam: Rodopi, 2011), 124.

24 Stuart Hall, 'Cultural identity and diaspora', 235. https://warwick.ac.uk/fac/arts/english/currentstudents/postgraduate/masters/modules/asiandiaspora/hallculturalidentityanddiaspora.pdf [accessed 6 October 2023].

25 See for example, Bernard Wasserstein, *Britain and the Jews of Europe, 1939–1945* (Oxford: Clarendon Press, 1979); Werner E. Mosse, Julius Carlebach, Gerhard Hirschfield, Aubrey Newman, Arnold Pauker and Peter Pulzer (eds), *Second Chance: Two Centuries of German-Speaking Jews in the United Kingdom* (Tübingen: J. C. B. Mohr, 1991); London, *Whitehall and the Jews*; Walter Laqueur, *Generation Exodus: The Fate of Young Jewish Refugees from Nazi Germany* (London: I. B. Tauris, 2004).

26 Linda McDowell, 'Moving stories: Precarious work and multiple migrations', *Gender, Place and Culture: A Journal of Feminist Geography* 25, 4 (2018): 471–88; Peter Gatrell, 'The question of refugees: Past and present', *Origins: Current Events in Historical Perspective* 10, 7 (2017). https://origins.osu.edu/article/question-refugees-past-and-present?language_content_entity=en [accessed 20 September 2023].

27 Migration Advisory Committee, 'Report on nursing shortage' (2016): 21. www.gov.uk/Government/news/migration-advisory-committee-mac-report-on-nursing-shortage [accessed 21 June 2017].

28 Gertrude Roberts, oral history interview by Alan Dein on 23 January 1982. Audio184. Oral History Collection, Jewish Museum, London.
29 Heidi Cowen (pseudonym) and Ruth Shire, oral history interview by Jane Brooks at Shire's home in the West Midlands on 13 February 2018. Personal archive.
30 Lee Fischer (Liesl Einstein), oral history interview by Jane Brooks on 12 October 2017. Personal archive.
31 Hortense Gordon, 'Marriage versus carreer' [sic]. Unpublished document given to me at our interview.
32 London, *Whitehall and the Jews*, 275.

Bibliography

Archives

Barbara Bates Center for the Study of Nursing History, Philadelphia
British Library
Friends Meeting House Library
Holocaust Memorial Museum, Washington, DC
Imperial War Museum
Jewish Museum, London
Jewish Museum, Manchester
King's College London Archives
Leo Baeck Institute Oral History Archive
London Metropolitan Archives
National Archives, Kew, London
People's History Museum, Manchester
Royal College of Nursing Archives
Tower Hamlets Local History Library and Archives
Wiener Library

Oral history interviews

Altschul, Annie, oral history interview at her home in Edinburgh. No date. Interview T8, Oral History Collection, RCN, Edinburgh.

Altschul, Annie, oral history interview at her home in Edinburgh by Jane Brooks on 7 August 2001. Personal archive.

Bown, Edith (Jacobowitz), oral history interview in Maidstone by Barbara Mortimer on 24 May 2008. Interview T379, Oral History Collection, RCN, Edinburgh.

Bruegel, Josephine, 'Reminiscences': oral history interview by Sylva Simsova between 1998 and 2001. OSP 2122, Wiener Holocaust Library, London.

Cowen, Heidi (pseudonym) and Shire, Ruth, oral history interview at Shire's home in the West Midlands by Jane Brooks on 13 February 2018. Personal archive.

Fink, Alice (Redlich), oral history interview by Lyn E. Smith in November 1997. Interview 1775, Sound Archive, Imperial War Museum, London.

Fischer, Lee (Einstein, Liesl), oral history interview by Jane Brooks on 12 October 2017. Personal archive.

Gordon, Hortense, oral history interview by Sharon Rapaport in London on 3 July 2004. Interview 65, Refugee Voices: Association of Jewish Refugees (AJR) Audio-Visual Testimony Archive, British Library, London.

Gordon, Hortense, oral history interview at her home in London by Jane Brooks on 27 October 2017. Personal archive.

Haar, Cilly (Brauer), oral history interview at her home in London by Jane Brooks on 4 September 2017. Personal archive.

Harding, Erna, oral history video interview in Walnut Creek by Peter Ryan on 11 April 2011. Gift of Jewish and Children's Services of San Francisco, the Peninsula, Marin and Sonoma Counties, United States Holocaust Memorial Museum (USHMM), Washington, DC.

Hector, Winifred, oral history interview at her home in London by Jane Brooks on 5 April 2000. Personal archive.

Heyman, Lotte, oral history interview at her home in Buckinghamshire by Barbara Mortimer on 15 September 2009. Interview T235, Oral History Collection, RCN, Edinburgh.

Hockey, Lisbeth, oral history interview at her home in Edinburgh by Susan McGann on 27 December 1987. Interview T26, Oral History Collection, RCN, Edinburgh.

Hockey, Lisbeth, oral history interview at her home in Edinburgh by Helen Sweet on 13 August 1996. Interview T221, Oral History Collection, RCN, Edinburgh.

Katz, Elisabeth (Rosenthal), oral history video interview by Sandra Bendayan on 4 August 1994. Gift of Jewish and Children's Services of San Francisco, the Peninsula, Marin and Sonoma Counties, USHMM, Washington, DC.

Kratz, Charlotte, oral history interview at her home in Eastbourne on 16 September 1988. Interview T37, Oral History Collection, RCN, Edinburgh.

Lefton, Esta, oral history interview by Susan McGann in North London on 16 February 2004. Interview T253, Oral History Collection, RCN, Edinburgh.

Linton, Susi, oral history interview by Rosalyn Livshin on 19 October 2004. Interview 78, Refugee Voices: AJR Audio-Visual Testimony Archive, British Library, London.

Loeffler, Susi, oral history interview by Jane Brooks from Australia on 18 January 2018, via Zoom. Personal archive. My grateful thanks to Susi's nephew Cameron Woodrow for introducing me to Susi.

Loeffler, Susi, 'Extract from draft: Appendix 4' (unpublished m/s July 2017), 3.

Lowton, Lenore (pseudonym), oral history interview at her home in the Midlands by Jane Brooks on 12 February 2018. Personal archive.

Menkes Wolloch, Edith, oral history interview at her home on 21 March 2006. Interview 2297, Austrian Heritage Collection (AHC) Oral History Archive, Leo Baeck Institute, Berlin and New York. https://digipres.cjh.org/delivery/DeliveryManagerServlet?dps_pid=IE2981299 [accessed 1 October 2023].

Nolan, Peter, personal communication on 22 September 2022 regarding Annie Altschul, via Zoom.

Pearl, Annaliese (Stift), oral history interview by Patrick Gyasi in Queens, New York on 29 May 2012. Interview 2087, AHC Oral History Archive, Leo Baeck Institute, Berlin and New York.

Price, Ruth (Schulvater), oral history interview at her home in Crowle, Worcestershire by Helen Lloyd on 29 July 2004. Interview 68, Refugee Voices: AJR Audio-Visual Testimony Archive, British Library, London.

Rayner, Claire, 'Frontline Females', BBC Radio 4 (11 April 1998). Participants: Monica Baly, Mary Bates, Glenys Branson, Constance Collingwood, Gertrude Cooper, Ursula Dowling, Brenda Fuller, Anne Gallimore, Monica Goulding, Daphne Ingram, Anita Kelly, Margaret Kneebone, Sylvia Mayo, Kay McCormack, Anne Moat, Phyllis Thoms and Margot Turner. H9872/2, British Library Sound Archive, London.

Roberts, Gertrude, oral history interview by Alan Dein on 23 January 1982. Interview 184. Oral History Collection, Jewish Museum, London.

Sacharin, Rosa (Goldschal), oral history interview by Barbara Mortimer on 28 April 2010. Interview T407, Oral History Collection, RCN, Edinburgh.

Schafer, Kitty (Kaufmann), oral history interview by Jane Brooks on 30 August 2017. Personal archive.

Scott Wright, Margaret, oral history interview by Rosalie Starzomski in Calgary, Canada on 10 February 1984. Audiovisual Recording Collection of the Learning Resource Centre, Faculty of Nursing, University of Calgary. My thanks to Geertje Boschma for sending me a copy of this interview.

Shire, Ruth, oral history interview by Jane Brooks at her home in the West Midlands on 13 February 2018. Personal archive.

Written testimony

Bown, Edith (Jacobowitz), 'Memories and reflections: A refugee's story' (1938). RCN Archives, Edinburgh.

Bruegel, Josephine, 'Memoirs', Wiener Holocaust Library, London. https://wiener.soutron.net/Portal/Default/en-GB/RecordView/Index/23314 [accessed 27 September 2023].

Charles, Susan (Ingelore Czarlinski) My thanks to Charles's family for sending me details of her life and relevant images.

Cohen, Gertrud Miriam Bettina Caroline Sylvia Camilla, A biographical database of European Medical Refugees in Great Britain, 1930s–1950s, Oxford: Oxford Brookes University. My thanks to Professor Paul Weindling at Oxford Brookes University, Oxford for providing me with access to his extensive archive of refugee nurses and doctors.

Dann, Gertrude, 'Memoir'. Leo Baeck Institute Memoir Collection (ME978), Leo Baeck Institute, Berlin and New York. https://digipres.cjh.org/delivery/DeliveryManagerServlet?dps_pid=IE9170107 [accessed 1 October 2023].

Dann-Treves, Lotte, 'Memoir'. Leo Baeck Institute Berlin Collection (M979), Leo Baeck Institute, Berlin and New York. https://digipres.cjh.org/delivery/DeliveryManagerServlet?dps_pid=IE8857024 [accessed 1 October 2023].

Haar, Cilly, *Then and Now: The Memoirs of Cilly Haar, nee Brauer*. There is no further information about this publication. It was presented to me by Haar on the occasion of the oral history interview.

Hodge, Margot (Pogorzelski), 'My Life, 1920–1943', 2004.633. Library and Archives, Rubenstein Institute, USHMM, Washington, DC.

Hoxter, Charlotte Leopold, 'How my parents Dr. Robert Hoxter and Luise Hoxter received their immigration permit to England.' My thanks to Hoxter's daughter for providing me with details of her mother's life and a range of documents relating to her escape and nursing.

Lewen, Ilse, A biographical database of European Medical Refugees in Great Britain, 1930s–1950s, Oxford Brookes University, Oxford.

Lewinsky, Susi, 'Memoirs, 1911–1940'. LBI Memoir Collection (ME1628): A32/6. Leo Baeck Institute Archive, Berlin and New York.

Loeffler, Susi, 'The Family Löffler: Part V – 1939: Escape of Susi' (unpublished ms, 2017). My thanks to Susi's nephew Cameron Woodrow for providing me with this history of the family.

Loeffler, Susi, 'Extract from draft: Appendix 4' (unpublished m/s July 2017). My thanks to Susi's nephew Cameron Woodrow for providing me with this history of the family.

Marflow, Margaret, 'For my Grandchildren' (2001). A biographical database of European Medical Refugees in Great Britain, 1930s–1950s, Oxford Brookes University, Oxford.

Moos, Gertrud (Trudie), 'I Remember: My Life Story' (printed 1995). A biographical database of European Medical Refugees in Great Britain, 1930s–1950s, Oxford Brookes University, Oxford.

Parkes, Marianne, 'The Past and other Pastimes' (no date). A biographical database of European Medical Refugees in Great Britain, 1930s–1950s, Oxford Brookes University, Oxford.

Radloff, Ann (Reeves) 'Going to Gooseberry Beach: Travels and adventures of a nursing Sister', Private Papers: Documents 147, Imperial War Museum, London.

Rawraway, Ruth, Testimonials, contracts of work, CV and personal communications with Ruth Rawraway's daughter. My thanks to her for providing me with access to this family archive.

Ross, Mia (Maria Fuchs), 'War memories.' My thanks to Mia's family for providing me with her memoirs.

Yarm School Assembly, A talk on the theme of 'Great Lives', 2 June 2014. A talk given by Eva Flatow's son, Dr David Gordon.

Primary published sources

Altschul, Annie, 'Report on a tour of the United States of America, Canada, and Australia to study psychiatric nursing, May 1960–April 1961', in Stephen Tilley (ed.), *Re-Reading Altschul: A Festchrift in Honour of Professor Emerita Annie Altschul, CBE, BA, MSc, RGN, RMN, RNT* (Penzance: Hypatia Trust, 2004).

Altschul, Annie T., 'Commitment to nursing', *Journal of Advanced Nursing* 4 (1979): 123–35.

Altschul, Annie T., 'Why higher education for nurses?: Issues and developments', *Nurse Education Today* 7 (1987): 10–16.

Anglo-Scott, 'Humanity begins at home', *Nursing Mirror and Midwives' Journal* (24 December 1938): 446.

Anonymous, 'The position of nursing: Past and present', *Lancet* (15 November 1930): 1090–3.

Anonymous, 'A shortage of nurses', *Daily Telegraph* (19 February 1932), 10.

Anonymous, 'Refugee scientists', *Lancet* (21 April 1934): 859–60.

Anonymous, 'Awake or dreaming?: The impressions of the German tour, June 1935', *Nursing Times* (13 July 1935): 684–6.

Anonymous, 'Cartoon – The College in 1935: Two new responsibilities – Occupational therapy & gas warfare', *Nursing Times* (21 December 1935): 1221. https://link.gale.com/apps/doc/OPRIIE463744181/WMNS?u=rcnur&sid=bookmark-WMNS&xid=47265fc4 [accessed 28 September 2023].

Anonymous, 'Germany's shortage', *Nursing Mirror and Midwives' Journal* (15 January 1938): 362.

Anonymous, 'Refugee doctors from Austria', *British Medical Journal* (9 July 1938): 79.
Anonymous, 'The London Jewish Hospital: New home for nurses. Lady Reading lays foundation-stone', *Jewish Chronicle* (22 July 1938): 29.
Anonymous, 'Nurse's German honour', *Nursing Mirror and Midwives' Journal* (20 August 1938): 478.
Anonymous, 'Helping the refugee nurse', *Nursing Mirror and Midwives' Journal* (10 December 1938): 357.
Anonymous, 'Reply to M.C.S.', *Nursing Mirror and Midwives' Journal* (11 February 1939): 695.
Anonymous, 'News in brief: Employment of aliens', *Nursing Times* (25 May 1940): 554.
Anonymous, 'Alien nurses dismissed', *Nursing Mirror and Midwives' Journal* (15 June 1940): 258.
Anonymous, 'To leave at once', *Nursing Times* (15 June 1940): 629.
Anonymous, 'Alien nurses', *Nursing Times* (22 June 1940): 653.
Anonymous, 'Alien nurses in hospitals', *Nursing Mirror and Midwives' Journal* (13 July 1940): 342.
Anonymous, 'Employment of aliens', *Nursing Times* (13 July 1940): 725.
Anonymous, 'Aliens may nurse again', *Nursing Mirror and Midwives' Journal* (9 November 1940): 121.
Anonymous, 'Ministry of Labour and National Service: The Nurses and Midwives (Registration for Employment) Order, 1943', *British Journal of Nursing* (April 1943): 44.
Anonymous, 'The Nurses' Act 1949: Its educational scope and potentialities', *Nursing Times* (8 July 1950): 13–15.
Anonymous, 'University of Edinburgh – Nurse Teaching Unit', *Nursing Times* (29 July 1955)
Anonymous, 'Nursing Teaching Unit, Edinburgh University', *Nursing Times* (2 December 1955): 1353.
Anonymous, 'Director, Nursing Teaching Unit, University of Edinburgh', *Nursing Times* (20 April 1956): 299.
Anonymous, 'PhD degree for nurses at Manchester University', *Nursing Times* (11 July 1974): 1055.
Bevin, Aneurin, Westwood, Joseph and Isaacs, George, 'Staffing the hospitals: An urgent need' (London: HMSO, 1945). Reprinted pamphlet, *International History of Nursing Journal* 3, 3 (1998): 6–15.
Bevington, Sheila M., *Nursing Life and Discipline: A Study Based on Over Five Hundred Interviews* (London: H. K. Lewis, 1943).
Brain, W. Russell, McAdam Eccles, W., Ellis, Arthur, Ellis, Richard W. B., Forsyth, David, Gillespie, R. D., Hunter, Donald, Hurst, Arthur, Hutchison, Robert, Moncrieff, Alan, Monkhouse, J. P., Poulton, E. P., Roaf, H. E., Ryle, John A., Stephen, Adrian, Wilson, C. P., Wynn, W. H.

(Medical Peace Campaign), 'The medical profession in Austria', *Nursing Times* (26 March 1938): 338.
Campbell, M. H., 'Guests of our nation', *Nursing Mirror and Midwives' Journal* (31 August 1940): 516.
Carling, Esther, 'Recruitment for nursing. To the Editor of The Lancet', *Lancet* (11 October 1930): 826.
Carter, Gladys B., 'British nurses with university degrees or diplomas', *Nursing Mirror* (1957): 1117–18.
Carter, Gladys B. and Pearce, Evelyn C., 'Reconsideration of nursing: Its fundamentals, purpose and place in the community, 4: Training of nurses in hospital', *Nursing Mirror and Midwives' Journal* (16 February 1946): 331–2.
Charles, Marion, 'From Nazi Germany to Clarence House', *Association of Jewish Refugees Magazine* (n.d.): 4–5. My thanks to Charles's family for donating this press clipping.
Darton, Lawrence, 'An account of the work of the Friends Committee for refugees and aliens, first known as the Germany Emergency Committee of the Society of Friends, 1933–1950.' Issued by the Friends Committee for Refugees and Aliens, 1954. Friends Meeting House Library, Euston Road, London.
G. M. Y., 'I: Christmastide with Frau Oberin Hubler', *Nursing Times* (21 December 1935): 1237.
Goodwin, Aubrey, '"Our Colleagues in Austria": To the Editor of The Lancet', *Lancet* (2 April 1938): 808.
Gordon, Hortense, 'Marriage versus carreer' [*sic*]. This is a short, typed piece that was given to me personally when I interviewed Gordon. I do not know if it was ever published, or if it was just for her family.
Gordon, Hortense, 'Supplement. Community forum 7 – Liaison: The vital link', *Nursing Mirror* (3 August 1983): i–iv.
Herz, U., 'Refugee nurse's plea', *Nursing Mirror and Midwives' Journal* (9 November 1940): 142.
Hillyers, G. V., 'Refugee nurses', *Nursing Times* (10 December 1938): 1310.
Hockey, Lisbeth, 'The Edinburgh University's Nursing Research Unit: The first four years', *Journal of Advanced Nursing* 1 (1976): 437–42.
Just an alien nurse, 'Alien nurse wishes to serve', *Nursing Mirror and Midwives Journal* (29 June 1940): 317.
Just an alien nurse, 'Aliens wish to serve', *Nursing Mirror and Midwives Journal* (3 August 1940): 415.
Lewis, L. H., 'Refugee nurses', *Nursing Mirror and Midwives' Journal* (7 January 1939): 513.
Logan, Winifred, 'Is education for a nursing elite?: Some highlights in nursing education in Europe and North America', *Nurse Education Today* 7 (1987): 5–9.

Lysaght, A. C., '"Our Colleagues in Austria": To the Editor of The Lancet', *Lancet* (16 April 1938); 914–15.
Mathieson, Alex, 'Chief nurse', *Mental Health Nursing* 19, 2 (1999): 28–9.
M. C. S., 'Refugee and training', *Nursing Mirror and Midwives' Journal* (11 February 1939): 695.
Minden, Eva, *How it all Started with the Shoes: Memoirs of a Career in Nursing from 1934–1951* (Baltimore, MD: Novice Publishers, 2021).
Owen, Grace M., 'Curriculum integration in nursing education: A concept or a way of life? A study of six courses integrating basic nursing education and health visiting in a single course', *Journal of Advanced Nursing* 2 (1977): 443–60.
Owen, Grace M., 'For better, for worse: Nursing in higher education', *Journal of Advanced Nursing* 13 (1988): 3–13.
Pearce, Evelyn C., *A General Textbook of Nursing: A Comprehensive Guide to the Final State Examinations* (London: Faber & Faber, 1937).
Pye, E. M., 'Midwifery training of refugees', *Nursing Mirror and Midwives' Journal* (10 June 1939): 380.
Pye, E. M., 'Text books for refugees', *Nursing Mirror and Midwives' Journal* (12 August 1939): 680.
Sacharin, Rosa M., *The Unwanted Jew: A Struggle for Acceptance* (Tullibody: Diadem Books, 2014).
Scott Wright, Margaret, 'Nursing and the universities', *Nursing Times* (15 February 1973): 222–7.
Scott Wright, Margaret, 'The nurse/graduate in nursing: Preliminary findings of a follow-up study of former students of the University of Edinburgh degree/nursing programme', *International Journal of Nursing Studies* 16 (1979): 205–14.
Sister, 'For the sake of humanity', *Nursing Mirror and Midwives' Journal* (26 November 1938): 305.
Socialist Medical Association, 'Memorandum on the nursing problem' (16 September 1947) www.sochealth.co.uk/1947/09/16/memorandum-nursing-problem.
Weir, E. M., 'Nurses with degrees', *Nursing Times* (30 May 1958): 629.
Wenger, M. L., 'Editorial: Nurse education and university courses', *Nursing Times* (7 December 1956): 1251–2.

Government and professional reports

Athlone Committee, Inter-Departmental Committee on Nursing Services, Interim Report (London: HMSO, 1939).
Lancet Commission on Nursing, *Final Report of The Lancet Commission on Nursing* (London: The Lancet Ltd, 1932).

Bibliography

Robbins Report, 'Higher Education: Report of the Committee appointed by the Prime Minister under the Chairmanship of Lord Robbins' (London: HMSO, 1963).

Royal College of Nursing, Chairman: Lord Horder, 'Nursing Reconstruction Committee: Section II, education and training' (London: Royal College of Nursing, 1943).

Theses

Brooks, Jane, '"Visiting Rights Only": The Early Experience of Nurses in Higher Education', PhD thesis, London School of Hygiene and Tropical Medicine, University of London, 2005.

Hatchett, Richard Paul, 'The History of Workforce Policy and Planning in British Nursing, 1939–1960', PhD thesis, London School of Hygiene and Tropical Medicine, University of London, 2005.

Rein, Howard Irving, 'A Comparative Study of the London German and the London Jewish Hospitals', PhD thesis, University of Southampton, 2016.

Secondary sources

Abrams, Lynn, 'Liberating the female self: Epiphanies, conflict and coherence in the life stories of post-war British women', *Social History* 39, 1 (2014): 14–35.

Ahonen, Pertii, 'Europe and refugees: 1938 and 2015–16', *Patterns of Prejudice* 52, 2–3 (2018): 135–48.

Aiken, Linda H., Sloane, Douglas, Griffiths, Peter, Rafferty, Anne Marie, Bruyneel, Luk, McHugh, Matthew, Maier, Claudia B., Moreno-Casbas, Teresa, Ball, Jane E., Ausserhofer, Dietmar and Sermeus, Walter: For the RN4CAST Consortium, 'Nursing skill mix in European hospitals: cross-sectional study of the association with mortality, patient ratings, and quality of care', *BMJ Quality & Safety* 26 (2017): 559–68.

Alter, Peter, 'Refugees from Nazism and cultural transfer to Britain', *Immigrants and Minorities* 30, 2/3 (2012): 190–210.

Anderson, Kathryn, Armitage, Susan, Jack, Dana and Wittner, Judith, 'Beginning where we are: Feminist methodology in oral history', *Oral History Review* 15, 1 (1987): 103–27.

Ash, Mitchell G., 'Women émigré psychologists and psychoanalysts in the United States', in Quack, Sibylle (ed.), *Between Sorrow and Strength: Women Refugees of the Nazi Period* (Cambridge: Cambridge University Press, 1995).

Baarnhielm, Sofie, Laban, Kees, Schouler-Ocak, Meryam, Rousseau, Cecile and Kirmayer, Laurence J., 'Mental health for refugees, asylum seekers and displaced persons: A call for a humanitarian agenda', *Transcultural Psychiatry* 54, 5–6 (2017): 565–74.

Bailey, Paul, 'Introduction', in Primo Levi, *The Drowned and the Saved* (London: Abacus, 2013).

Bajohr, Frank, *'Aryanisation' in Hamburg: The Economic Exclusion of Jews and the Confiscation of their Property in Nazi Germany* (New York: Berghahn Books, 2002).

Baly, Monica E., *Nursing and Social Change* (London: Routledge, 1995).

Barnett, Ruth, 'The acculturation of the Kindertransport children: Intergenerational dialogue on the Kindertransport experience', *Shofar: An Interdisciplinary Journal of Jewish Studies* 23, 1 (2004): 100–8.

Beaven, Brad and Griffiths, John, 'The blitz, civilian morale and the city: Mass-Observation and working-class culture in Britain, 1940–41', *Urban History* 26, 1 (1999): 71–88.

Ben-Sefer, Ellen, 'Surviving survival: Nursing care at Bergen-Belsen 1945', *Australian Journal of Advanced Nursing* 26, 3 (2009), 101–10.

Ben-Sefer, Ellen and Shields, Linda, 'Courage under adversity: Luba Bielicka-Blum (1906–1973) and the nursing school of the Warsaw Ghetto', *Health and History: Journal of the Australian and New Zealand Society for the History of Medicine* 18, 2 (2016): 27–39.

Benson, Evelyn R., 'Nursing in Germany: A historical study of Jewish presence', *Nursing History Review* 3 (1995): 189–200.

Benz, Wolfgang and Andrea Hammel, 'Emigration as rescue and trauma: The historical context of the Kindertransport', *Shofar: An Interdisciplinary Journal of Jewish Studies* 23, 1 (2004): 2–7.

Berghahn, Marion, *Continental Britons: German-Jewish Refugees from Nazi Germany* (Oxford: Berg, 1988).

Berghahn, Marion, 'Women émigrés in England', in Sibylle Quack (ed.), *Between Sorrow and Strength: Women Refugees of the Nazi Period* (Cambridge: Cambridge University Press, 1995), 69–81.

Bivins, Roberta, 'Picturing race in the British National Health Service, 1948–1988', *Twentieth Century British History* 28, 1 (2017): 83–109.

Black, Gerry, 'The struggle to establish the London Jewish Hospital: Lord Rothschild versus the barber', *Jewish Historical Studies* 32 (1990-2): 337–53.

Bliss, Julie and While, Alison, 'Team work and collaboration: The position of district nursing, 1948–1974', *International History of Nursing Journal* 5, 3 (2000): 22–9.

Bloxham, Donald and Tony Kushner (eds), *The Holocaust: Critical Historical Approaches* (Manchester: Manchester University Press, 2005).

Bond, Brian, 'The calm before the storm: Britain and the "Phoney War" 1939–40', *RUSI Journal* 135, 1 (1990): 61–7.

Bourke, Joanna, *The Second World War: A People's History* (Oxford: Oxford University Press, 2001).
Boyd, Julia, *Travellers in the Third Reich: The Rise of Fascism Through the Eyes of Everyday People* (London: Elliott & Thompson, Kindle edition, 2017).
Bradshaw, Anne, *The Nurse Apprentice, 1860–1977* (London: Routledge, 2001).
Bramadat, Ina J. and Chalmers, Karen I., 'Nursing education in Canada: Historical "progress" – contemporary issues', *Journal of Advanced Nursing* 14 (1989): 719–26.
Braybon, Gail and Summerfield, Penny, *Out of the Cage: Women's Experiences in Two World Wars* (London: Pandora, 1987).
Bretherton, Inge, 'The origins of attachment theory: John Bowlby and Mary Ainsworth', *Developmental Psychology*, 28, 5 (1992): 759–75.
Brooks, Jane, 'Managing the burden: Nursing older people in England, 1955–1980', *Nursing Inquiry* 18 (2011): 226–34.
Brooks, Jane, 'The bombing Blitz of London and Manchester, England, 1940 to 1944', in Keeling, Arlene W. and Mann Wall, Barbra (eds), *Nurses and Disasters: Global, Historical Case Studies* (New York: Springer, 2015).
Brooks, Jane, '"The nurse stoops down…for me": Nursing the liberated persons at Bergen-Belsen', in Brooks, Jane and Hallett, Christine E. (eds), *One Hundred Years of Wartime Nursing Practices* (Manchester: Manchester University Press, 2015).
Brooks, Jane, *Negotiating Nursing: British Army Sisters and Soldiers in the Second World War* (Manchester: Manchester University Press, 2018).
Brooks, Jane, 'From "unwanted Jew" to "a brighter professional future": Kinder girls and the nursing profession in wartime Britain', *Jewish Historical Studies: Transactions of the Jewish Historical Society of England* 51 (2019): 68–85.
Brooks, Jane, '"My questionable status as a friendly enemy alien": British responses to Jewish refugee nurses, 1933–1948', *Nursing History Review* 29 (2021): 202–22.
Bruley, Sue, *Women in Britain since 1900* (Basingstoke: Palgrave, 1999).
Brush, Barbara, 'Refuge and rescue: Jewish nurse refugees and the International Council of Nurses, 1947–1965', *Nursing History Review* 7 (1999): 113–25.
Bud, Robert, *Penicillin: Triumph and Tragedy* (Oxford: Oxford University Press, 2007).
Bunkle, Phillida, 'The 1944 Education Act and Second Wave Feminism', *Women's History Review* 25, 5 (2016): 791–811.
Burletson, Louise, 'The state, internment and public criticism in the Second World War', in David Cesarani and Tony Kushner (eds), *The Internment of Aliens in Twentieth Century Britain* (London: Frank Cass, 1993), 102–24.

Caestecker, Frank and Moore, Bob (eds), *Refugees from Nazi Europe and the Liberal European States* (New York: Berghahn Books, 2010).

Calder, Angus, *The Myth of the Blitz* (London: Random House, 1991).

Caruth, Cathy, *Unclaimed Experience: Trauma, Narrative, and History* (Baltimore, MD: Johns Hopkins University Press, 1996).

Cesarani, David (ed.), *The Final Solution: Origins and Implementation* (London: Routledge, 1994).

Cesarani, David, *Final Solution: The Fate of the Jews, 1933–1949* (London: Pan Macmillan, Kindle edition, 2017).

Chalmers, Beverley, 'Jewish women's sexual behaviour and sexualized abuse during the Nazi Era', *Canadian Journal of Human Sexuality* 24, 2 (2015): 184–96.

Chavez, Christina, 'Conceptualizing from the inside: Advantages, complications, and demands on insider positionality', *Qualitative Report*, 13, 3 (2008): 474–94.

Clark, Mary Marshall, 'Case study: Field notes on catastrophe: Reflections on the September 11, 2001, oral history and memory narrative project', in Ritchie, Donald A. (ed.), *The Oxford Handbook of Oral History* (Oxford: Oxford University Press, 2011).

Cohen, Susan, 'Crossing borders: Academic refugee women, education and the British Federation of University Women during the Nazi era', *History of Education* 39, 2 (2010): 175–82.

Cohen, Susan, *Rescue the Perishing: Eleanor Rathbone and the Refugees* (London: Vallentine Mitchell, 2015).

Cooke, Miriam and Woollacott, Angela, 'Introduction', in Cooke, Miriam and Woollacott, Angela (eds), *Gendering War Talk* (Princeton, NJ: Princeton University Press, 1993).

Craig-Norton, Jennifer, 'Contesting the Kindertransport as a "model" refugee response', *European Judaism* 50, 2 (2017): 24–33.

Craig-Norton, Jennifer, *The Kindertransport: Contesting Memory* (Bloomington: Indiana University Press, 2019).

Craig-Norton, Jennifer, 'Refugees at the margins: Jewish domestics in Britain, 1938–45', *Shofar: An Interdisciplinary Journal of Jewish Studies* 37, 3 (2019): 295–330.

Craig-Norton, Jennifer, 'Servitude, displacement and trauma: Jewish refugee domestics in Britain, 1938–45', in Michaels, Paula A. and Twomey, Christina (eds), *Gender and Trauma since 1900* (London: Bloomsbury, 2021).

Craig-Norton, Jennifer, '"We had the most marvellous time": Jewish refugee domestics' narratives of internment in Britain during the Second World War', *Jewish Historical Studies: Transactions of the Jewish Historical Society of England* 52, 1 (2021): 37–55.

Craven, Hannah, 'Horror in our time: Images of the concentration camps in the British media, 1945', *Historical Journal of Film, Radio and Television* 21, 3 (2001): 205–53.
Cree, Vivienne, Morrison, Fiona, Mitchell, Mary and Gulland, Jackie, 'Navigating the gendered academy: Women in social work academia', *Social Work Education* 39, 5 (2020): 650–64.
Crook, Sarah, 'In conversation with the women's liberation movement: Intergenerational histories of second wave feminism', British Library, 12 October 2013, *History Workshop Journal* 77, 1 (2014): 339–42.
Curio, Claudia, 'Were unaccompanied child refugees a privileged class of refugees in the liberal states of Europe?', in Caestecker, Frank and Moore, Bob (eds), *Refugees from Nazi Europe and the Liberal European States* (New York: Berghahn Books, 2010).
Davidson, Jillian, 'German-Jewish women in England', in Mosse, Werner E., Carlebach, Julius, Hirschfield, Gerhard, Newman, Aubrey, Pauker, Arnold and Pulzer, Peter (eds), *Second Chance: Two Centuries of German-Speaking Jews in the United Kingdom* (Tubingen: J. C. B. Mohr, 1991).
Davies, Angela. 'Belonging and "unbelonging": Jewish refugee and survivor women in 1950s Britain', *Women's History Review* 26, 1 (2016): 130–46.
Davies, Celia, 'Continuities in the development of hospital nursing in Britain', *Journal of Advanced Nursing* 2 (1976): 479–93.
D'Cruze, Shani, 'Women and the family', in Purvis, June (ed.), *Women's History Britain, 1850–1945* (London: UCL Press, 1995).
Decker, Karola, 'Divisions and diversity: The complexities of medical refuge in Britain, 1933–1948', *Bulletin of the History of Medicine* 77, 4 (2003): 850–73.
Delap, Lucy, *Knowing their Place: Domestic Service in Twentieth-Century Britain* (Oxford: Oxford University Press, 2011).
Denham, Michael, J., 'Doreen Norton OBE, MSc, SRN, FRCN (1922–2007): Pioneer who revolutionised pressure sore management and geriatric nursing to international acclaim', *Journal of Medical Biography* 24, 2 (2016): 201–6.
Dickinson, Tommy, *Curing Queers: Mental Nurses and their Patients, 1935–74* (Manchester: Manchester University Press, 2015).
Dingwall, Robert, Rafferty, Anne Marie and Webster, Charles, *An Introduction to the Social History of Nursing* (London: Routledge, 1988).
Dwork, Deborah, *Children with a Star: Jewish Youth in Nazi Europe* (New Haven, CT: Yale University Press, 1991).
Dyhouse, Carol, 'Troubled identities: Gender and status in the history of the mixed colleges in English universities since 1945', *Women's History Review* 12, 2 (2003): 169–94.

Dyhouse, Carol, *Students: A Gendered History* (London: Routledge, 2006).
Evans, Richard J., *The Third Reich in Power, 1933–1939* (London: Penguin, 2005).
Evans, Stephen G. and Delaney, Keith B., 'The V1 (Flying Bomb) attack on London (1944–1945): The applied geography of early cruise missile accuracy', *Applied Geography* 99 (2018):44–53.
Ewart, Henrietta, '"Coventry Irish": Community, class, culture and narrative in the formation of a migrant identity, 1940–1970', *Midland History* 36, 2 (2011): 225–44.
Ferguson, Marion C., 'Nursing at the crossroads. Which way to turn? A look at the model of a nurse practitioner', *Journal of Advanced Nursing* 1 (1976): 237–42.
Ferguson, Rona, 'Autonomy, tension and trade-off: Attitudes to doctors in the history of district nursing', *International History of Nursing Journal* 6, 1 (2001): 10–17.
Fieseler, Beate, Hampf, Michaela M. and Schwarzkopf, Jutta, 'Gendering combat: Military women's status in Britain, the United States and the Soviet Union during the Second World War', *Women's Studies International Forum* 47 (2014): 115–26.
Fisher, Roy, 'Gender, class and school teacher education from the mid-nineteenth century to 1970: Scenes from a town in the North of England', *History of Education* 48, 6 (2019): 806–18.
Flynn, Karen, 'Proletarianization, professionalization and Caribbean immigrant nurses', *Canadian Woman Studies* 18, 1 (1998): 57–60.
Flynn, Karen, *Moving Beyond Borders: A History of Black Canadian and Caribbean Women in the Diaspora* (Toronto: University of Toronto Press, 2011).
Flynn, Karen and Henwood, Cindy-Lou, 'Nothing to write home about Caribbean Canadian daughters, mothers and migration', *Journal of the Association for Research on Mothering* 2, 2 (2000): 118–29.
Ford, Steve, 'Exclusive: High level of racial discrimination faced by nurses revealed', *Nursing Times* (2 October 2019). www.nursingtimes.net/news/workforce/exclusive-high-level-of-racial-discrimination-faced-by-nurses-revealed-02-10-2019 [accessed 20 September 2023].
Friedlander, Saul, *Nazi Germany and the Jews: Volume I, The Years of Persecution, 1933–1939* (London: Phoenix, 1997).
Ganor, Sheer, 'Forbidden words, banished voices: Jewish refugees at the service of the BBC propaganda to wartime Germany', *Journal of Contemporary History* 55, 1 (2020): 97–119.
Gardiner, Juliet, *The Blitz: The British Under Attack* (London: Harper Press, 2010).
Gatrell, Peter, *The Making of the Modern Refugee* (Oxford: Oxford University Press, 2015).

Gatrell, Peter, 'The question of refugees: Past and present', *Origins: Current Events in Historical Perspective* 10, 7 (2017). https://origins.osu.edu/article/question-refugees-past-and-present?language_content_entity=en [accessed 20 September 2023].

Georges, Jane and Benedict, Susan, 'Nursing gaze of the Eastern Front in World War II: A feminist narrative', *Advances in Nursing Science* 31, 2 (2008): 139–52.

Gershon, Karen (ed.), *We Came as Children: A Collective Autobiography of Refugees* (London: Papermac, 1989).

Gilbert, Martin, *Kristallnacht: Prelude to Destruction* (London: Harper Perennial, 2006).

Gilbert, Martin, *The Second World War: A Complete History* (London: Phoenix, 2009).

Gillespie, Veronica, 'Working with the "Kindertransports"', in Oldfield, Sybil (ed.), *This Working-Day: Women's Lives and Culture(s) in Britain, 1914–1945* (London: Taylor & Francis, 1994).

Gold, Dina, *Stolen Legacy: Nazi Theft and the Quest for Justice at Krausenstrasse 17/18, Berlin* (Chicago: American Bar Association Publishing, 2016).

Gopfert, Rebekka and Hammel, Andrea, 'Kindertransport: History and memory', *Shofar: An Interdisciplinary Journal of Jewish Studies* 23, 1 (2004): 21–7.

Gorsky, Martin, 'The British National Health Service 1948–2008: A review of the historiography', *Social History of Medicine* 21, 3 (2008): 437–60.

Gorsky, Martin, Mohan, John and Willis, Tim, 'Hospital contributory schemes and the NHS debates 1937–46: The rejection of social insurance in the British welfare system', *Twentieth Century British History* 16, 2 (2005): 170–92.

Grayzel, Susan R., *At Home and Under Fire: Air Raids and Culture in Britain from the Great War to the Blitz* (Cambridge: Cambridge University Press, 2012).

Greenlees, Janet, 'To care and educate: The continuity within Queen's Nursing in Scotland', *Nursing History Review* 26 (2018): 97–110.

Greenspan, Henry, 'The unsaid, the incommunicable, the unbearable, and the irretrievable', *Oral History Review* 41, 2 (2014): 229–43.

Grenville, Anthony, *Jewish Refugees from Germany and Austria in Britain, 1933–1970* (London: Vallentine Mitchell, 2010).

Grenville, Anthony and Reiter, Andrea (eds), *Political Exile and Exile Politics in Britain after 1933* (Amsterdam, NL: Rodopi, 2011).

Glynn, Sean, 'Irish immigration to Britain, 1911–1951: Patterns and policy', *Irish Economic and Social History* (1981): 50–69. https://journals.sagepub.com/doi/10.1177/033248938100800104 [accessed 25 September 2023].

Gunn, Jennifer L., 'Meeting rural health needs: Interprofessional practice or public health', *Nursing History Review* 24 (2016): 90–7.

Haire, Emily Jane, 'A debased currency? Using memoir: Material in the study of Anglo-French Intelligence Liaison', *Intelligence and National Security* 29, 5 (2014): 758–77.

Hajkova, Anna, 'Medicine in Theresienstadt', *Social History of Medicine* 33, 1 (2018): 79–105.

Hall, Stuart, 'Cultural identity and diaspora', 235. hallculturalidentityanddiaspora.pdf (warwick.ac.uk) [accessed 23 September 2023].

Hallam, Julia, *Nursing the Image Media, Culture and Professional Identity* (London: Routledge, 2000).

Hallett, Christine E., 'The "Manchester scheme": A study of the Diploma in Community Nursing, the first pre-registration nursing programme in a British university', *Nursing Inquiry* 12, 4 (2005): 287–94.

Hallett, Christine, E., 'Colin Fraser Brockington (1903–2004) and the revolution in nurse-education', *Journal of Medical Biography* 16 (2008): 89–95.

Hallett, Christine E., *Veiled Warriors: Allied Nurses of the First World War* (Oxford: Oxford University Press, 2014).

Hardman, Lesley H. and Goodman, Cecily, *The Survivors: The Story of the Belsen Remnant* (London: Vallentine Mitchell, 1958).

Harley, Sir Thomas, MBE, MC, 'The early problems of the NHS', *International History of Nursing Journal* 3, 3 (1998): 30–5.

Harrisson, Tom, *Living Through the Blitz* (London: Penguin, 1976).

Haste, Helen, 'Asset, alien or asylum seeker? Immigration and the United Kingdom', *Prospects* 36, 3 (2006): 327–41.

Hathaway, James C. and Foster, Michelle, 'Alienage', in Hathaway, James C. and Foster, Michelle (eds), *The Law of Refugee Status* (Cambridge: Cambridge Core, 2014). https://www.cambridge.org/core/books/law-of-refugee-status/alienage/D1BEC5D910910E9AF870DBA82641D9ADb [accessed 29 September 2023].

Hawkins, Sue, *Nursing and Women's Labour in the Nineteenth Century: The Quest for Independence* (London: Routledge, 2010).

Hayes, Nick, 'Did we really want a National Health Service? Hospitals, patients and public opinions before 1948', *English Historical Review* 127, 526 (2012): 625–61.

Hayes, Nick, '"Our hospitals"? Voluntary provision, community and civic consciousness in Nottingham before the NHS', *Midland History* 37, 1 (2012): 84–105.

Hertzog, Esther, 'Introduction: Studying the Holocaust as a feminist', in Hertzog, Esther (ed.), *Life, Death and Sacrifice: Women and Family in the Holocaust* (Jerusalem: Gefen Publishing House, 2008).

Hicks, Carolyn, 'Barriers to evidence-based care in nursing: Historical legacies and conflicting cultures', *Health Services Management Research* 11, 3 (1998): 137–47.

Hilton, Claire, 'A Jewish contribution to British psychiatry: Edward Mapother, Aubrey Lewis and their Jewish refugee colleagues at the Bethlem and Maudsley Hospital and Institute of Psychiatry, 1933–66', *Jewish Historical Journal* 41 (2007): 209–29.

Hirsch, Marianne and Spritzer, Leo, 'Gendered translations: Claude Lanzmann's *Shoah*', in Cooke, Miriam and Woollacott, Angela (eds), *Gendering War Talk* (Princeton, NJ: Princeton University Press, 1993).

Hirsch, Tal Litvak, Lazar, Alon and Braun-Lewensohn, Orna, 'Sense of coherence during female Holocaust survivors' formative years', *Journal of Loss and Trauma* 21, 5 (2016): 360–71.

Holmes, Colin, 'Enemy aliens?', *History Today* (September 1990): 26.

Holmes, Colin, *A Tolerant Country?: Immigrants, Refugees and Minorities in Britain* (London: Faber & Faber, 1991).

Holmes, Rose, 'Love, labour, loss: Women, refugees and the servant crisis in Britain, 1933–1939', *Women's History Review* 27, 2 (2017): 288–309.

Holmes, Rose, 'The politics of compassion: The Refugee Children's Movement and caring for the Kinder', *Jewish Historical Studies* 51, 1 (2020): 51–67. https://doi.org/10.14324/111.444.jhs.2020v51.005 [accessed 27 September 2023].

Homer, Stephanie, 'The resilience of the refugee: How Kindertransport memoirs complicate understandings of "resilience"', *Transactions of the Jewish Historical Society of England* 51 (2019): 105–18.

Honigsbaum, Frank, *The Division in British Medicine: A History of the Separation of General Practice from Hospital Care, 1911–1968* (London: Kogan Page, 1979).

Howard, Joanne M. and Brooking, Julia I., 'The career paths of nursing graduates from Chelsea College, University of London', *International Journal of Nursing Studies* 24, 3 (1987): 181–9.

Howse, Carrie, '"The ultimate destination of all nursing": The development of district nursing in England, 1880–1925', *Nursing History Review* 15 (2007): 65–94.

Hutchinson, Kitty, 'Memories of the founding of the NHS in 1948', *International History of Nursing Journal* 3, 4 (1998): 34–5.

Jefferson, Laura, Bloor, Karen and Maynard, Alan, 'Women in medicine: Historical perspectives and recent trends', *British Medical Bulletin* 114 (2015): 5–15.

Jones, Esyllt, 'Nothing too good for the people: Local labour and London's interwar health centre movement', *Social History of Medicine* 25, 1 (2011): 84–102.

Jones, Helen, 'National, community and personal priorities: British women's responses to refugees from the Nazis, from the mid-1930s to early 1940s', *Women's History Review* 21,1 (2012): 121–51.

Josephs, Zoe, *Survivors: Jewish Refugees in Birmingham, 1933–1945* (Birmingham: Meridian Books, 1988).

Kaplan, Marion, 'Prologue: Jewish women in Nazi Germany before emigration', in Quack, Sibylle (ed.), *Between Sorrow and Strength: Women Refugees of the Nazi Period* (Cambridge: Cambridge University Press, 1995).

Kaplan, Marion, *Between Dignity and Despair: Jewish Life in Nazi Germany* (New York: Oxford University Press, 1998).

Kapp, Yvonne, and Mynatt, Margaret, *British Policy and the Refugees, 1939–1941* (London: Frank Cass, 1997).

Kearns, Ade, Whitley, Elise, Egan, Matt, Tabbner, Catherine and Tannahill, Carol, 'Healthy migrants in an unhealthy city? The effects of time on the health of migrants living in deprived areas of Glasgow', *International Migration and Integration* 18 (2017): 675–98.

Kemp, Joan, 'Graduates in nursing: A report of a longitudinal study at the University of Hull', *Journal of Advanced Nursing* 13 (1988): 281–7.

Kirby, Stephanie, 'A splendid scope for professional practice: Leading the London County Council Nursing Service, 1929–1948', *Nursing History Review* 14 (2006): 31–57.

Kochan, Miriam, 'Women's experience of internment', in David Cesarani and Tony Kushner (eds), *The Internment of Aliens in Twentieth Century Britain* (London: Frank Cass, 1993).

Kushner, Tony, 'Asylum or servitude? Refugee domestics in Britain, 1933–1945', *Bulletin of the Society for the Study of Labour History* 53, 3 (1988): 19–27.

Kushner, Tony, *The Persistence of Prejudice: Antisemitism in British Society during the Second World War* (Manchester: Manchester University Press, 1989).

Kushner, Tony, 'An alien occupation – Jewish refugees and domestic service in Britain, 1933–1948', in Mosse, Werner E., Carlebach, Julius, Hirschfield, Gerhard, Newman, Aubrey, Pauker, Arnold and Pulzer, Peter (eds), *Second Chance: Two Centuries of German-Speaking Jews in the United Kingdom* (Tübingen: J. C. B. Mohr, 1991).

Kushner, Tony, 'Clubland, cricket tests and alien internment, 1939–40', in Cesarani, David and Kushner, Tony (eds), *The Internment of Aliens in Twentieth Century Britain* (London: Frank Cass, 1993).

Kushner, Tony, *The Holocaust and the Liberal Imagination: A Social and Cultural History* (Oxford: Blackwell, 1994).

Kushner, Tony, 'Finding refugee voices', in Grenville, Anthony and Reiter, Andrea (eds), *Political Exile and Exile Politics in Britain after 1933* (Amsterdam: Rodopi, 2011).

Kushner, Tony, *Journeys from the Abyss: The Holocaust and Forced Migration from the 1880s to the Present* (Liverpool: Liverpool University Press, 2017).

Kushner, Tony and Cesarani, David, 'Alien internment in Britain during the twentieth century: An introduction', in David Cesarani and Tony Kushner (eds), *The Internment of Aliens in Twentieth Century Britain* (London: Frank Cass, 1993).

Kushner, Tony, Cesarani, David, Reilly, Jo and Richmond, Colin, 'Approaching Belsen: An introduction', in Reilly, Jo, Cesarani, David, Kushner, Tony and Richmond, Colin (eds), *Belsen in History and Memory* (London: Frank Cass, 1997).

LaCapra, Dominick, *Writing History, Writing Trauma* (Baltimore, MD: Johns Hopkins University Press, 2001).

Langer, Lawrence L., *Holocaust Testimonies: The Ruins of Memory* (New Haven, CT: Yale University Press, 1991).

Laqueur, Walter, *Generation Exodus: The Fate of Young Jewish Refugees from Nazi Germany* (London: I. B. Tauris, 2004).

Lattek, Christine, 'Bergen-Belsen: From "privileged" camp to death camp', in Reilly, Jo, Cesarani, David, Kushner, Tony and Richmond, Colin (eds), *Belsen in History and Memory* (London: Frank Cass, 1997).

Lavsky, Hagit, 'British Jewry and the Jews in post-Holocaust Germany: The Jewish Relief Unit, 1945–1950', *Journal of Holocaust Education* 4, 1 (1995): 29–40.

Leverton, Bertha and Lowensohn, Shmuel, *I Came Alone: The Stories of the Kindertransports* (Sussex: Book Guild, 1990).

Levi, Primo, *The Drowned and the Saved* (London: Abacus 2013).

Lipman, Vivian D., 'Anglo-Jewish attitudes to the refugees from Central Europe 1933–1939', in Mosse, Werner E., Carlebach, Julius, Hirschfield, Gerhard, Newman, Aubrey, Pauker, Arnold and Pulzer, Peter (eds), *Second Chance: Two Centuries of German-Speaking Jews in the United Kingdom* (Tübingen: J. C. B. Mohr, 1991).

Loewenau, Aleksandra, 'Between resentment and aid: German and Austrian psychiatrist and neurologist refugees in Great Britain since 1933', *Journal of the History of the Neurosciences* 25, 3 (2016): 348–62.

London, Louise, 'British immigration controls procedures and Jewish refugees, 1933–1939', in Mosse, Werner E., Carlebach, Julius, Hirschfield, Gerhard, Newman, Aubrey, Pauker, Arnold and Pulzer, Peter (eds), *Second Chance: Two Centuries of German-Speaking Jews in the United Kingdom* (Tübingen: J. C. B. Mohr, 1991).

London, Louise, *Whitehall and the Jews, 1933–1948: British Immigration Policy, Jewish Refugees and the Holocaust* (Cambridge: Cambridge University Press, 2000).

MacNalty, Arthur Salusbury, 'Influence of war on family life', in Marchant, Sir James (ed.), *Rebuilding Family Life in the Post-War World: An Enquiry with Recommendations* (London: Odhams Press, 1945).

Markides, Kyriakos S. and Rote, Sunshine, 'The healthy immigrant effect and aging in the United States and other Western countries', *Gerontologist* 59, 2 (2018): 205–14.

Marwick, Arthur, *War and Social Change in the Twentieth Century: A Comparative Study of Britain, France, Germany, Russia and the United States* (London: Macmillan, 1974).

McCarthy, Helen, 'Women, marriage and paid work in post-war Britain', *Women's History Review* 26, 1 (2017): 46–61.

McDowell, Linda, 'Moving stories: Precarious work and multiple migrations', *Gender, Place and Culture: A Journal of Feminist Geography* 25, 4 (2018): 471–88.

McGann, Susan, Crowther, Anne and Dougall, Rona, *A History of the Royal College of Nursing, 1916–90: A Voice for Nurses* (Manchester: Manchester University Press, 2009).

McIntosh, Tania, '"I'm not a tradesman": A case study of district midwifery in Nottingham and Derby, 1954–1974', *Social History of Medicine* 27, 2 (2014): 221–40.

Mitchell, Gemma, 'Minister rejects plea to waive NHS fee for overseas nurses', *Nursing Times* (14 November 2018). https://www.nursingtimes.net/author/gemma-mitchell-3/page/128/ [accessed 20 September 2023].

Molnar, Michael, 'Portrait of an alien enemy', *Psychoanalysis and History* 10, 2 (2008): 169–83.

Mooney, Graham and Reinarz, Jonathan, 'Hospital and asylum visiting in historical perspective: Themes and issues', in Mooney, Graham and Reinarz, Jonathan, *Permeable Walls: Historical Perspectives on Hospital and Asylum Visiting* (Amsterdam: Rodopi, 2009).

Morley, Joel, 'The memory of the Great War and morale during Britain's phoney war', *Historical Journal* 63, 2 (2020): 437–67.

Morris, Mary (ed. Acton, Carol), *A Very Private Diary: A Nurse in Wartime* (London: Weidenfeld & Nicolson, 2014).

Mortimer, Barbara, *Sisters: Extraordinary True-Life Stories from Nurses in World War Two* (London: Hutchinson, 2012).

Moshenska, Gabriel, 'Moaning Minnie and the doodlebugs: Soundscapes of air warfare in Second World War Britain.' https://discovery.ucl.ac.uk/id/eprint/1549850/1/Moshenska_Moaning%20Minnie%20and%20the%20Doodlebugs.pdf [accessed 20 September 2023].

Mosse, Werner E., Carlebach, Julius, Hirschfield, Gerhard, Newman, Aubrey, Pauker, Arnold and Pulzer, Peter, *Second Chance: Two Centuries of German-Speaking Jews in the United Kingdom* (Tübingen: J. C. B. Mohr, 1991).

Nelson, Sioban, 'The fork in the road: Nursing history versus the history of nursing', *Nursing History Review* 10 (2002): 175–88.

Neushul, Peter, 'Fighting research: Army participation in the clinical testing and mass production of penicillin during the Second World War', in Cooter, Roger, Harrison, Mark and Sturdy, Steve (eds), *War, Medicine and Modernity* (Stroud: Sutton Publishing, 1998).

Niederland, Doron, 'Areas of departure from Nazi Germany and the social structure of the emigrants', in Mosse, Werner E., Carlebach, Julius, Hirschfield, Gerhard, Newman, Aubrey, Pauker, Arnold and Pulzer, Peter (eds), *Second Chance: Two Centuries of German-Speaking Jews in the United Kingdom* (Tübingen: J. C. B. Mohr, 1991).

Noakes, Lucy, *Women in the British Army: War and the Gentle Sex, 1907–1948* (London: Routledge, Kindle edition, 2006).

Noakes, Lucy, '"Serve to save": Gender, citizenship and Civil Defence in Britain, 1937–41', *Journal of Contemporary History* 47, 4 (2012):734–53.

Nolan, Peter 'Annie Altschul's legacy to 20th century British mental health nursing', *Journal of Psychiatric and Mental Health Nursing* 6 (1999): 267–72.

Ofer, Dalia and Weitzman, Leonore J., *Women in the Holocaust* (New Haven, CT: Yale University Press, 1998).

Oldfield, Sybil, '"It is usually she": The role of British women in the rescue and care of the Kindertransport Kinder', *Shofar: An Interdisciplinary Journal of Jewish Studies, Special Issue: Kindertransporte 1938/39 – Rescue and Integration* 23, 1 23, 1 (2004): 57–70.

Ong, Walter, *Orality and Literacy: The Technologizing of the Word*. 30th Anniversary Edition with John Hartley (London: Routledge, 2002).

Paperno, Irina, 'What can be done with diaries', *Russian Review* 63, 4 (2004): 561–73.

Pattinson, Juliette, *Behind Enemy Lines: Gender, Passing and the Special Operations Executive in the Second World War* (Manchester: Manchester University Press, 2007).

Phillimore, Jenny and Goodson, Lisa, 'Problem or opportunity? Asylum seekers, refugees, employment and social exclusion in deprived urban areas', *Urban Studies* 43, 10 (2006): 1715–36.

Pickering, Barbara A., 'Women's voices as evidence: Personal testimony is pro-choice films', *Argumentation and Advocacy: The Journal of the American Forensic Association* 40 (Summer 2003): 1–22.

Pistol, Rachel, '"Heavy is the responsibility for all the lives that might have been saved in the pre-war years": British perceptions of refugees, 1933–1940', *European Judaism* 40, 2 (2017): 42–9.

Pope, Rex, 'British demobilization after the Second World War', *Journal of Contemporary History* 30 (1995): 65–81.

Powley, Edward H., 'Reclaiming resilience and safety: Resilience activation in the critical period of crisis', *Human Relations* 62, 9 (2009): 1289–1326.

Prysor, Glyn, 'The "fifth column" and the British experience of retreat, 1940', *War in History* 12, 4 (2005): 418–47.

Pulzer, Peter, 'Jews and nation-building in Germany 1815–1918', *Baeck Institute Year Book* 41, 1 (1996): 199–214.

Quack, Sibylle (ed.), *Between Sorrow and Strength: Women Refugees of the Nazi Period* (Cambridge: Cambridge University Press, 1995).

Radu, Loredana, 'More or less Europe? The European leaders' discourses on the refugees crisis', *Romanian Journal of Communication and Public Relations* 18, 2 (2016): 21–37.

Rafferty, Anne Marie, *The Politics of Nursing Knowledge* (London: Routledge, 1996).

Reilly, Jo, 'Cleaner, carer and occasional dance partner?: Writing women back into the liberation of Bergen-Belsen', in Reilly, Jo, Cesarani, David, Kushner, Tony and Richmond, Colin (eds), *Belsen in History and Memory* (London, Frank Cass, 1997).

Reynolds, Robert, 'Trauma and the relational dynamics of life-history interviewing', *Australian Historical Studies* 43 (2012): 78–88.

Ring, Nicola, 'A personal and historical investigation of the career trends of UK graduate nurses qualifying between 1970 and 1989', *Journal of Advanced Nursing* 40, 2 (2002): 199–209.

Ritchie, Donald A. (ed.), *The Oxford Handbook of Oral History* (Oxford: Oxford University Press, 2011).

Rolfe, Gary and Gardner, Lyn, 'Towards a geology of evidence-based practice—A discussion paper', *International Journal of Nursing Studies* 43 (2006): 903–13.

Romain, Gemma, 'The *Anschluss*: The British response to the refugee crisis', *Journal of Holocaust Education* 8, 3 (1999): 87–102.

Roper, Michael, 'Splitting in unsent letters: Writing as a social practice and a psychological activity', *Social History* 26, 3 (2001): 318–39.

Rose, Sonya O., *Which People's War?: National Identity and Citizenship in Wartime Britain 1939–1945* (Oxford: Oxford University Press, 2003).

Rowbotham, Sheila, *A Century of Women: The History of Women in Britain and the United States* (London: Penguin, 1999).

Royal College of Nursing, 'London nurses experience the most racism', *Nursing Standard* 33, 8 (2018): 6. www.nursingtimes.net/news/work

force/exclusive-high-level-of-racial-discrimination-faced-by-nurses-revealed-02-10-2019/ [accessed January 2020].

Ryan, Louise, 'Migrant women, social networks and motherhood: The experiences of Irish nurses in Britain', *Sociology* 41, 2 (2007): 295–312.

Salvage, Jane, *The Politics of Nursing* (Oxford: Butterworth-Heinemann, 1985).

Sarkar, Mahua, 'Between craft and method: Meaning and inter-subjectivity in oral history analysis', *Journal of Historical Sociology* 25, 4 (2012): 578–600.

Schwartz, Agatha and Takševa, Tatjana, 'Between trauma and resilience: A transnational reading of women's life writing about wartime rape in Germany and Bosnia and Herzegovina', *Aspasia: The International Yearbook of Central, Eastern, and Southeastern European Women's and Gender History* 14 (2020): 124–43.

Schwartz, Rabbi Sidney, *Judaism and Justice: The Jewish Passion to Repair the World* (Woodstock: Jewish Lights Publishing, 2006).

Segal, Lore, *Other People's Houses: A Novel* (London: Sort of Books, 2018).

Shacknove, Andrew E., 'Who is a refugee?', *Ethics* 95, 2 (1985): 274–84.

Sharf, Andrew, *The British Press and Jews under Nazi Rule* (London: Oxford University Press, 1964).

Sharf, Andrew, 'Noah Barou Memorial Lecture: "Nazi racialism and the British Press, 1933–1945"', delivered at University College London (London: World Jewish Congress, 16 December 1963).

Sheftel, Anna and Zembrzycki, Stacey, 'Only human: A reflection on the ethical and methodological challenges of working with "difficult" stories', *Oral History Review* 37, 2 (2010): 191–214.

Sheftel, Anna and Zembrzycki, Stacey, 'Who's afraid of oral history? Fifty years of debates and anxiety about ethics', *Oral History Review* 43, 2 (2016): 338–66.

Shephard, Ben, 'The medical relief effort at Belsen', in Bardgett, Suzanne and Cesarani, David (eds), *Belsen 1945: New Historical Perspectives* (London: Vallentine Mitchell), 2006.

Shephard, Ben, *After Daybreak: The Liberation of Belsen, 1945* (London: Pimlico, 2005).

Shkimba, M. and Flynn, Karen, '"In England we did nursing": Caribbean and British nurses in Great Britain and Canada, 1950–70', in Barbara Mortimer and Susan McGann (eds), *New Directions in Nursing History: International Perspectives* (London: Routledge, 2004).

Shlain, Margalit, 'Nursing in the Theresienstadt Ghetto', *Nashim: A Journal of Jewish Women's Studies & Gender Issues* 36, 5780 (2020): 60–85.

Simsova, Sylva, 'Who were the pre-Second World War refugees from Czechoslovakia?', in Brinson, Charmian and Malet, Marian (eds), *Exile in and from Czechoslovakia during the 1930s and 1940s*, Yearbook of the Research Centre for German and Austrian Exile Studies: Volume II (Leiden: Brill, 2009).

Sinclair, Helen C., 'Graduate nurses in the United Kingdom: Myth and reality', *Nurse Education Today* 7 (1987): 24–9.

Snow, Stephanie, 'The art of medicine, the NHS at 70: The story of our lives', *Lancet* 392 (2018): 22.

Snow, Stephanie and Whitecross, Angela F., 'Making history together: The UK's National Health Service and the story of our lives since 1948', *Contemporary British History* (2022) DOI: 10.1080/13619462.2022.2045199.

Spencer, Stephanie, 'Women's dilemmas in postwar Britain: career stories for adolescent girls in the 1950s', *History of Education* 29, 4 (2000): 329–42.

Starns, Penny, *Nurses at War: Women on the Frontline, 1939–45* (Stroud: Sutton Publishing, 2000).

Staub, Ervin, *The Roots of Evil: The Origins of Genocide and Other Group Violence* (Cambridge: Cambridge University Press, 1989).

Steinert, Johannes-Dieter, 'British relief teams in Belsen concentration camp: Emergency relief and the perception of survivors', *Holocaust Studies: A Journal of Culture and History* 12, 1–2 (2006): 62–78.

Stephenson, Jo, 'How nurses of the Windrush generation confounded bias', *Nursing Standard* 36, 7 (2021): 39–41.

Steppe, Hilde, 'Nursing in Nazi Germany', *Western Journal of Nursing Research* 14, 6 (1992): 697–800.

Stevens, Robert, *From University to Uni: The Politics of Higher Education in England since 1944* (London: Politico's, 2004).

Stewart, John, '"For a healthy London": The Socialist Medical Association and the London County Council in the 1930s', *Medical History* 42 (1997): 417–36.

Stewart, John, 'Angels or aliens? Refugee nurses in Britain 1938–1942', *Medical History* 47 (2003): 149–72.

Stewart, John, '"The finest municipal hospital service in the world"?: Contemporary perceptions of the London County Council's hospital provision, 1929–39', *Urban History* 32, 2 (2005): 237–44.

Stewart, John, *The Battle for Health: A Political History of the Socialist Medical Association* (London: Routledge Revivals, 2018).

Stoller, Sarah, 'Forging a politics of care: Theorizing household work in the British Women's Liberation Movement', *History Workshop Journal* 85 (2018): 95–119.

Stone, Robyn I., 'The migrant direct care workforce: An international perspective', *Generations: Journal of the American Society on Aging* 40, 1 (2016): 99–105.

Summerfield, Penny, *Reconstructing Women's Wartime Lives: Discourse and Subjectivity in Oral Histories of the Second World War* (Manchester: Manchester University Press, 1998).

Summerfield, Penny, '"They didn't want women back in that job": The Second World War and the construction of gendered work histories', *Labour History Review* 63, 1 (1998): 83–104.

Summerfield, Penny, 'Culture and composure: Creating narratives of the gendered self in oral history interviews', *Cultural and Social History* 1 (2004): 65–93.

Summers, Anne, *Female Lives, Moral States: Women, Religion and Public Life in Britain, 1800–1930* (Newbury: Threshold Press, 2000).

Summers, Anne, *Christian and Jewish Women in Britain, 1880–1940: Living with Difference* (London: Palgrave Macmillan, 2017).

Sweet, Helen M. with Dougall, Rona, *Community Nursing and Primary Healthcare in Twentieth-Century Britain* (London: Routledge, 2008).

Taylor, Becky, Stewart, John and Powell, Martin, 'Central and local government and the provision of municipal medicine, 1919–39', *English Historical Review* 122, 496 (2007): 397–426.

Thane, Pat, 'Afterword: Challenging women in the British professions', *Women's History Review* 29, 4 (2020): 748–58.

Tilley, Stephen (ed.) *Re-Reading Altschul: A Festchrift in Honour of Professor Emerita Annie Altschul, CBE, BA, MSc, RGN, RMN, RNT* (Penzance: Hypatia Trust, 2004).

Tilley, Stephen, 'Three nurses: Stories of refugee nurses in Scotland', *Scottish Review* (March 2018): 1–5.

Timms, Edward, 'The ordeals of Kinder and evacuees in comparative perspective', *Yearbook of the Research Centre for German and Austrian Exile Studies* 13 (2012): 125–40.

Tosh, John, *The Pursuit of History* (London: Pearson Education, 2002).

Traynor, Michael, 'A historical description of the tensions in the development of modern nursing in nineteenth-century Britain and their influence on contemporary debates about evidence and practice', *Nursing Inquiry* 14, 4 (2007): 299–305.

Twells, Alison, '"Went into raptures": Reading emotion in the ordinary wartime diary, 1941–1946', *Women's History Review* 25,1 (2016): 143–60.

Tydor Baumel, Judith, *Double Jeopardy: Gender and the Holocaust* (London: Vallentine Mitchell, 1998).

Tydor Baumel, Judith, '"You said the words you wanted me to hear but I heard the words you couldn't bring yourself to say": Women's first-person accounts of the Holocaust', *Oral History Review* 27, 1 (2000): 17–56.

Tydor Baumel-Schwartz, Judy, 'The rescue of Jewish girls and teenage women to England and the USA during the Holocaust: A gendered perspective', *Jewish History* 26 (2012): 223–45.

van Rahden, Till, 'Jews and the ambivalences of civil society in Germany, 1800–1933: Assessment and reassessment', *Journal of Modern History* 77 (2005): 1024–47.

Vojvoda, Dolores, Weine, Stevan M., McGlashan, Thomas, Becker, Daniel F. and Southwick, Steven M., 'Posttraumatic stress disorder symptoms in Bosnian refugees 3½ years after resettlement', *Journal of Rehabilitation Research and Development* 45, 3 (2008): 421–6.

von Villiez, Anne, 'The emigration of women doctors from Germany under National Socialism', *Social History of Medicine* 22, 3 (2009): 553–67.

Wallach, Kerry, *Passing Illusions: Jewish Visibility in Weimar Germany* (Ann Arbor: University of Michigan Press, 2017).

Wasserstein, Bernard, *Britain and the Jews of Europe, 1939–1945* (London: Clarendon Press, 1979).

Webster, Charles, 'Conflict and consensus: Explaining the British health service', *Twentieth Century British History* 1, 2 (1990): 115–51.

Webster, Charles, 'The elderly and the early National Health Service', in Pelling, Margaret and Smith, Richard M. (eds), *Life, Death and the Elderly: Historical Perspectives* (London: Routledge, 1991).

Webster, Charles, 'Nursing as the early crisis of the NHS', *International History of Nursing Journal* 3, 3 (1998): 36–43.

Webster, Charles, *The National Health Service: A Political History* (Oxford: Oxford University Press, 2002).

Webster, Wendy, 'Enemies, allies and transnational histories: Germans, Irish, and Italians in Second World War Britain', *Twentieth Century British History* 25, 1 (2014): 63–86.

Weindling, Paul, 'The impact of German medical scientists on British medicine: A case study of Oxford, 1933–45', in Ash, Mitchell G. and Sollner, Alfons (eds), *Forced Migration and Scientific Change: Émigré German-speaking Scientists and Scholars after 1933* (Cambridge: Cambridge University Press, 1996).

Weindling, Paul, 'Medical refugees and the modernisation of British medicine, 1930–1960', *Social History of Medicine* 22, 3 (2009): 489–511.

Weindling, Paul, 'Refugee nurses in Great Britain, 1933–1945: From a place of safety to a new homeland', in Grant, Susan (ed.), *Russian and Soviet Healthcare from an International Perspective* (London: Palgrave Macmillan, 2017).

Weir, Rosemary, *A Leap in the Dark: The Origins and Development of the Department of Nursing Studies, The University of Edinburgh* (Penzance: Jamieson Library, 1996).

Weir, Rosemary, *Educating Nurses in Scotland: A History of Innovation and Change, 1950–2000* (Penzance: Hypatia Trust, 2004).

White, Rosemary, *Social Change and the Development of the Nursing Profession: A Study of the Poor Law Nursing Service, 1848–1948* (London: Henry Kimpton, 1978).

White, Rosemary, 'The Nurses' Act, 1949: 2 – Service priorities', *Nursing Times* 78, 5 (1982): 48–50.

White, Rosemary, *The Effects of the National Health Service on the Nursing Profession, 1948–1961* (London: King's Fund Publishing Office, 1985).

Wiederhorn, Jessica, 'Case study: "Above all, we need the witness": The oral history of Holocaust survivors', in Ritchie, Donald A. (ed.), *The Oxford Handbook of Oral History* (Oxford: Oxford University Press, 2011).

Wieler, Joachim, 'Destination social work: Émigrés in a women's profession', in Quack, Sibylle (ed.), *Between Sorrow and Strength: Women Refugees of the Nazi Period* (Cambridge: Cambridge University Press, 1995).

Wiese, Christian and Betts, Paul (eds), *Years of Persecution, Years of Extermination: Saul Friedlander and the Future of Holocaust Studies* (London: Continuum, 2010).

Williams, Bill, *Jews and other Foreigners: Manchester and the Rescue of the Victims of European Fascism, 1933–40* (Manchester: Manchester University Press, 2011), 1.

Willott, John and Stevenson, Jacqueline, 'Attitudes to employment of professionally qualified refugees in the United Kingdom', *International Migration* 51, 5 (2013): 120–32.

Yanklowitz, Shmuly, *The Soul of Jewish Social Justice* (Jerusalem: Urim Publications, 2014).

Yeates, Nicola, 'A dialogue with "global care chain" analysis: Nurse migration in the Irish context', *Feminist Review* 77 (2004):79–95.

Ziemann, Benjamin, 'Weimar was Weimar: Politics, culture and the employment of the German Republic', *German History* 28, 4 (2010): 542–71. https://doi.org/10.1093/gerhis/ghq114 [accessed 27 September 2023].

Zweiniger-Bargielowska, Ina, *Women in Twentieth-Century Britain* (Harlow: Pearson Education, 2001).

Index

Reference to images are in *italics*; references to notes are indicated by n.

Abrams, Lynn 24
Ahonen, Pertii 6
Air Raid Precautions (ARP) 128, 147–8
air raids 157
Aliens War Service Department 133
Allied Forces 128
Alter, Peter 50, 105
Altschul, Annie 1, 8, 21, 24, 26, 93, *198*
  dismissal 135, 140
  mental health training 110
  Mortimer narratives 14
  NHS 184–5
  post-war degree 193, 194–5
  psychiatric work 155–6
  re-employment 143
  research work 197
  war declaration 130
  war work 146
Anderson, Sir John 105
antibiotics *see* penicillin
antisemitism 7, 42, 43–4, 220–1, 225–6
  Austria 42
  Britain 104–5, 136
  education 48
  Nazis 11, 25, 45–6

Northern Ireland 151–2
nurses 98
apprenticeships *see* training
ARP *see* Air Raid Precautions
Aryans 47, 48
Association of Nurses 89
Athlone, Lord 88, 89
ATS *see* Auxiliary Training Service
Auschwitz 158, 172
Austria 24–5, 49; *see also* Vienna
Auxiliary Training Service (ATS) 10, 113

Bailey, Paul 192
Baker, Dorothy 199
Baly, Sister Monica 150
Barbican Mission 57
Baumel, Judith Tydor 23, 80n.137, 154
Beaven, Brad 146
Benedict, Susan 18
Ben-Sefer, Ellen 122n.100
Bergen-Belsen 26, 176–81, 206n.36
  liberation 158, 172, 174, 204n.16
Berghahn, Marion 57, 59, 70–1, 91, 130, 153

Index

Bevington, Sheila: *Nursing Life and Discipline* 89
Black, Gerry 109
Blitz 142, 145–9
Bloomsbury House 25, 91–2, 140–1
Bond, Brian 128
Booth Hall Children's Hospital (Manchester) 85, 95, 107, 144
border controls 49, 70
Bown, Edith 14, 22, 49, 93, 156
  alienation of 151–2, 153, 155
  Holocaust news 174–5
  Kindertransport 52, 53, 58, 59
  memoirs 18, 19
  Northern Ireland 105–6
  ward work 149
Bown, Gert (Gerald) 52, 53, 58
Boyd, Julia: *Travellers in the Third Reich* 98
Brexit 5
Britain *see* Great Britain
British Expeditionary Force 134, 135, 220
British Federation of University Women 97
British Medical Association 101, 189
Brockington, Fraser 200
Brook, Charles 111
Bruegel, Josephine 1, 42, 93, 97
  air raids 157
  Bloomsbury House 91
  dismissal 134–5, 139–40
  nursing visa 69
  re-employment 143
  training 67–8, 111
Bruley, Sue 60
Buchenwald 49

Caestecker, Frank: *Refugees from Nazi Germany* 15–16
Calder, Angus 145
Campbell, M. H. 96

Canada 187
Canterbury, Archbishop of 108
Caribbean nurses 8, 224
Carling, Dr Esther 87
Carter, Gladys 89–90, 193, 197
  A New Deal for Nurses 191
Caruth, Cathy 24
Catholic Teachers' College (Liverpool) 63
Central British Fund for World Jewish Relief 94
Central Co-Ordinating Committee for Refugees 91
Central Council for Jewish Refugees 96–7, 132–3, 139
Cesarani, David 12, 17, 44–5, 140, 174
Chadwick, Trevor 51
Chalmers, Beverley 55
Chamberlain, Neville 50
Charles III, King 26
Charles, Susan 12, 26
children 85, 150, 190–1
  Bergen-Belsen 179–80
  Blitz period 145, 146
  parental visits 165n.98
  see also education; Kindertransport
Christianity 57
Churchill, Winston 203n.10
civilians 128, 148
Civil Nursing Reserve 128
Clark, Mary Marshall 24
class *see* middle-classes
Cockayne, Elizabeth 104
Cohen, Susan 52, 105
Cohn, Bettina 183
College of Nursing 88, 90
Committee of the Central Office for Refugees 4, 10
community nursing 189–90
concentration camps 22, 24, 49; *see also* Bergen-Belsen

conscription 2
Cooper, E. N. 9–10, 141
COVID-19 5–6
Cowen, Heidi 20, 49, 55–6, 112, 226
Craig-Norton, Jennifer 25
   domestic service 3–4, 7, 14–15, 43, 60, 219
   Kindertransport 22, 52, 59–60, 193, 223–4
   The Kindertransport: Contesting Memory 15
Craven, Hannah 177
Crew, Francis A. E. 196–7
curfews 130
Curio, Claudia 52, 57
Czechoslovakia 12, 24–5, 67–8
Czech Refugee Trust Fund 134, 139–40

Dachau 49
Dann, Gertrude 42, 61–2
Dann, Lotte 42, 43
Darton, Laurence 68–9, 172
Davidson, Jillian 16
Davies, Angela 16
Davies, Celia 191
Dawson of Penn, Lord 100–1
days off 95–6, 117n.49
Death Marches 177
Decker, Karola 102
dentists 4, 46–7, 102, 132–3
Department *see* Nursing and Midwifery Department
depersonalisation 35n.82
diaries 18–19
Diary of Anne Frank, The 18
Dimbleby, Richard 158
dismissals 132–5, 139–41
district nurses 189–90
doctors 4, 97, 100–3, 189
   dismissals 132–3
   practise ban 46–7
   see also general practioners

Domestic Bureau of the Council of German Jewry 60–1, 62, 64
domestic service 3–4, 219
   escape route 41, 60–6
   exploitation 14–15
   mass dismissals 129
   suitability 28n.2, 43
   and visas 1, 7, 10, 16
Domestic Service Bureau 91
Dovercourt 56, 57
Dreadnaught Hospital (Greenwich) 70
Dubs, Lord Alfred 52
Dunkirk 134
Dwork, Deborah: *Children with a Star* 24
Dyhouse, Carol 193

East Croydon Hospital 92
economics 88–9, 98
Edinburgh University 196–7, 199, 199–200
education 42–3, 48–50, 190–4, 222; *see also* universities
Education Act (1944) 181–2
Eichmann, Adolf 192
Eisenhower, Gen Dwight D. 171
emigration 44–6, 70–1
enemy alien status 129–30
Ensing, Elsie 196
Epson Hospital (Surrey) 143
escape 1–2, 6–7, 11–12, 22, 41
   British routes 50–1
   methods 25
   nursing visas 66–70
   see also domestic service; Kindertransport
Essinger, Anna 58

Ferguson, Marion 26, 194, 199
Fieseler, Beate 171
fifth columnists 9

Index

Fink, Alice 26, 109–10, 158
  Bergen-Belsen 176–81
  enemy alien status 130
  internment 138–9
  midwifery 156
  war work 135
First World War 3, 132
Firth of Forth 134
Fischer, Lee 7, 12, 85, 93, 226
  Booth Hall Hospital 95, 107
  domestic service 64–5
  Kindertransport 58, 59
  ward work 150
  war work 144, 146–7
Fisher, Roy 193
Flatow, Eva 1, 42, 130, 141–3
Flynn, Karen 224
foster homes 56, 57–9
France 9, 26, 132, 135
Freemantle, Sir Francis 115n.13
Freud, Anna 132
Freud, Sigmund 132
Frey, Miss 92, 141
Friedlander, Saul 46
Friends Committee for Refugees and Aliens 172

Ganor, Sheer 129
Gardiner, Juliet 146
gender 2, 4, 16–17, 25, 96–7; see also men; women
General Nursing Council 14, 67, 103, 141
general practitioners (GPs) 189–90
Georges, Jane 18
George VI, King 100
German Jewish Aid Committee 80n.141, 90
German University (Prague) 67–8
Germany 8, 24–5, 42–3; see also Nazi Germany
Gestapo 39, 45, 69
ghettos 25, 122n.100, 154, 174

Gilbert, Martin 158
Gillespie, Veronica 56
Glasgow Royal Infirmary 168n.138
Gold, Aviva 93, 94, 133–4
Gold, Dina 46
Gopfert, Rebekka 52
Gordon, Hortense 1, 22–3, 27, 42, 226
  domestic service 63
  education 49
  health visitor work 189, 190
  married life 188
  midwifery 185–6
  training 103
  ward work 150
Gorsky, Martin 183
governesses 63
Grayzel, Susan 147–8
Great Britain 5, 70–1, 128
  class structure 43
  Holocaust awareness 173–4, 203n.10
  immigration 25
  visa restrictions 49–50
Greenlees, Janet 186–7
Greenspan, Henry 152, 154, 155, 176
Grenville, Anthony 221
Grier, Lynda 201
Griffiths, John 146

Haar, Cilly 2, 19, 27, 154–5, 188
  domestic service 62–3
  war nursing 144–5
Hahn-Warburg, Lola 39
Hallam, Julia 7–8
Hall, Stuart 225
Hammel, Andrea 52
Harding, Erna 2, 43, 44
Hardman, Lesley 177
Harefield Hospital (London) 143
Harrison, Tom 146
Haste, Helen 130, 132

Hastings, Somerset 111
health visitors 189
Hertzog, Esther 17
Hillyers, G. V. 9, 92, 94–5
Hilton, Claire 45
Hirsch, Tal Litvak 56
Hitler, Adolf 12–13, 24, 41, 50, 149
  antisemitism 44, 45–6
  assassination attempt 157
  education policies 48
  nurses 100
  suicide 171
Hoare, Sir Samuel 101
Hockey, Lizbeth 1, 8–9, 21, 26, 93, *131*
  alienation of 152–3
  dismissal 135, 140
  domestic service 63
  GP relationships 189
  Mortimer narratives 14
  NHS 182–3, 184, 185
  post-war degree 193
  research work 196, 197, 199, 201
  support 108–9
  war declaration 130
  ward work 150
  war work 145–6, 147, 148
Hodge, Margot 2, 19, 142
  internment 136, 137, 138
  nursing visa 66, 67
  war declaration 129, 130, 135
holiday camps 56, 57
holidays 95–6, 117n.49
Holmes, Colin 105, 129, 221
  A Tolerant Country? 15–16
Holocaust 1, 6, 8, 172, 173–6
  Bergen-Belsen 176–81
  British reaction 203n.10
  camp liberations 158–9
  family stories 154–5
  Hitler's ideology 12–13
  personal testimonies 17–18
  survivors 55, 192–3, 202
  women 16
Home Office 4, 61, 91, 102
  border control 49–50
Do It Now (film) 148
Homer, Stephanie 153
Honigsbaun, Frank 111
Horder, Lord 89
Horsburgh, Florence 10
hospitals 25–6
Hostile Environment 5
Hoxter, Charlotte 108
Hutchinson, Kitty 184
Hutter, Doryt (Rita) 224
Hutter, Otto 224

Immigration Health Surcharge 5–6
Interdepartmental Committee on Nursing Services 88–9
internment 129, 135–9, 140, 220
Irish nurses 8
Isle of Man 136–9, 142, 220
isolation 105–7

Jewish Committee for Relief Abroad (JCRA) 177, 178
Jewish Hospital (Berlin) 39, 66, 71n.1
Jewish Hospital (Frankfurt) 66–7
Jewish Hospital (London) 86, 108
Jewish Relief Unit (JRU) 177, 178
Jews 104, 112–13
  civil service ban 46–7
  East End community 109
  education 25, 48–50
  emigration plans 44–5
  European destruction 173–6
  pre-National Socialism 41–4, 70
  war declaration 129–30
  wartime Britain 136
  see also antisemitism; Holocaust; refugees
Jodl, Gen Alfred 171

Jones, Helen 57, 98
junior nurses 90

Kaplan, Marion 16–17, 47
Kapp, Yvonne 47, 105
Katz, Elisabeth 2, 48, 66–7, 92, 142
  internment 137–8
  war declaration 129, 130
  war work 145
Keighley and District Victoria
  Hospital (W. Yorks) 106, 149
Keitel, FM Wilhelm 171
Kindertransport 10, 12, 15, 41,
  51–60, 223–4
  reunions 77n.93
  selection for 22
King's College Hospital (London)
  103–4
Kinnair, Dame Donna 6
Kirby, Stephanie 186
Kramer, Josef 177
Kratz, Charlotte 1, 26, 104, 193–4,
  195, 199–201
Kristallnacht see November
  pogrom
Kushner, Tony 50, 51, 173–4
  antisemitism 98, 104–5, 136
  domestic service 14–15, 61, 129,
  223
  internment 138, 139, 140
  Journeys from the Abyss 5

Lambeth Hospital (London) 144–5
Lamb, Margaret 197
Lancet (magazine) 101–2
Lancet Commission 87–8
Land Army 10
Lang, Miss 20, 112–13
Laqueur, Walter 10, 42, 48
Law for the Restoration of the
  Professional Civil Service 46–7
LCC *see* London County Council
letters 18

Leverson, Jane 177, 178
Levi, Primo 22, 35n.88
  The Lost and the Saved 192
Lewen, Ilse 183
Lewinsky, Susi 45–6, 69–70
Linton, Susi 63–4, 91, 175
Lipman, Vivian 102
Local Government Act (1929) 110
Loeffler, Susi 12, 134, 140, 143, 176
Kinderstransport 53, 59, 60
London County Council (LCC)
  hospitals 86–7, 141, 186, 219
  support 109, 110–11
London Hospital, Whitechapel 86,
  108–9
London, Louise 61, 102, 221
  *Whitehall and the Jews,
  1933–1948* 15–16
loss 22–4
Lowton, Leonore 59
Luftwaffe 146

Manchester University 199–201
Marflow, Margaret 1, 19, 45, 92,
  130
marriage 27, 82n.158, 187–8
Mass Observation project 128, 146
matrons 4, 8, 86, 96, 107, 219
Maudsley Hospital (London) 102,
  110, 156, 197
McDowell, Linda 7
McGann, Susan 191, 196
Medical Practitioners Union 101
medical profession *see* dentists;
  doctors
medicine 1, 68, 188
memoirs 18–20
men 2, 3, 17
  internment 136
  Kindertransport 224
  November pogrom 11, 41
  sexual advances 61
  social status 47

middle-classes 3, 8, 16, 43
  domestic service 60, 61
  German Jews 42
Middlesex County Council 109, 112
midwives 4, 96–7, 186–7
migration 5–9, 25, 225–6
Miller Hospital, Greenwich 109–10
Mill Hill Hospital (London) 155–6
Millisle (Northern Ireland) 58, 79n.125
Minden, Eva 26, 53–5, 176–81
mistakes 89
Moore, Bob: *Refugees from Nazi Germany* 15–16
Moos, Trudie 1, 9, 19, 42, 43–4
  air raids 157
  Bloomsbury House 92
  enemy alien status 130
  Holocaust revelations 159
  internment 138
  NHS 183
  post-war work 191–2
  retirement 193
  training 103–4, 150–1
  war work 146, 148
Morley, Joel 128
Mortimer, Barbara: *Sisters: Memories from the Courageous Nurses of World War Two* 14
motherhouse (*Mutterhaus*) 98, 119n.67
Munich Agreement 50
municipal hospitals 86
munitions factory work 10, 113
Mynatt, Margaret 47, 105

National Health Service (NHS) 2, 5–6, 182–7, 222
  inauguration of 172
  Irish nurses 8
  post-war 26
  staff requirements 181
  treatment differences 209n.67
National Socialism *see* Nazi Germany
naturalisation 26, 40–1, 221
Nazi Germany 11, 19–20, 25, 50
  developing horror of 44–50
  gender 16–17
  Isle of Man 137
  Russia 98, 99
  see also Gestapo
Nelson, Siobhan 13
Netherlands 132
NHS *see* National Health Service
Niederland, Doron 44
Nightingale, Florence 168n.138
Nolan, Peter 24, 143, 156
North Africa 13
Northern Ireland 58, 105–6, 151–2
North Sea 134
Norton, Doreen 196
November pogrom 11, 25, 33n.66, 41, 49, 54
Nuremberg Laws 48
Nurse and Midwifery Department 25
Nurses Act (1949) 187
Nurses' Home 2, 7, 108
nursing 1–3, 187–90
  degrees 194–6, 199–201, 202–3, 222–3
  dismissals 132–3
  education work 190–4
  escape route 41
  Kindertransport 223–4
  NHS 182–7
  post-war 181–2
  racial issues 7–8
  recruitment 9–10, 25–6, 90–103
  refugees 4–5, 93–8, 100, 219
  status of 87–90

Index

visas 66–70
war work 10–11
see also war nurses
Nursing and Midwifery
  Department 9, 91, 92,
  140–1
Nursing Mirror (journal) 95, 96,
  98, 100, 133, 141
nursing press 86
Nursing Times (journal) 94–5, 98,
  100, 133

oral history 20–1, 24

Palestine 134
Parkes, Marianne 19, 104, 136
Park Prewitt Hospital (Basingstoke)
  104
Parry, Elizabeth 91
Passover 112–13
passports 53–4, 69
patriarchy 17
Pattinson, Juliette 130
Peace Campaign 103
Pearce, Evelyn: *A General Text
  Book of Nursing* 90
Pearl, Annaliese 1, 130, 181
penicillin 145, 149–50, 167n.136
Peplau, Hildegard: *Interpersonal
  Relations* 197
Pfillering, Ruth 192, 202
philanthropy 3, 98
'phoney war' 128–30, 132
Polish medical students 105
Poor Law 110
Powley, Edward H. 152
Price, Ruth 43, 45, 49
Princess Elizabeth Children's
  Hospital (London) 111
Princess Margaret Rose Hospital
  (Edinburgh) 93, 94, 133–4
prisoners of war 171, 176–7, 221
Prysor, Glyn 135–6

psychiatry 102, 141–2, 155–6,
  197
Pye, E. M. 92, 96

Quakers 63, 68–9, 177
Queen Mary's Hospital, Carshalton
  144
Queen's Institute for District
  Nurses 189
Queen's Nursing Institute (QNI)
  196

racism see anti-semitism
Radloff, Ann 35n.82
Rafferty, Anne Marie 88
Ramsden, Gertrude 196
Rawraway, Ruth 2, 39–41
RCN see Royal College of Nursing
Reconstruction Committee 89
Red Cross 154–5
Refugee Children's Movement
  56–7
refugees 4–5, 13–17
  alienation of 151–5
  British citizenship 221–2
  discrimination of 7–8
  dismissals 132–5, 139–41
  doctors 100–3
  escape routes of 11–13
  gender 2
  German invasion fears 148–9
  internment 135–9
  modern-day crisis 5, 225–6
  nursing 93–8, 100, 219, 224–5
  personal testimonies 17–24
  precarity of 6–7
  recruitment of 9–11, 90–103
  re-employment 141–5
  social conscience of 8–9
  survivor's guilt 192–3
  voluntary hospitals 103–5
  war declaration 129–30, 132
  see also escape

Reilly, Jo 179
Rein, Howard 108
remuneration 89
Ring, Nicola 194
Robbins Report 193, 194, 195
Roberts, Gertrude 2, 43, 45, 175–6, 226
  war work 146, 153, 154
Roper, Michael 19
Rose, Sonya O. 104, 136, 220
Ross, Mia 19, 106–7, 154
  domestic service 65
  Kindertransport 53
  passport 54
  ward work 149–50
Royal Air Force 143
Royal Cancer Hospital, Fulham 134
Royal College of Nursing (RCN) 6, 89, 196
Royal College of Physicians and Surgeons 101
Royal Free Hospital (London) 104, 150–1, 157
Russia 13, 98, 99, 149

SA (Sturmabteilung) 53
Sacharin, Rosa 14, 19, 93, 158
  education 48
  Kindertransport 56, 57, 58–9
  psychology 156
  retirement 193
  support 107–8
  teaching 190–1
Sachsenhausen 49
Sarkar, Mahua 24
Schafer, Kitty 2, 11–12, 41–2, 91–2, 107
  internment 138
  training 127
  war work 144
Schonfeld, Rabbi Solomon 51
Scott Wright, Marjorie 196, 197
Second World War 12, 157–9, 171

'phoney' 128–30, 132
  see also Nazi Germany; war nurses
secular schools 42, 48, 49
Segal, Lore 62
servants see domestic service
Sex Discrimination Act (1975) 188
Sheftel, Anna 152, 155
Shephard, Ben 177
Shields, Linda 122n.100
Shire, Ruth 20, 112–13
Simpson, Marjorie 196
Simsova, Sylva 97
Sington, Derrick 158
SMA see Socialist Medical Association
Smith, Alwyn 200
Snow, Stephanie 183
Socialist Medical Association (SMA) 86, 111–12, 181, 185
social justice 8
social workers 64
Society of Apothecaries 101
Special Operations Executive 129–30
spies 9, 133, 135
SS (Schutzstaffel) 53
Staines Emergency Hospital 20, 112
Starns, Penny 150
Staub, Ervin 47
Stephany, Mr 94
Stephenson, Elsie 197
Stewart, John 4, 14, 90–1, 111, 227
St James's Hospital (Leeds) 66, 142
St Luke's Hospital (Bradford) 67, 142
St Mary's Hospital, Islington 142–3
Strong, Rebecca 168n.138
St Thomas's Hospital (London) 4, 9, 39, 92, 168n.138
suicides 24, 192
Summerfield, Penny 20, 188
  Reconstructing Women's Wartime Lives 14

Summers, Anne 3, 61
survivors 24, 53, 55, 176, 192–3
Sutton and Cheam Hospital (Surrey) 104

Tosh, John 19
tourism 98
training 7, 10, 67, 86
  entry requirements 95
  isolation of 105–7
  Royal Free Hospital 150–1
  Strong 168n.138
  support 107–13
  teachers 190–1
  voluntary hospitals 103–5
  war years 143
transmigration 56, 60, 71, 95, 219
trauma 22–4
Turk, Dr Martha 94

United Nations Relief and Rehabilitation Administration (UNRRA) 180
United States of America (USA) 12, 26, 80n.137, 187
universities 187–8, 193–7, 199–201, 202–3, 222–3
University College London 134
University of London 101
upper-class women 3

V1 bombs (doodlebugs) 157–8
V2 missiles 157–8
Vienna 41–2
Vietnam War 24
Villier, Anne von 97
violence 48, 65
Voluntary Aid Detachment recruits (VADs) 3
voluntary hospitals 86, 89, 103–5

Wallach, Kerry 42
ward sisters 90

war nurses 26, 155–7, 171–2
  alienation of 151–5
  Blitz 145–9
  re-employment 141–5
  ward work 149–51
Warriner, Doreen 51
Warsaw Ghetto 122n.100
war work 2, 10–11, 129–30
Wasserstein, Bernard 172
  Britain and the Jews of Europe 15
Webster, Charles 184, 185
Webster, Wendy 147
Weindling, Paul 14, 102, 110, 183, 227
Weir, Rosemary 190
Whipps Cross Hospital (Leytonstone) 111
Whitecross, Angela 183
White, Rosemary 183
Wiederhorn, Jessica 18
Wieler, Joachim 8
Winterton, Lord 101
Winton, Nicholas 51, 57
Wolloch, Edith Menkes 7, 46, 130
women 14, 16
  of colour 13
  degradation of 154
  doctors 97
  employment 181–2, 188–9
  internment 136–7
  Nazi abuses 55
  Nazi developments 47
  strip-searching of 11, 69
  undercover work 129–30
  war work 148, 171
Women's Voluntary Services (WVS) 148
Wright, C. J. 174

York Hill Hospital (Glasgow) 107–8

Zembrzycki, Stacey 152, 155

EU authorised representative for GPSR:
Easy Access System Europe, Mustamäe tee 50,
10621 Tallinn, Estonia
gpsr.requests@easproject.com

www.ingramcontent.com/pod-product-compliance
Lightning Source LLC
Chambersburg PA
CBHW051605230426
43668CB00013B/1992